TRANSSEPTAL CATHETERIZATION

AND INTERVENTIONS

TRANSSEPTAL
CATHETERIZATION
AND INTERVENTIONS

EDITORS

RANJAN THAKUR MD, MPH, MBA, FHRS
Professor of Medicine and Director, Electrophysiology Fellowship,
Thoracic and Cardiovascular Institute, Sparrow Health System,
Michigan State University, Lansing, Michigan

ANDREA NATALE MD, FACC, FHRS
Executive Medical Director, Texas Cardiac Arrhythmia Institute,
St. David's Medical Center, Austin, Texas; Consulting Professor, Division
of Cardiology, Stanford University, Stanford, California; Clinical Associate
Professor of Medicine, Case Western Reserve University, Cleveland, Ohio;
Senior Clinical Director, EP Services, California Pacific Medical Center,
San Francisco, California; Director of Interventional EP, Scripps Green,
San Diego, California

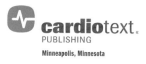
cardiotext.
PUBLISHING
Minneapolis, Minnesota

Cardiotext Publishing, LLC
3405 W. 44th Street
Minneapolis, Minnesota 55410
USA
www.cardiotextpublishing.com

Any updates to this book may be found at:
www.cardiotextpublishing.com/titles/detail/9780979016417

Comments, inquiries, and requests for bulk sales can be directed to the publisher at:
info@cardiotextpublishing.com.

Cover image (large): With kind permission from Springer Science+Business Media: *Journal of Interventional Cardiac Electrophysiology,* Complicated transseptal puncture during intervention catheter ablation on atrial fibrillation concomitant with straight back syndrome, 19, 2007, 41-43, Tao H, Dong J, Yu R, Ma C.

Unless otherwise stated, all figures and tables in this book are used courtesy of the authors.

Cover and book design by Ann Delgehausen, Trio Bookworks

Library of Congress Control Number: 2010924267

ISBN: 978-0-9790164-1-7

Printed in Canada

15   14   13   12   11   10   1   2   3   4   5   6   7   8   9   10

To my wife, Niti, for her love, support, and encouragement,
to our son, Jay—my friend and inspiration,
and to my mother

Ranjan Thakur

To my wife, Marina, and
our daughters, Veronica and Eleonora

Andrea Natale

Contents

CONTRIBUTORS

Editors

RANJAN THAKUR **MD, MPH, MBA, FHRS**
Professor of Medicine and Director, Electrophysiology Fellowship, Thoracic and
Cardiovascular Institute, Sparrow Health System, Michigan State University, Lansing,
Michigan

ANDREA NATALE **MD, FACC, FHRS**
Executive Medical Director, Texas Cardiac Arrhythmia Institute, St. David's Medical Center,
Austin, Texas; Consulting Professor, Division of Cardiology, Stanford University, Stanford,
California; Clinical Associate Professor of Medicine, Case Western Reserve University,
Cleveland, Ohio; Senior Clinical Director, EP Services, California Pacific Medical Center,
San Francisco, California; Director of Interventional EP, Scripps Green, San Diego, California

Contributors

SAWSAN M. AWAD **MD**
Rush Center for Congenital and Structural Heart Disease, Section of Cardiology,
Department of Pediatrics, Rush University Medical Center, Chicago, Illinois

CONOR D. BARRETT **MD**
Massachusetts General Hospital Heart Center and Harvard Medical School,
Boston, Massachusetts

J. DAVID BURKHARDT MD
Texas Cardiac Arrhythmia Institute at St. David's Medical Center, Austin, Texas

DAVID CALLANS MD
Division of Cardiovascular Medicine, Electrophysiology,
University of Pennsylvania, Philadelphia, Pennsylvania

QI-LING CAO MD
Associate Professor and Director of the Echocardiography Research Lab, Rush Center
for Congenital and Structural Heart Disease, Section of Cardiology, Department of Pediatrics,
Rush University Medical Center, Chicago, Illinois

SHIH-ANN CHEN MD
Division of Cardiology, Department of Medicine, Taipei Veterans General Hospital,
Taipei, Taiwan; Institute of Clinical Medicine, and Cardiovascular Research Institute,
National Yang-Ming University, Taipei, Taiwan

TAHMEED CONTRACTOR MD
Department of Medicine, Division of Internal Medicine, Michigan State University,
East Lansing, Michigan

RICHARD J. CZOSEK MD
Senior Fellow in Cardiac Electrophysiology, Children's Hospital, Boston, Massachusetts;
Fellow in Pediatrics, Harvard Medical School, Boston, Massachusetts

LUIGI DI BIASE MD
Texas Cardiac Arrhythmia Institute at St. David's Medical Center, Austin, Texas; Department
of Cardiology, University of Foggia, Foggia, Italy; Department of Biomedical Engineering,
University of Texas, Austin, Texas

GREGORY K. FELD MD
Professor of Medicine, University of California, San Diego, School of Medicine;
Director, Cardiac Electrophysiology Program, UCSD Medical Center, San Diego, California

ZIYAD M. HIJAZI MD, MPH, FSCAI, FACC, FAAP
Director of the Rush Center for Congenital and Structural Heart Disease;
Pediatric Cardiology Section Chief and Professor of Pediatrics and Internal Medicine,
Rush University Medical Center, Chicago, Illinois

SIEW YEN HO   PhD, FRCPath, FESC

Consultant and Professor of Cardiac Morphology, Royal Brompton Hospital
and Imperial College, London, United Kingdom

RODNEY P. HORTON   MD, FACC

Texas Cardiac Arrhythmia Institute at St. David's Medical Center, Austin, Texas;
Adjunct Professor, Cockrell School of Engineering, Department of Biomedical Engineering,
University of Texas, Austin, Texas

MING-HSIUNG HSIEH   MD

Division of Cardiovascular Medicine, Taipei Medical University–Wan Fang Hospital,
Taipei, Taiwan

YU-FENG HU   MD

Division of Cardiology, Department of Medicine, Taipei Veterans General Hospital,
Taipei, Taiwan; Institute of Clinical Medicine, and Cardiovascular Research Institute,
National Yang-Ming University, Taipei, Taiwan

PIERRE JAÏS   MD

Hôpital Cardiologique du Haut-Lévêque, Bordeaux-Pessac, France

ATUL KHASNIS   MD

Fellow, Center for Vasculitis Care and Research, Department of Rheumatic and Immunologic
Diseases, Cleveland Clinic, Cleveland, Ohio

SÉBASTIEN KNECHT   MD

Hôpital Cardiologique Haut-Lévêque, Bordeaux-Pessac, France;
Université Victor Segalen Bordeaux 2, Bordeaux, France; CHU Brugmann, Bruxelles, Belgium

BRADLEY P. KNIGHT   MD, FACC, FHRS

Director of Cardiac Electrophysiology, Bluhm Cardiovascular Institute of Northwestern;
Professor of Medicine, Feinberg School of Medicine, Northwestern University,
Chicago, Illinois

MICHAEL KÜHNE   MD

Attending physician, AF Clinic, Cardiology/Electrophysiology,
University Hospital Basel, Switzerland

PETER LEONG-SIT MD
Assistant Professor of Medicine, Arrhythmia Service, London Health Sciences Hospital, London, Ontario, Canada

MOUSSA MANSOUR MD
Director, Cardiac Electrophysiology Laboratory; Director, Atrial Fibrillation Program, Massachusetts General Hospital Heart Center and Harvard Medical School, Boston, Massachusetts

ISABELLE NAULT MD
Hôpital Haut Lévêque, Bordeaux-Pessac, France; Institut Universitaire de Cardiologie et de Pneumologie de Québec, Québec, Canada

HAKAN ORAL MD
Frederick G. L. Huetwell Professor of Cardiovascular Medicine and Director, Cardiac Electrophysiology Service, University of Michigan Health System, Ann Arbor, Michigan

KHYATI PANDYA MD
Cardiologist (India); Fellow, Division of Pediatric Cardiology, Rainbow Babies and Children's Hospital, Cleveland, Ohio

MEHUL B. PATEL MD
Bay Pines VA Medical Center, Division of Cardiology, Bay Pines, Florida

VIVEK Y. REDDY MD
Director, Cardiac Arrhythmia Service, and Leona M. and Harry B. Helmsley Charitable Trust Professor of Medicine in Cardiac Electrophysiology, Mount Sinai School of Medicine, New York, New York

JOHN ROSS JR. MD
Professor of Medicine, Division of Cardiology, Department of Medicine, School of Medicine and Medical Center, University of California San Diego (UCSD), La Jolla, California

JAVIER E. SÁNCHEZ MD
Texas Cardiac Arrhythmia Institute at St. David's Medical Center, Austin, Texas

SAMIN K. SHARMA **MD, FACC**
Professor of Medicine (Cardiology) and Director, Cardiac Catheterization Lab,
Mount Sinai Medical Center, New York, New York

MICHAEL M. SHEHATA **MD**
Cedars-Sinai Heart Institute, Electrophysiology Section, Cedars-Sinai Medical Center,
Los Angeles, California

KALYANAM SHIVKUMAR **MD, PhD**
Professor of Medicine and Radiology, and Director, UCLA Cardiac Arrhythmia Center
and EP Programs, David Geffen School of Medicine at UCLA, Ronald Reagan
UCLA Medical Center, Los Angeles, California

SHELDON M. SINGH **MD**
Cardiac Arrhythmia Service, Mount Sinai School of Medicine, New York, New York

MATTHEW P. SMELLEY **MD**
Section of Cardiology, Department of Internal Medicine, University of Chicago,
Chicago, Illinois

JOHN K. TRIEDMAN **MD**
Senior Associate, Cardiac Electrophysiology Division, Children's Hospital Boston;
Associate Professor of Pediatrics, Harvard Medical School, Boston, Massachusetts

EDWARD P. WALSH **MD**
Chief, Cardiac Electrophysiology Division, Children's Hospital Boston; Professor of Pediatrics,
Harvard Medical School, Boston, Massachusetts

YAN WANG **MD**
Cardiovascular Division, Tongji Hospital, Tongji Medical College
of Huazhong University of Science & Technology, Wuhan, People's Republic of China

Foreword

Transseptal Left Heart Catheterization: The Past — The Present — The Future

Eugene Braunwald MD

Distinguished Hersey Professor of Medicine
Harvard Medical School
Boston, Massachusetts, USA

In the 1950s, the most frequently performed cardiac operation worldwide was mitral valvotomy for rheumatic mitral stenosis. Assessment of the hemodynamic severity of the stenosis, and perhaps even more important, determination of the presence and severity of accompanying mitral regurgitation, were critical to the selection of patients for this new and sometimes risky procedure. For this assessment, direct measurement of left atrial and left ventricular pressures were necessary. A variety of techniques for access to the left side of the heart emerged in the early and mid-1950s. These involved percutaneous puncture—more or less blind—of the left atrium or ventricle and included advancing a needle into the suprasternal notch through the great vessels and (hopefully) the left atrium, and then passing a polyethylene catheter through the needle and into the left ventricle. Other approaches included a posterior transthoracic puncture of the left atrium, and transbronchial left atrial puncture by passing a needle

through a rigid bronchoscope. Measuring left ventricular pressure directly became critical when aortic valve surgery came along in the late 1950s and early 1960s. Needle puncture of the ventricle using a subxiphoid or apical approach were widely employed. All of these (and a few other) techniques were developed and carried out by cardiovascular surgeons. All were hazardous and some, especially transbronchial left heart catheterization, which was carried out through a rigid bronchoscope, were extremely uncomfortable for patients.

Our group of cardiologists and cardiovascular surgeons working in the intramural program of the National Heart Institute (now the Heart, Lung and Blood Institute) was deeply involved in the use of some of these techniques and recognized their deficiencies. In 1958, John Ross, a fellow trainee, stepped up to the plate and developed transseptal left heart catheterization (TSLHC) in experimental animals. One of the most thrilling events in my professional life occurred in 1959, when I observed Ross carry out the first transseptal puncture of the left atrium in the Institute's catheterization laboratory. Ross, Glenn Morrow (the Chief of Cardiac Surgery), and I knew that something very important had just occurred. Ross taught me how to manipulate the sheath and needle and soon we were in the "see one, do one, teach one" mode.

Following our early publications (see Figure P.1), cardiologists from across the world visited our catheterization laboratory to learn how to perform TSLHC. The technique proved to be relatively safe, it did not involve surgeons, the patients were not uncomfortable, and it allowed detailed assessment of left heart hemodynamics in patients who were in a steady basal state. In addition to facilitating cardiovascular diagnosis, we found that this approach was extremely useful in the conduct of physiologic and pharmacologic studies. By the mid-1960s, TSLHC had become the

dominant technique for measuring left heart pressures worldwide.

By the late 1960s, however, the picture changed again. Retrograde catheterization of the left ventricle became possible for cardiologists using the percutaneous Seldinger technique (named for the Swedish radiologist who developed this approach). As a consequence, the use of TSLHC declined as rapidly as it had grown only a decade earlier.

But TSLHC did not die, it merely hibernated for about two decades. It awoke in the late 1980s, when access to the left atrium again became of critical importance, this time to allow radiofrequency ablation of left-sided accessory pathways responsible for drug refractory supraventricular tachycardias. It really picked up steam in the 1990s when catheter ablation of atrial fibrillation became a reality. TSLHC became the preferred method of access to the left atrium and pulmonary veins in the cure of this common

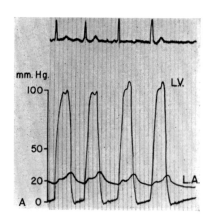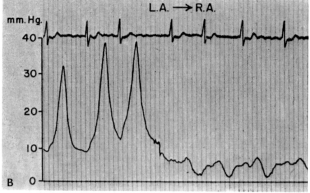

FIGURE P.1   **A.** Simultaneous left atrial and left ventricular pressures obtained in a patient with mitral stenosis and atrial fibrillation. The left atrial pressure was obtained by transseptal puncture and the left ventricular pressure by percutaneous puncture through the anterior chest wall. **B.** Pressure tracing obtained as the needle was withdrawn from the left atrium (L.A.) across the interatrial septum into the right atrium (R.A.) in a patient with mitral regurgitation. Ross J Jr, Braunwald E, Morrow AG. Transseptal left atrial puncture: new technique for the measurement of left atrial pressure in man. *Am J Cardiol* 1959;3:653-655.

arrhythmia. At present, TSLHC is being carried out for this indication far more frequently worldwide than it ever was during the 1960s.

What about the future of TSLHC? Just as it morphed from a diagnostic tool for the hemodynamicist into a therapeutic modality for the clinical cardiac electrophysiologist, it is again becoming important in the *treatment* of valvular heart disease. This also began in the 1980s—with balloon valvuloplasty for mitral stenosis. It is now expanding by allowing the insertion of a clip for the edge-to-edge repair of the valve leaflets in the treatment of mitral regurgitation. Clinical trials are being conducted to evaluate transseptal implantation of prosthetic aortic valves, as well as closure of the left atrial appendage. Another recent application is in percutaneous left ventricular assistance carried out by inserting a wide-bore catheter transseptally into the left atrium and pumping the blood so obtained into a cannula inserted into a systemic artery.

The technique of TSLHC has improved over the last half century, and it is now aided by transesophageal and intracardiac echocardiography. Surprisingly, the basic equipment—that is, the needle and sheath—is not much changed from what we used in the early days, except that it is now adapted for specific purposes. TSLHC is here to stay; it already plays an important role in the repertoire of both interventional cardiologists and clinical electrophysiologists, and it will play an increasingly important role in the future.

Transseptal Catheterization and Interventions is the first book on this subject. The editors, Drs. Thakur and Natale, as well as their talented authors, should be congratulated for providing such an excellent and eminently readable volume. The applications of this approach to the left side of the heart are growing, and both the technique and the equipment are evolving. I can't wait for the next edition.

PREFACE

Transseptal catheterization was introduced half a century ago by Drs. John Ross Jr., Constantin Cope, and Eugene Braunwald as a technique for measuring left atrial pressure. Valvular heart disease was common at that time, even in the Western world, and our understanding of cardiovascular physiology was in a nascent stage. Due to the potential for complications, particularly in inexperienced hands, the technique became cloaked in danger and intrigue in the 1960s. In the 1970s, echocardiography and Doppler assessment of valvular lesions and pressure measurements became available; transseptal catheterization became somewhat redundant and the procedure fell out of favor. Modern interventional cardiologists became interested in this technique with the advent of percutaneous mitral valvuloplasty, which was introduced in the mid-1980s. Shortly thereafter, cardiac electrophysiologists became interested in the technique for ablation of left-sided accessory pathways and left atrial tachy-

cardias. The development of catheter ablation for atrial fibrillation and new therapeutic interventions for the interventional cardiologist began a resurgence of the technique.

It is surprising that this important technique has not been the subject of a textbook until now. Readers and those learning the technique for the first time have had to search the literature for the pertinent information on their own. This textbook provides important discussion about topics relevant for all readers interested in safely performing transseptal catheterization, from embryology and anatomy of the interatrial septum to detailed discussions about the various methods, and illustrations of difficult cases, complications, and new technologies for improving safety and efficacy. Some readers will find specific chapters of particular interest to them: transseptal technique in pediatric cardiology (chapter 9), emerging applications in interventional cardiology (chapters 11 and 12) and left atrial appendage closure (chapter 13) will be of interest to interventionalists as well as electrophysiologists.

Transseptal Catheterization and Interventions will be especially useful for interventional cardiologists and electrophysiologists in training or in practice, in both adult and pediatric cardiology, who are not yet fully conversant in this technique. Of course, teachers responsible for educating a new generation of interventionalists will find it useful for pedagogical purposes. Laboratory staff and nurses working in catheterization and electrophysiology laboratories will also find the book useful. Other readers, such as those working in the related medical device industry, will find this to be a necessary reference.

We are indebted to our colleagues around the world who have contributed their time and expertise to making this endeavor possible. The next generation of cardiologist who performs this technique will owe a great deal to the inventors and investigators who have developed a body of literature on the subject and to the teachers in these pages who make the material so readily accessible. Indeed, the readers stand on all of their shoulders and we sincerely hope that they will see further.

Every subject of interest is always evolving, so by no means is this textbook a final word on the subject. As far as we can tell, transseptal catheterization will be an essential tool for delivering therapeutic interventions for years to come. We encourage our readers to share their experiences with us: difficult cases, interesting anatomies, novel ways of doing things. We would be delighted to receive their comments and analyses as well as images (still or video files), so that we may share those with the readers in subsequent editions of this book.

This project owes its success to Steven Korn at Cardiotext Publishing, who first embraced the idea of a textbook on transseptal catheterization, and to Mike Crouchet, president of Cardiotext Publishing, who has offered unwavering support. We are also indebted to the production staff at Cardiotext, but particularly to Ann Delgehausen (of Trio Bookworks) and Caitlin Crouchet for their countless efforts and attention to detail.

Finally, we want to acknowledge our families for their love and support—they are truly our inspiration and we dedicate this work to them.

Ranjan Thakur
Lansing, MI
thakur@msu.edu

Andrea Natale
Austin, TX
andrea.natale@stdavids.com

HISTORY OF TRANSSEPTAL CATHETERIZATION

GREGORY K. FELD, JOHN ROSS JR.

Transseptal left heart catheterization, originally developed in experimental animal studies and then later in humans, was reported in 1959 by John Ross Jr, MD, at the National Institutes of Health (NIH).[1-4] It was first used to measure left heart pressures as a diagnostic method and later as a research tool to study left heart dynamics in human diseases such as heart failure, heart valve dysfunction, and hypertrophic obstructive cardiomyopathy.[4,5,*] In 1960, the needle used for transseptal catheterization (Figure 1.1) was slightly modified with a smaller needle tip by Edwin Brockenbrough, MD, a trainee in the NIH cardiovascular research program, for use with a larger catheter passed percutaneously by the Seldinger method.[7] Subsequently the procedure became widely used as a diagnostic method to assess left atrial and left ventricular pressures in both adult and pediatric patients with valvular and congenital heart disease who were being considered as candidates for surgical repair procedures.[8-10] With the developments of right heart, balloon, and thermodilution (Swan-Ganz) catheterization to estimate left atrial pressures[11] and retrograde left ventricular catheterization, transseptal catheterization became less widely practiced in the 1970s and early 1980s, except

---

* Our experiments on transseptal catheterization in dogs were successfully completed in 1957-58, and demonstrated healing of the puncture site; these results were presented at a surgical meeting[2] and later published in 1959.[1,2] After the experimental studies in animals, followed by studies in human cadavers, our initial studies in 12 patients were published in 1959.[3] Left atrial and left ventricular pressures were measured without complication using a special needle (a longer version than the one used in experimental animals) which had a curved distal end, a reverse bevel needle tip,

Transseptal Catheterization and Interventions.
© 2010 Ranjan Thakur MD and Andrea Natale MD, eds.
Cardiotext Publishing, ISBN 978-0-9790164-1-7.

in those centers performing procedures, such as mitral balloon valvulotomy, which require transseptal puncture.

During the 1980s, however, at a time when clinical cardiac electrophysiology was primarily a diagnostic specialty, the use of electrical fulguration for atrioventricular (AV) node ablation, septal accessory pathway ablation, and ventricular tachycardia ablation was described,[12-13] rapidly advancing cardiac electrophysiology into an interventional specialty. Fortunately, considering the limitations of high-energy shocks for ablation, including the high failure rates and risks of complications from this technique,[12-13] radiofrequency energy for catheter ablation was described.[14] This led to an explosion in the use of catheter ablation to cure a variety of cardiac arrhythmias, including AV reentry,[15-16] AV nodal reentry,[17] atrial flutter,[18-19] atrial tachycardia,[20] and ventricular tachycardia.[21]

In many cases, however, the successful application of radiofrequency energy via catheter for curative ablation required access to the left atrium and left ventricle. This was particularly true for left-sided accessory pathways,[15-16] left ventricular tachycardia,[21] atrial fibrillation and atypical atrial flutter.[22] While often this could be accomplished by retro-

grade arterial catheterization across the aortic and mitral valves, usually from the femoral artery or rarely from the radial artery, in many cases easier access could be achieved by a transseptal catheterization approach. Thus, for the treatment of a variety of supraventricular and ventricular tachyarrhythmias there was a gradual resurgence in the use of transseptal catheterization in the field of interven-

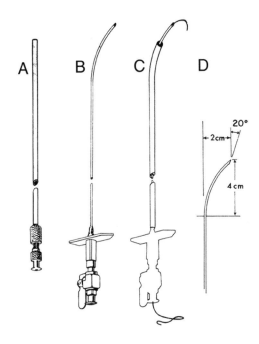

FIGURE 1.1   *Original Transseptal Equipment for Human Use*

A. Cournand catheter (with removable hub) through which the needle is inserted. **B, D.** The transseptal needle has a specified curve and bevel, with an attached arrow-handle for controlled rotation. **C.** The 17-gauge needle allows passage of a small catheter for pressure measurements in the left atrium and left ventricle. It also allows for injection of indicator dye into the left ventricle with brachial arterial sampling, for calculation of the cardiac output. Reproduced with permission from Ross J Jr., Braunwald E, Morrow AG. Left heart catheterization by the transseptal route: a description of the technic and its applications. *Circulation* 1960;22:927-934.

and an arrow at the hub for rotating the needle tip (Figure 1.1). This needle was originally fabricated by the NIH machine shop and later manufactured by Becton-Dickinson, Inc and marketed as the Ross needle. C. Cope published a preliminary report in 1959[6] in which he described lack of success in animal experiments, as well as attempted transseptal catheterization in two patients. Using a percutaneous approach from the right leg, a catheter was positioned in the right atrium and a long needle was passed through the catheter, which was used for septal puncture. This was followed by attempted insertion of the catheter over the needle into the left atrium (in one of the two patients, this procedure was unsuccessful).

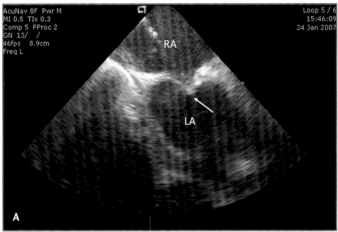

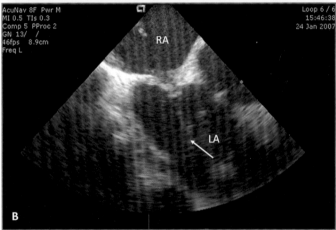

FIGURE 1.2   *Intracardiac Echocardiography (ICE) During Transseptal Catheterization Using the AcuNav Steerable Ultrasound Catheter*

A. ICE image demonstrating tenting of interatrial septum by transseptal needle (arrow) prior to puncture into the left atrium. **B.** ICE image demonstrating transseptal needle puncture of the interatrial septum with the tip of the needle in the left atrium and bubble contrast in the left atrium resulting from saline flush of the needle (arrow).

ways in patients with Wolff-Parkinson-White syndrome and refractory supraventricular tachycardia,[23-25] in the occasional patient with failed right-sided slow or fast pathway ablation for AV nodal reentrant tachycardia,[26-27] in those with failed right-sided AV node ablation for refractory atrial fibrillation,[28] and in those with left ventricular tachycardia in whom access to the left ventricle is required for both mapping and ablation.[29-30] Large numbers of transseptal catheterization procedures have been performed at numerous institutions worldwide over the last several decades, including many in electrophysiology laboratories, with very high success and very low complication rates,[31] even if performed on an outpatient basis.[32] The most serious potential risks from transseptal catheterization include cardiac or aortic perforation with pericardial effusion and tamponade, which may require percutaneous pericardial catheter drainage and, occasionally, surgical intervention.

tional cardiac electrophysiology, beginning in the 1980s; this use increased dramatically in the 2000s as ablation of atrial fibrillation became widely practiced.

Thus, in the cardiac electrophysiology laboratory, transseptal catheterization has become particularly useful for obtaining access to the left atrium for radiofrequency catheter ablation of left-sided accessory path-

While the technique of transseptal catheterization remains largely unchanged since it was originally described and modified,[1-4] several new technologies have made the approach considerably easier and potentially less risky, and are routinely employed today in many clinical electrophysiology laboratories. These new technologies include trans-esophageal echocardiography,[33] now largely replaced by intracardiac echocardiography (ICE),[34-37] to guide transseptal puncture, transseptal puncture performed using radio-frequency energy applied to a modified trans-septal needle (NRG RF Transseptal Needle, Baylis Medical Company, Inc, Montreal QC, Canada), or use of a needle-tipped guidewire (SafeSept Transseptal Guidewire, Pressure Products, Inc, San Pedro, CA) passed through a standard Brockenbrough transseptal needle into the left atrium through a variety of pre-shaped transseptal sheaths (Fast-Cath, St. Jude Medical, Inc, St. Paul, MN). With the use of ICE, typically performed with a steer-able 8 F or 10 F intracardiac ultrasound cath-eter (AcuNav, Siemens Medical Solutions USA, Inc, Malvern, PA), contrast injection to stain the septum is no longer required, since micro-bubbles in the saline flush provide adequate echo-contrast to ensure successful left atrial access, reducing the risk of cardiac perforation with the transseptal needle (Fig-ure 1.2). The radiofrequency transseptal nee-dle[38] and the needle-tipped guidewire further reduce the risk of inadvertent needle perfora-tion of the left atrial lateral wall or roof dur-ing transseptal catheterization. For ablation of left-sided accessory pathways, a numbered series of transseptal sheaths (eg, SL1, SL2 [Daig Corp, Minnetonka, MN]) with differ-ent lengths of the distal-shaped segment was developed that, when extended just beyond the sheath, position the ablation catheter at specific locations around the mitral valve annulus (Fast-Cath, St. Jude Medical, Inc, St. Paul, MN).

With the recognition that electrical isolation of the pulmonary veins with radio-frequency catheter ablation may cure atrial fibrillation,[39] an entirely new procedure in interventional cardiac electrophysiology was launched in the late 1980s, namely the ablation of atrial fibrillation. This approach required transseptal catheterization of the left atrium and, in most cases, double transsep-tal catheterization (Figure 1.3) because both a circular mapping catheter and an ablation catheter need to be introduced into the left atrium to ensure successful isolation of the pulmonary veins. This can be accomplished either by performing two separate transseptal punctures[33-37] or a single transseptal punc-ture[40] through which an ablation catheter is guided either by ICE or fluoroscopy after withdrawing the sheath (through which the initial puncture was made) back into the right atrium while retaining a guidewire in the left atrium. Once the ablation catheter is passed through the transseptal puncture into the left atrium, the retained sheath can be passed over the guidewire back into the left atrium, through which the circular mapping cath-eter can then be deployed in the left atrium for mapping the pulmonary veins. Both approaches may be guided by ICE, and recent advances in 3-D echo may further enhance success and reduce the risks of the procedure. Studies suggest that long-term complications are similar with either approach, and while the single transseptal puncture approach may result in patency of the puncture site for a lon-ger period of time than the double transseptal puncture approach, closure eventually occurs with either approach.[41]

Another aspect of transseptal catheter-ization that has evolved with the advent of atrial fibrillation ablation has been the use of intensified anticoagulation regimens for pre-vention of thromboembolic events, includ-ing maintaining an activated clotting time (ACT) >350 seconds during ablation[42-43] and front-loading with heparin before transseptal puncture, as well as consideration of trans-septal catheterization and ablation while fully anticoagulated with warfarin with an INR of 2-3.[44] Detection of left atrial thrombus before

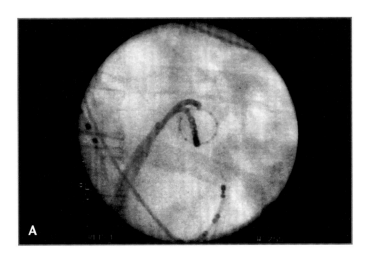

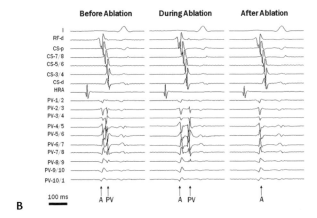

FIGURE 1.3   *Fluoroscopic View and Endocardial Recordings Demonstrating Method for Segmental Ostial Ablation and Pulmonary Vein Isolation*

A. Right anterior oblique (RAO) fluoroscopic view of double transseptal (single puncture) approach for mapping of the pulmonary vein with a Lasso catheter and segmental antral pulmonary vein ablation with an 8 mm tipped catheter. **B.** Surface electrocardiogram (ECG) (lead I) and endocardial electrograms recordings from the radiofrequency ablation catheter (RF-d), coronary sinus catheter (CSp-d), high right atrial catheter (HRA), and Lasso catheter (PV1-10), demonstrating the presence of both atrial (A) and pulmonary vein (PV) potentials before ablation, the delay of the PV potentials during ablation, and the elimination of the PV potentials after ablation.

reduce the risk of thromboembolic events.

Since the methods for ablation of atrial fibrillation vary significantly, from segmental antral pulmonary vein isolation (Figure 1.3) to circumferential pulmonary vein ablation and isolation with or without additional linear ablation (Figure 1.4), different transseptal sheaths have been employed to achieve the goals of these ablation procedures, including fixed-curve sheaths, such as the Fast-Cath SL1 sheath (St. Jude Medical, Inc, St. Paul, MN), and steerable sheaths, such as the Agilis sheath (St. Jude Medical, Inc, St. Paul, MN). In addition, robotic systems, such as the Sensei X (Hansen Medical, Inc, Mountain View, CA), have recently been introduced, which control large, steerable sheaths, such as the Artisan sheath (14 F) (Hansen Medical, Inc, Mountain View, CA), through which any radiofrequency ablation catheter can be positioned for ablation of atrial fibrillation.[47] The type of catheters used for ablation of atrial fibrillation vary widely as well, but most commonly include either a standard (4-5 mm tipped) or large-

or during radiofrequency ablation of atrial fibrillation has also been enhanced by the use of ICE,[44-45] which may be an important tool to

tipped (8-10 mm tipped) ablation catheter, an internally perfused ablation catheter (Chilli II, Boston Scientific, Inc, Natick, MA) or an

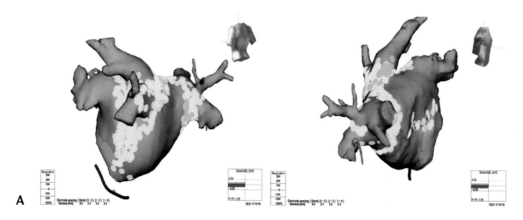

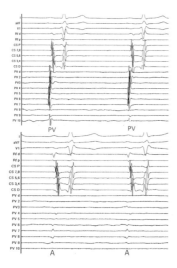

FIGURE 1.4 *Three Dimensional CT Image of the Left Atrium and Pulmonary Veins Demonstrating Circumferential Pulmonary Vein Ablation Plus Additional Left Atrial Linear Ablation, and Endocardial Recordings Demonstrating Resultant Pulmonary Vein Isolation*

A. ESI NavX (St. Jude Medical, Inc, Minnetonka, MN) image with imported and registered 3-D computed tomography (CT) angiogram of the left atrium and pulmonary veins (PV) from the left posterior oblique (LPO) and right anterior oblique (RAO) views, showing left and right circumferential pulmonary vein ablation lines, plus left atrial linear ablation at the roof and mitral isthmus (yellow and green dots). **B.** Surface electrocardiogram (ECG) leads (I, aVF, and V1) and endocardial electrograms recordings from the radiofrequency ablation catheter (RF-d and p), coronary sinus catheter (CSp-d), and the Lasso catheter (PVd-10) demonstrating the presence of pulmonary vein (PV) potentials before right circumferential PV ablation (upper panel) and their elimination after ablation (lower panel) with only a residual far-field atrial (A) potential.

externally perfused ablation catheter (ThermoCool, Biosense Webster, Inc, Diamond Bar, CA). These ablation catheters generally are 8 F or smaller in diameter and fit through the standard fixed-curve or steerable transseptal sheaths commonly used today. In addition, a circular mapping catheter (Lasso, Biosense Webster, Inc, Diamond Bar, CA) is usually passed through a second transseptal sheath to map the pulmonary veins, or occasionally a balloon mapping catheter (EnSite Array, St. Jude Medical, Inc, St. Paul, MN) passed into the left atrium for 3-D mapping, in the event of evidence that a non-pulmonary vein focus is triggering atrial fibrillation.[48] Due to the tendency for atrial fibrillation to recur

despite apparently initially successful ablation, repeat procedures may be difficult due to septal scarring,[49] requiring radiofrequency[38] or guidewire-needle assistance for transseptal catheterization. In addition, unusual vascular anatomy has resulted in the development of alternative approaches for transseptal catheterization, such as a superior vena caval approach, in the event of congenital or surgical interruption of the inferior vena cava.[50] A future intervention requiring transseptal catheterization, likely to be employed by electrophysiologists (as well as interventional cardiologists), is the deployment of the left atrial appendage occluder device (WATCH-MAN, Atritech, Inc, Plymouth, MN) to prevent systemic thromboembolic events, such as stroke, in patients with persistent or recurrent atrial fibrillation despite attempted ablation or antiarrhythmic drug therapy who wish to discontinue use of warfarin or who have relative or absolute contraindications to the use of warfarin.[51]

In summary, the basic approach to transseptal catheterization has changed little since its first description in 1959.[52] However, its clinical application has dramatically expanded, particularly in the field of cardiac electrophysiology, as recently reviewed by Babaliaros et al.[53] Furthermore, advances in imaging technology and adjunctive devices have increased the ease with which transseptal catheterization can be performed, and arguably its safety as well.

References

1. Ross J Jr. Transseptal left heart catheterization: a new method of left atrial puncture. *Ann Surg* 1959;149:395-401.
2. Ross J Jr. Catheterization of the left heart through the interatrial septum: a new technique and its experimental application. *Surg Forum* 1959;9:297-300.
3. Ross J Jr., Braunwald E, Morrow AG. Transseptal left atrial puncture: a new method for the measurement of left atrial pressure in man. *Am J Cardiol* 1959;3:653-655.
4. Ross J Jr., Braunwald E, Morrow AG. Left heart catheterization by the transseptal route: a description of the technic and its applications. *Circulation* 1960;22:927-934.
5. Ross J Jr, Braunwald E, Morrow AG. Transseptal left heart catheterization: a new diagnostic method. *Prog Cardiovasc Dis* 1960;2:315-318.
6. Cope C. Technique for transseptal catheterization of the left atrium; preliminary report. *J Thorac Surg* 1959;37:482-486.
7. Brockenbrough EC, Braunwald E. A new technique for left ventriculography and transseptal left heart catheterization. *Am J Cardiol* 1960;6:1062-1064.
8. Braunwald E, Brockenbrough EC, Ross J Jr., Morrow AG. Left heart catheterization in infants and children. *Pediatrics* 1962;30:253-261.
9. Brockenbrough EC, Braunwald E, Ross J Jr. Transseptal left heart catheterization: a review of 450 studies and description of an improved technique. *Circulation* 1962;25:15-21.
10. Ross J Jr. Considerations regarding the technique for transseptal left heart catheterization. *Circulation* 1966;34:391-399.
11. Swan HJ, Ganz W, Forrester J, Marcus H, Diamond G, Chonette D. Catheterization of the heart in man with use of a flow-directed balloon-tipped catheter. *N Engl J Med* 1970;283:447-451.
12. Scheinman MM. Catheter techniques for ablation of supraventricular tachycardia. *N Engl J Med* 1989;320:460-461.
13. Morady F, Scheinman MM, Di Carlo LA Jr, et al. Catheter ablation of ventricular tachycardia with intracardiac shocks: results in 33 patients. *Circulation* 1987;75:1037-1049.
14. Huang SK, Bharati S, Lev M, Marcus FI. Electrophysiologic and histologic observations of chronic atrioventricular block induced by closed-chest catheter desiccation with radiofrequency energy. *Pacing Clin Electrophysiol* 1987;10:805-816.
15. Jackman WM, Wang XZ, Friday KJ, et al. Catheter ablation of accessory atrioventricular pathways (Wolff-Parkinson-White

syndrome) by radiofrequency current. *N Engl J Med* 1991;324:1605-1611.

16. Calkins H, Sousa J, el-Atassi R, et al. Diagnosis and cure of the Wolff-Parkinson-White syndrome or paroxysmal supraventricular tachycardias during a single electrophysiologic test. *N Engl J Med* 1991;324:1612-1618.

17. Jackman WM, Beckman KJ, McClelland JH, et al. Treatment of supraventricular tachycardia due to atrioventricular nodal reentry, by radiofrequency catheter ablation of slow-pathway conduction. *N Engl J Med* 1992;327:313-318.

18. Feld GK, Fleck RP, Chen PS, et al. Radiofrequency catheter ablation for the treatment of human type 1 atrial flutter: identification of a critical zone in the reentrant circuit by endocardial mapping techniques. *Circulation* 1992;86:1233-1240.

19. Cosio FG, López-Gil M, Goicolea A, Arribas F, Barroso JL. Radiofrequency ablation of the inferior vena cava-tricuspid valve isthmus in common atrial flutter. *Am J Cardiol* 1993;71:705-709.

20. Tracy CM, Swartz JF, Fletcher RD, et al. Radiofrequency catheter ablation of ectopic atrial tachycardia using paced activation sequence mapping. *J Am Coll Cardiol* 1993;21:910-917.

21. Morady F, Harvey M, Kalbfleisch SJ, el-Atassi R, Calkins H, Langberg JJ. Radiofrequency catheter ablation of ventricular tachycardia in patients with coronary artery disease. *Circulation* 1993;87:363-372.

22. European Heart Rhythm Association (EHRA); European Cardiac Arrhythmia Society (ECAS); American College of Cardiology (ACC); American Heart Association (AHA); Society of Thoracic Surgeons (STS); Calkins H, Brugada J, Packer DL, et al. HRS/EHRA/ECAS expert consensus statement on catheter and surgical ablation of atrial fibrillation: recommendations for personnel, policy, procedures and follow-up. A report of the Heart Rhythm Society (HRS) Task Force on catheter and surgical ablation of atrial fibrillation. *Heart Rhythm* 2007;4:816-861. Published correction (a professional title of a coauthor) appears in *Heart Rhythm* 2009;6:148.

23. Lesh MD, Van Hare GF, Scheinman MM, Ports TA, Epstein LA. Comparison of the retrograde and transseptal methods for ablation of left free wall accessory pathways. *J Am Coll Cardiol* 1993;22:542-549.

24. Vora AM, McMahon S, Jazayeri MR, Dhala A. Ablation of atrial insertion sites of left-sided accessory pathways in children: efficacy and safety of transseptal versus transaortic approach. *Pediatr Cardiol* 1997;18:332-338.

25. Law IH, Fischbach PS, LeRoy S, et al. Access to the left atrium for delivery of radiofrequency ablation in young patients: retrograde aortic vs transseptal approach. *Pediatr Cardiol* 2001;22:204-209.

26. Sorbera C, Cohen M, Woolf P, Kalapatapu SR. Atrioventricular nodal reentry tachycardia: slow pathway ablation using the transseptal approach. *Pacing Clin Electrophysiol* 2000;23:1343-1349.

27. Kobza R, Hindricks G, Tanner H, Kottkamp H. Left-septal ablation of the fast pathway in AV nodal reentrant tachycardia refractory to right septal ablation. *Europace* 2005;7:149-153.

28. Fenrich AL Jr, Friedman RA, Cecchin FC, Kearney D. Left-sided atrioventricular nodal ablation using the transseptal approach: clinico-histopathologic correlation. *J Cardiovasc Electrophysiol* 1998;9:757-760.

29. Schwartzman D, Callans DJ, Gottlieb CD, Marchlinski FE. Catheter ablation of ventricular tachycardia associated with remote myocardial infarction: utility of the atrial transseptal approach. *J Interv Card Electrophysiol* 1997;1:67-71.

30. Pratola C, Baldo E, Notarstefano P, Tiziano T, Ferrari R. Feasibility of the transseptal

approach for fast and unstable left ventricular tachycardia mapping and ablation with a non-contact mapping system. *J Interv Card Electrophysiol* 2006;16:111-116.

31. De Ponti R, Zardini M, Storti C, Longobardi M, Salerno-Uriarte JA. Trans-septal catheterization for radiofrequency catheter ablation of cardiac arrhythmias: results and safety of a simplified method. *Eur Heart J* 1998; 19:943-950.

32. Sorbera C, Dhakam S, Cohen M, Woolf P, Agarwal Y. Safety and efficacy of outpatient transseptal radiofrequency ablation of atrio-ventricular accessory pathways. *J Interv Card Electrophysiol* 1999;3:173-175.

33. Tucker KJ, Curtis AB, Murphy J, et al. Transesophageal echocardiographic guidance of transseptal left heart catheterization during radiofrequency ablation of left-sided accessory pathways in humans. *Pacing Clin Electrophysiol* 1996;19:272-281.

34. Epstein LM, Smith T, TenHoff H. Nonfluoroscopic transseptal catheterization: safety and efficacy of intracardiac echocardiographic guidance. *J Cardiovasc Electrophysiol* 1998;9:625-630.

35. Daoud EG, Kalbfleisch SJ, Hummel JD. Intracardiac echocardiography to guide transseptal left heart catheterization for radiofrequency catheter ablation. *J Cardiovasc Electrophysiol* 1999;10:358-363.

36. Andrikopoulos GK, Tzeis S, Tsilakis D, Kranidis A, Manolis AS. Intracardiac echocardiography-facilitated ablation of a left-lateral bypass tract in a patient with atrial septal aneurysm. *Hellenic J Cardiol* 2008;49:437-440.

37. Lakkireddy D, Rangisetty U, Prasad S, et al. Intracardiac echo-guided radiofrequency catheter ablation of atrial fibrillation in patients with atrial septal defect or patent foramen ovale repair: a feasibility, safety, and efficacy study. *J Cardiovasc Electrophysiol* 2008;19:1137-1142.

38. Sherman W, Lee P, Hartley A, Love B. Transatrial septal catheterization using a new radiofrequency probe. *Catheter Cardiovasc Interv* 2005;66:14-17.

39. Haïssaguerre M, Jaïs P, Shah DC, et al. Spontaneous initiation of atrial fibrillation by ectopic beats originating in the pulmonary veins. *N Engl J Med* 1998;339:659-666.

40. Lim KK, Sugeng L, Lang R, Knight BP. Double transseptal catheterization guided by real-time 3-dimensional transesophageal echocardiography. *Heart Rhythm* 2008;5: 324-325.

41. Fagundes RL, Mantica M, De Luca L, et al. Safety of single transseptal puncture for ablation of atrial fibrillation: retrospective study from a large cohort of patients. *J Cardiovasc Electrophysiol* 2007;18:1277-1281.

42. Ren JF, Marchlinski FE, Callans DJ, et al. Increased intensity of anticoagulation may reduce risk of thrombus during atrial fibrillation ablation procedures in patients with spontaneous echo contrast. *J Cardiovasc Electrophysiol* 2005;16:474-477.

43. Wazni OM, Rossillo A, Marrouche NF, et al. Embolic events and char formation during pulmonary vein isolation in patients with atrial fibrillation: impact of different anticoagulation regimens and importance of intracardiac echo imaging. *J Cardiovasc Electrophysiol* 2005;16:576-581.

44. Wazni OM, Beheiry S, Fahmy T, et al. Atrial fibrillation ablation in patients with therapeutic international normalized ratio: comparison of strategies of anticoagulation management in the periprocedural period. *Circulation* 2007;116:2531-4.

45. Maleki K, Mohammadi R, Hart D, Cotiga D, Farhat N, Steinberg JS. Intracardiac ultrasound detection of thrombus on transseptal sheath: incidence, treatment, and prevention. *J Cardiovasc Electrophysiol* 2005;16:561-565.

46. Okuyama Y, Kashiwase K, Mizuno H, et al. Development of thrombus on a transseptal

sheath in the left atrium during attempted electrical pulmonary vein isolation for the treatment of paroxysmal atrial fibrillation. *Europace* 2006;8:191-192.

47. Saliba W, Reddy VY, Wazni O, et al. Atrial fibrillation ablation using a robotic catheter remote control system: initial human experience and long-term follow-up results. *J Am Coll Cardiol* 2008;51:2407-2411.

48. Schneider MA, Ndrepepa G, Zrenner B, et al. Noncontact mapping-guided catheter ablation of atrial fibrillation associated with left atrial ectopy. *J Cardiovasc Electrophysiol* 2000;11:475-479.

49. Tomlinson DR, Sabharwal N, Bashir Y, Betts TR. Interatrial septum thickness and difficulty with transseptal puncture during redo catheter ablation of atrial fibrillation. *Pacing Clin Electrophysiol* 2008;31:1606-1611.

50. Lim HE, Pak HN, Tse HF, et al. Catheter ablation of atrial fibrillation via superior approach in patients with interruption of the inferior vena cava. *Heart Rhythm* 2009;6:174-179.

51. Nageh T, Meier B. Intracardiac devices for stroke prevention. *Prev Cardiol* 2006;9:42-48.

52. Ross J Jr. Transseptal left heart catheterization: a fifty year odyssey. *J Am Coll Cardiol* 2008;51:2107-2115

53. Babaliaros VC, Green JT, Lerakis S, Lloyd M, Block PC. Emerging applications for transseptal left heart catheterization: old techniques for new procedures. *J Am Coll Cardiol* 2008;51:2116-2122.

2

Embryology and Anatomy of the Atrial Septum

Siew Yen Ho

Increasingly, transcatheter interventional procedures require access to the left heart chambers via the atrial septum. To ensure that these procedures are successful and to reduce the risk of complications, a detailed knowledge and understanding of the atrial septum, which separates the left and right atrial chambers, is crucial. While morphologists can view the heart from all angles and display the atrial septum to best advantage, their views sometimes differ from those commonly used by interventional electrophysiologists. Adopting McAlpine's attitudinal approach for describing the locations of the heart's structures can improve our understanding of its anatomy.[1] Nevertheless, there remains the issue of speaking a common language. The terminology used when describing cardiac embryogenesis is confusing because, histori-cally, the same structures have been given different names, and eponyms are rather common.[2] Furthermore, the conversion of Latin terms into English, while laudable for readers who are fluent in English, can be confusing for others.

Echoing Whitmore's sentiments in "Terminologia Anatomica: New Terminology for the New Anatomist" that terminology must accommodate all users, I hope the terminology used in this chapter will suit cardiologists, morphologists, and scientists alike.[3] Latinate terms will be offered in association with their commonly used English equivalents. The first part of this chapter is a review of the embryologic development of the atrial septum. As this section is meant to enhance the understanding of structures in the definitive heart, I will use attitudinal orientations as much as possible when describing those locations. The bending and growth of the heart tube during development continually shifts these structures, however, so their loca-

Transseptal Catheterization and Interventions.
© 2010 Ranjan Thakur MD and Andrea Natale MD, eds.
Cardiotext Publishing, ISBN 978-0-9790164-1-7.

tions can be described only in general terms. Traditionally, embryologists use *ventral, dorsal, cephalad,* and *caudad* as their compass points because those terms can be applied to both bipeds and quadrupeds. I prefer the terms *anterior, posterior, superior,* and *inferior,* respectively, which are more compatible with descriptions of the human postnatal heart.

Developmental Anatomy

At the early stages of cardiac development, the embryonic heart tube is more or less straight with a venous pole at the inferior end and an arterial pole at the superior end. The tube is attached posteriorly along its length by mesocardium to the body of the embryo. This tube gives rise to the ventricles and, through the process of looping, detaches much of its length from the mesocardium. During the looping process, the inferior pole, which is also the inlet part of the tube, expands to form the atrial component, concomitant with the expansion of the superior pole, the outlet portion, through recruitment of extracardiac cells. Wide venous channels, which carry blood from both the right and left sides of the embryo back to the heart, connect to the developing atrial portion. The paired veins form the so-called horns of the sinus venosus. The common cardinal veins (ducts of Cuvier) drain from each side of the embryo into the sinus, as do the umbilical veins from the placenta and the vitelline veins from the yolk sac.

At the fourth week of development, there are no anatomical borders between the sinus venosus and the primitive atrium. The sinus venosus portion becomes asymmetrical as the left horn diminishes in size and is incorporated into the developing left atrioventricular junction, while the right horn grows rapidly. The left horn, which ultimately receives only

the left duct of Cuvier, persists as the coronary sinus. Consequently, the entire systemic venous component opens to the right portion of the primitive atrium, which, in turn, continues to the developing atrioventricular junction at the atrioventricular canal (Figure 2.1a).

While the primitive atrium is developing, endocardial cushions form within the canal in preparation for the remodelling of the atrioventricular junction and cardiac septation (Figure 2.1b). Two cushions, the superior and inferior cushions, project into the lumen; they meet in the middle, dividing the common orifice of the canal into right and left orifices. The union of the endocardial cushions is thought to form the septum intermedium, but the cushions are not the only contributors to septation of the atrioventricular canal (discussed below).

The remaining systemic veins remodel. The vitelline and umbilical veins become a single vessel, the inferior caval vein (inferior vena cava). Thus, the venous component, which includes the entrances of three veins, the inferior caval vein and the right and left ducts of Cuvier, opens into the posterior aspect of the primitive atrium. Valve-like structures develop to the right and left sides of the venous component to demarcate its junction with the atrium, allowing anatomical distinction between the sinus venosus and the primitive atrium. These valves, described as the right and left venous valves, fuse at their superior and inferior extremities (Figure 2.1a). The right venous valve continues into the posterosuperior wall of the atrium, forming the septum spurium, which, as the name suggests, is a false septum because it reaches its fullest development during the third month and then diminishes to become the sagittal bundle in the formed heart. The posteroinferior wall of the sinus venosus folds inward to form the so-called sinus septum (eustachian ridge); this fold divides the right venous valve into

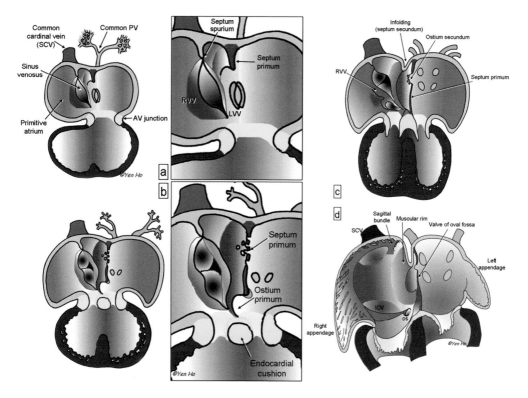

FIGURE 2.1　　*Development of the Atrial Septum*
　　A. At approximately day 30, the right (RVV) and left (LVV) venous valves guard the entrance of the sinus venosus to the primitive atrium. The septum primum begins to form. At the same time, the common pulmonary vein (PV) connects with the atrium. The PV's portal is guarded by right and left ridges (green). **B.** As the septum primum grows toward the endocardial cushions, its superior portion breaks down to form the ostium secundum at approximately day 32. The leading edge of the septum primum carries the right pulmonary ridge. The left ridge regresses as the pulmonary vein becomes incorporated into the atrium. **C.** An infolding of the atrial wall develops to the right of the septum primum as the septum primum fuses to the endocardial cushions. The left venous valve disappears. The posterior wall of the sinus venous folds inward and divides the right venous valve (RVV). **D.** The primitive atrium is partitioned into right and left atrial chambers, each with its own atrial appendage. ICV = inferior caval vein; SCV = superior caval vein.

two portions (Figure 2.1c). The valvar remnants become the eustachian and Thebesian valves, which guard the orifices of the inferior caval vein and the coronary sinus, respectively. The tendinous commissure between the two venous valves extends through the sinus septum, which later becomes the antero-inferior rim of the foramen ovale and a border for the triangle of Koch (discussed below). As the sinus venosus becomes incorporated into the primitive atrium, the left and right sides of

the primitive atrium expand to form the atrial appendages. In the definitive heart, the right border between the sinus venosus and the atrial appendage is marked internally by the crista terminalis (terminal crest).

At the time when the primitive atrium begins to be partitioned, approximately day 30 of development, the lungs are just beginning to bud from the trachea, and a venous channel forms in the posterior mesocardium behind the heart. The venous channel becomes the common pulmonary vein that collects the pulmonary venous plexus into the posteroinferior part of the primitive atrium. The entrance of the common pulmonary vein is slightly to the left of the atrial midline, and it is bound on the right and left sides by ridges of persisting posterior mesocardium that protrude into the atrial cavity (Figure 2.1a). The right ridge, described as the spina vestibuli by His, develops to be more prominent and contributes to cardiac septation.[4]

The first sign of atrial septation is the appearance of the septum primum (primary septum) as a crescent of muscle in the atrial roof (Figures 2.1a, 2.1b). The inferior part of the septum primum is continuous with the spina vestibuli (vestibular spine, dorsal mesenchymal protrusion).[5] This extends further and further into the cavity of the primitive atrium toward the endocardial cushions that are in the process of fusing to divide the atrioventricular canal into right and left portions. During this time, approximately day 32 of development, the atrioventricular canal expands rightward in readiness for connecting the developing right atrium to the distal part of the looped heart tube, which is to become the future right ventricle (Figure 2.1b). The leading margin of the septum primum is edged by mesenchyme (cells of mesodermal origin), which is thought to be derived from embryonic endocardium.[6,7] The gap between the free edge of the septum primum and the fused superior and inferior atrioventricular endocardial cushions is the ostium primum (foramen primum or primary atrial foramen). With the incorporation of additional mesodermal tissue, the spina vestibuli expands, and, by approximately day 42 of development, combines with the septum primum and the endocardial cushions to ultimately close the ostium primum.[8] This process carries the inferior ends of the venous valves anteriorly, and muscularization

of the expanded spina vestibuli reinforces the base of the septum primum. The upper portion of the septum primum remains thin and persists as the flap valve of the definitive foramen ovale (Figure 2.1d). However, before the ostium primum can be fully obliterated, the upper portion of the septum primum, close to its origin at the atrial roof, breaks down to form the ostium secundum (foramen secundum, foramen ovale secundum, or secondary atrial foramen) (Figure 2.1c). The ostium secundum is important for the continuation of adequate blood flow to the left side of the heart after cardiac septation.

At approximately day 37 of development, the common pulmonary vein divides into left and right branches and becomes incorporated into the developing left atrium to form its posterior wall. The left pulmonary ridge disappears. Remodelling of the portion of roof of the atrium between the left venous valve that guards the entrance of the superior caval vein (superior vena cava) and the septum primum begins. To the right of the septum primum, the atrial wall folds inward to form the posterior, superior, and anterosuperior margins of the muscular rim (limbus fossa ovalis). This infolding is the septum secundum; it acts like a door frame, allowing the septum primum, or the "door," to close against it after birth. The curved shape of the leading edge of the septum secundum demarcates the foramen ovale, which is analogous to the doorway. In the developed heart, this edge is described as the limbus (rim) of the foramen ovale. Unfortunately, as we shall see in a later section, there is some confusion regarding the term *foramen ovale* (oval foramen, fossa ovalis/oval fossa). The anterosuperior part of the infolding, together with the septum primum, separates the orifice of the superior caval vein from the orifice of the right superior pulmonary vein. The atrial walls expand inferiorly and posteriorly while the atrioventricular junction develops to incorporate the insulating fibrofatty tissue plane of the atrioventricular groove. This remodelling carries the newly muscularized spina vestibuli forward to form the anteroinferior margin of the muscular rim and the triangle of Koch.[8] While the primitive atrium develops, the heart tube bends upon itself, ultimately bringing the outlet portion in front of the atria. The rapid growth of the atria and their appendages results in the anterior atrial walls appearing to embrace the outlet (Figure 2.1d). As the heart grows bigger, the ventricles become larger than the atria, and the aorta becomes the great artery that is closest to the anterior walls of the atria.

As discussed above, the septum primum serves as a one-way valve during fetal life, allowing placental blood from the right atrium to pass into the left atrium and into systemic circulation. In normal hearts, the septum primum is larger than the foramen ovale, and it overlaps the muscular rim (limbus). When pressure in the left atrium increases after birth, the septum primum shuts off the passageway, effecting functional closure of the foramen ovale. Anatomic closure occurs when fibrosis at the margins of the muscular rim renders the valve adherent. Adhesion is not always complete around the circumference of the rim, however. The anterosuperior margin quite often remains non-adherent, leaving a potential passage for right-to-left shunting even though the septum primum is overlapping the limbus. This crevice is described as probe patency of the foramen ovale (discussed below).

In fetal life, the valve of the foramen ovale (septum primum) is thin and membrane-like, comprising a few myocytes sandwiched between two thin layers of endocardium. Its myocardial component increases progressively as the fetus grows. At birth, the endocardium remains a thin lining. However, a dramatic increase in the thickness of the valve occurs soon after birth and continues until 1 year of age. Following this period, the thickness increases only slightly throughout life.[9] The myocardial component forms a bilaminar arrangement of orthogonally-oriented myocytes interspersed with fibrous tissue, and the myocytes become enlarged.[10,11] It has been suggested that this arrangement may contribute to maintenance of left septal atrial flutter.[10] However, the major contribution to increased thickness is endocardial proliferation characterized by fibroelastosis that tends to be thicker on the right side of the septum primum.[9] In adult hearts, it is common to find fibrofatty tissue sandwiched between endocardium and myocardium on both sides of the valve.[11]

The Definitive Atrial Septum

Location of the Septum

When the heart is viewed from the front, the right atrial cavity is right and anterior whereas the left atrial cavity is mainly posterior and slightly left of the right atrium. Thus, the plane of the atrial septum does not coincide with the anterior-posterior sagittal plane. Instead, it runs at an angle of approximately 65° from right posterior to left anterior, similarly to how it appears on transesophageal echocardiography (Figure 2.2a). With this orientation, the septal plane is more or less *en face* when viewed in the radiographic right-anterior oblique projection (Figure 2.2b). When the left atrium is enlarged, the angle is increased. Seen in this projection, however, the septum appears much more extensive than it is. The true septal area for safe access between the atrial chambers occupies a considerably smaller area.

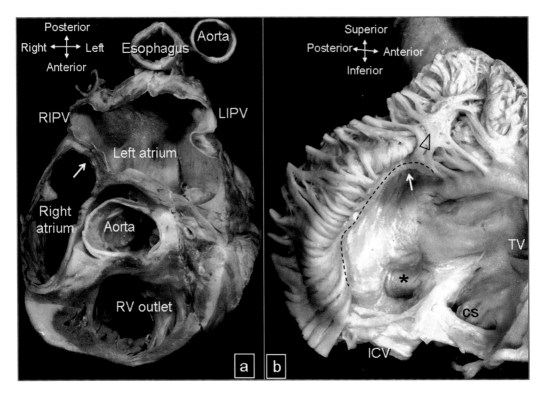

FIGURE 2.2   *Location of the Atrial Septum*
A. Transverse orthogonal section showing the plane of the atrial septum (white arrow). Note the location of the aortic root immediately anterior to the septal plane. **B.** The right atrium is opened to display the septal aspect. The asterisk (*) marks the floor of the oval fossa, and the arrow indicates the orifice of the superior caval vein. Note the terminal crest (dotted line) and sagittal bundle (triangle). CS = coronary sinus; ICV = inferior caval vein; LIPV = left inferior pulmonary vein; RIPV = right inferior pulmonary vein; RV = right ventricle; TV = tricuspid valve.

Access to the Right Atrial Aspect

Whether approaching the atrial septum via the inferior caval vein or the superior caval veins, the catheter may occasionally be hindered. The most common substrate for obstruction is the configuration of the eustachian valve, which is derived from the right venous valve. The left venous valve rarely persists. When it does, it is in the form of an insignificant flap or ridge.

Guarding the orifice of the inferior caval vein, the morphology of the eustachian valve ranges from a small crescent-shaped flap (or absence) to a large fenestrated flap and a filigreed network (Figure 2.3).[12] In a study of 100 heart specimens, 24 hearts had large fenestrated valves.[12] Thin strands in fenestrated and filigreed valves may be sites of thrombus formation. In rare cases, this matrix of fine fibers, known as the Chiari network, is very extensive. The originally described Chiari network stretched from in front of the superior caval orifice to the inferior caval orifice and was thought to have derived in part from the septum spurium.[12] This anatomical remnant is present in 2%-3% of the population and has no purpose, nor is it pathological. It may be seen on a 2-D echocardiographic study

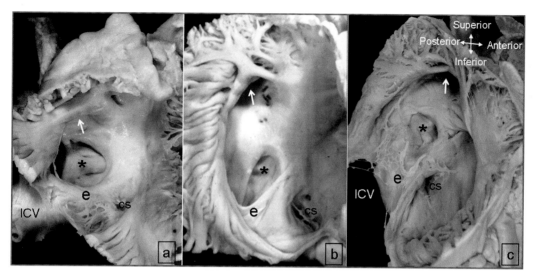

FIGURE 2.3   *Morphological Variants of the Eustachian Valve*

The septal aspect of the right atrium is displayed in approximately right anterior-oblique view to show variations in morphology of the eustachian valves. **A.** In place of a valve, there is a muscular ridge. **B.** The valve is like a crescentic flap. **C.** The valve is an extensive Chiari network. CS = coronary sinus; ICV = inferior caval vein; e = eustachian valve.

and is characterized by whip-like motion and attachment near the inferior vena cava. It should be distinguished from pathological masses in the right atrium: vegetations, thrombi, and myxoma. In very rare cases, the network forms a membrane, which effectively divides the right atrium into two. The Chiari network is not readily visualized on imaging. When encountering a Chiari network, the interventionist should heed the potential risk of inadvertently dislodging thrombi or tearing off fragments of the delicate valve when the catheter becomes entangled.

Structure of the Septum

The true septum is the structure that can be removed without exiting the atrial chambers. Strictly speaking, the atrial septum is limited to the floor of the oval fossa (septum primum) and its immediate muscular anteroinferior rim, which is confluent with the apical part of Koch's triangle.[13] From the right atrial aspect,

the valve forming the floor of the fossa usually appears as a crater-like depression surrounded by a muscular rim (Figure 2.4). The valve is thin; its thickness ranges from 0.5 mm to 1.5 mm in adult heart specimens.[9,14] It tends to be slightly thinner in hearts with atrial enlargement and thicker in those with valvar disease, but the presence of atrial fibrillation or atrial septal defect does not affect the thickness.[9,14,15] In some hearts the valve is thinner and aneurysmal in appearance as it herniates into the atrial chambers through the cardiac cycle. Most cardiologists accept a 1-cm excursion on echocardiography as a septal aneurysm. Occasionally, the valve is extremely floppy so that when pushed with the tip of a catheter it may even extend to the lateral wall of the left atrium, risking exit into the pericardial space when the "septum" is punctured.

The size and location of the fossa varies widely from patient to patient (Figure 2.4). In a study using intracardiac echocardiography and fluoroscopy, Hanaoko and colleagues

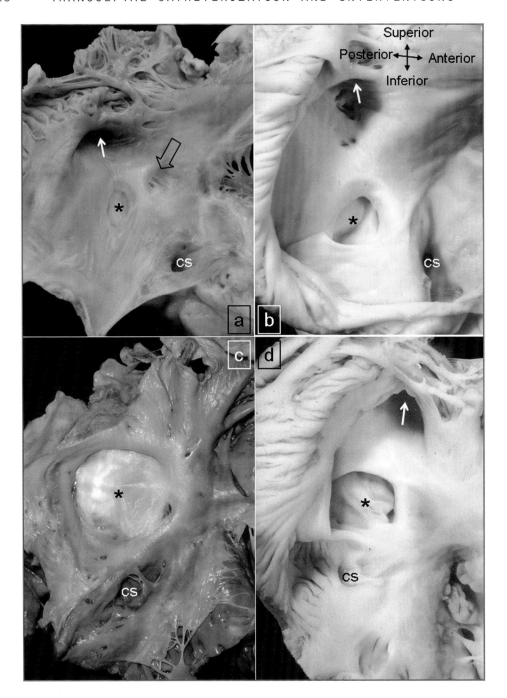

FIGURE 2.4   *Morphological Variants of the Oval Fossa*

The right atrium of 4 hearts displayed in similar orientation as in Figure 2.3 to illustrate the variations in oval fossa, shown here by asterisks (*). The white arrows point to the orifice of the superior caval vein. **A.** The valve of the oval fossa is small, and the muscular rim around the fossa is not distinctive. The area anterior to the anterior part of the rim contains several pits and crevices (open arrow). **B.** The muscular rim around the valve is prominent. Note the presence of small pits near the orifice of the superior caval vein. **C.** The valve is large and thin (transilluminated). The muscular rim is well defined. **D.** The valve is aneurysmal, herniating into the right atrium in this display. cs = coronary sinus.

found a superior-inferior dimension range of 10 mm to 31 mm and an anterior-posterior dimension range of 4.8 mm to 14.2 mm.[16] The size of the fossa may be reduced in hearts that have an enlarged coronary sinus, such as those associated with persistence of the left superior caval vein. Furthermore, as a study by Schwinger and colleagues using trans-esophageal echocardiography showed, the muscular rim around the fossa is not always prominent.[14] In 82% of the patients in that study, there was a detectable change in topography when going from the muscular rim to the valve of the fossa. This change allows the interventionist to feel a "jump" as the tip of the catheter drops onto the valve (Figures 2.4b, 2.4c, 2.4d). The thin valve can then be "tented" when pushed toward the left atrium. The remainder of patients in Schwinger et al showed only gradual thinning toward the fossa (Figure 2.4a).

In addition to this difficulty in finding the true septum, the fossa is not consistently located in the middle of the septal aspect when viewed from the right atrium.[16] When the fossa is located more anteriorly, the risk of encountering the aortic root when performing septal puncture increases. A more posterior location raises the risk of entering the posterior interatrial groove and the peri-cardial space. It is important, therefore, to understand what constitutes the septal aspect of the atria, for no anatomic borders exist between the muscular rim and the remaining atrial wall.

A cursory look from the right atrium gives the impression of an extensive septal structure. In particular, anterosuperior to the oval fossa, the seemingly vast expanse of the "atrial septum" is actually the right atrial wall that overlies the aortic root (Figures 2.5a, 2.5b). Known as the aortic mound because it projects into the right atrium, this region often contains small pits and crevices

that may lodge the tip of a catheter or perforating device and give the false impression of the catheter having "tented" the septum when attempting to cross the fossa ovalis (Figure 2.4a). Unfortunately, any transgression through this wall will exit the heart into the transverse pericardial sinus and through that space into the aortic root (Figure 2.2a). Placing a marker in the aortic root or over the His bundle may be helpful in determining whether one is puncturing too anteriorly.

Sections through the septal area demonstrate that much of the muscular rim is not true septum (Figure 2.6). The peripheral structures are the infolded right atrial wall, anterosuperiorly, superiorly, posteriorly, and inferiorly. The superior and posterior parts of the rim, often called the septum secundum, is mainly the infolded right atrial wall between the base of the superior caval vein and the insertion of the right pulmonary veins to the left atrium (Figure 2.6). From the epicardial aspect, this infolding is known to surgeons as Waterston's groove. Through it the left atrium can be accessed without entering the right atrium. Posteroinferiorly, the rim is continuous with the wall of the inferior caval vein. Filling the epicardial side of the muscular rim's fold is fatty tissue, which forms the interatrial groove or septal raphe. The anterosuperior part of the groove often contains the sinus node artery, which ascends from the right coronary artery to the sinus node at the superior cavoatrial junction. The extent of fatty tissue varies, but in the normal heart excessive amounts of fatty tissue can give the erroneous impression of lipomatous septal hypertrophy. In young adults, the upper limit of normal fat deposit is defined as 1.5 cm in transverse dimension on echocardiography.[17]

The anteroinferior rim is continuous with the eustachian ridge (sinus septum) and the vestibule leading to the tricuspid valve. This area, previously dubbed the muscular

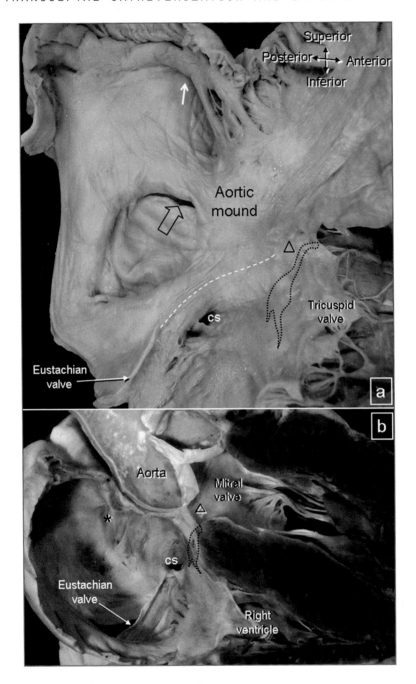

FIGURE 2.5   *PFO and Proximity to Aortic Root*

A. This right atrial view shows probe patency of the foramen ovale (open arrow). The white broken line marks the posterior border of the triangle of Koch. At the apex of triangle is the membranous septum (Δ). The shape outlined by dots represents the atrioventricular node and the penetrating atrioventricular bundle. The atrial wall anterior to the oval fossa is known as the aortic mound. The white arrow marks the orifice of the superior caval vein. **B.** This longitudinal section through the membranous septum (Δ) shows the relationship between the aortic mound and the aortic root. The oval fossa (*) lies more posteriorly. Note the location of the atrioventricular node (dotted shape). The atrioventricular conduction bundle is sandwiched between the membranous septum and the muscular ventricular septum. CS = coronary sinus.

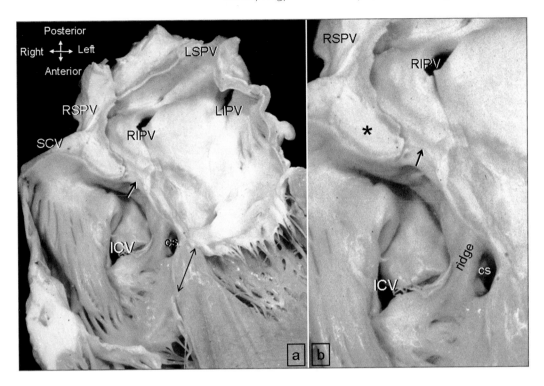

FIGURE 2.6   *Structure of the Atrial Septum*

This longitudinal cut through the 4 cardiac chambers profiles the atrial septum.
A. The valve of the oval fossa (short arrow) is surrounded by a muscular rim. The hingelines of the mitral and tricuspid valves are offset (double-headed arrows). **B.** This magnified view shows the infolded atrial wall filled with epicardial fat (*). The eustachian ridge lies between the orifices of the inferior caval vein (ICV) and coronary sinus (cs). Note the orifices of the right pulmonary veins are adjacent to the plane of the atrial septum. LIPV = left inferior pulmonary vein; LSPV = left superior pulmonary vein; RIPV = right inferior pulmonary vein; RSPV = right superior pulmonary vein; SCV = superior caval vein.

atrioventricular septum, is a "sandwich" comprising the right atrial wall, fatty tissue of the inferior atrioventricular groove, and the wall of the left ventricle. In location, this area separates the right atrium from the left ventricle; the separation is due to a disparity in the levels of attachment between the mitral and the tricuspid valves (Figure 2.6a). The artery supplying the atrioventricular node passes within the fatty tissue plane. The atrial part of the "sandwich" contains the atrioventricular node, which lies within a millimeter or so of the endocardial surface. The anatomical landmark for the location of the atrioventricu-

lar node is the triangle of Koch in the right atrium (Figure 2.5a). This triangular area is delineated posteriorly by the course of the tendon of Todaro, which is the continuation of the commissure between the eustachian and Thebesian valves that traverses within the sinus septum.[18] The tendon inserts superiorly into the central fibrous body at the apex of the triangle (Figure 2.5a). The anterior border of the triangle is marked by the hingeline of the septal leaflet of the tricuspid valve. The base of the triangle is marked by the orifice of the coronary sinus, and the vestibule between that orifice and the tricuspid valve is known

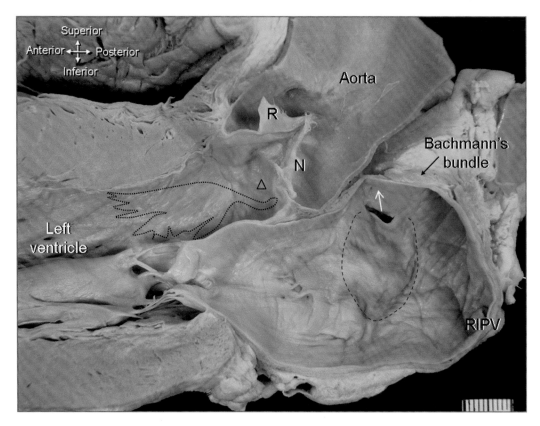

FIGURE 2.7   *Left Aspect of Atrial Septum*

This longitudinal cut through the left heart shows the left atrial aspect of the valve of the oval fossa (broken line). There is probe patency of the foramen ovale that allows a probe to be passed from the right atrium into the left atrium. Upon entering the left atrium, the probe points to the anterior wall that has a close relationship with the aortic root. In this preparation, the Bachmann bundle has been cut in cross section. The dotted shape represents the atrioventricular conduction bundle and the left bundle branch. The anatomical landmark for the bundle is the membranous septum (Δ) sited inferior to the closure line between right (R) and noncoronary (N) aortic valve leaflets. RIPV = right inferior pulmonary vein.

to interventionists as the paraseptal isthmus, which is a target for ablation of the slow pathway in atrioventricular nodal reentrant tachycardia.[19] The compact atrioventricular node resides near the apex of the triangle, and the penetrating bundle of His extends from it into the central fibrous body. From there, the atrioventricular conduction bundle passes onto the crest of the ventricular septum to lie close to the subaortic outflow tract, immediately below the membranous septum (Figure 2.5b). Here, the anatomical landmark is the area between

the hingelines of the right and non-coronary leaflets of the aortic valve (Figure 2.7).

Patent Foramen Ovale

As long as the blood pressure in the left atrium exceeds that in the right atrium, the valve that comprises the floor of the fossa closes shut against the rim. For the valve to close, it must be large enough to overlap the rim completely. Anatomical closure of the fossa is accomplished when the valve becomes adherent to the rim. In approximately 25% to 34% of the population, the seal is incomplete, leaving a crevice at the anterosuperior quadrant of the rim that can allow a probe to be passed obliquely from the right atrium through what is commonly known as a patent foramen ovale, or PFO (Figures 2.5a, 2.7).[20] This term, however, can be confusing. It is sometimes mistakenly given to an opening at the site of the original foramen ovale (ostium secundum), or so-called secundum ASD (atrial septal defect), where the valve is inadequate to overlap the rim so that the foramen ovale is not obliterated (discussion below). In heart specimens, the probe-patent foramen ovale ranges from 1 mm to 10 mm in diameter.[20,21] The length of the tunnel through which the probe passes depends on the extent of overlap between the flap valve and the rim.[21,22] Morphologically, there are two forms of patent foramen ovale.[21] The first is the valve-competent form in which, under normal circumstances, the valve is large enough to overlap the muscular rim, much like a door closing against a door frame. Although forming a perfect seal, some of these valves are aneurysmal and bow into the right and left atrial chambers with the respiratory phases. The second form is the valve-incompetent form. It probably results from the stretching of the muscular rim during atrial dilatation and/or retraction of the aneurysmal valve. This stretching allows the flap valve to herniate markedly leftward or rightward, reducing the extent of overlap. It is not clear if this form is due to deficiency of valvar tissues and, thus, is a true defect of the oval fossa ("secundum defect") or whether it is a deficiency of the muscular rim.

On the left atrial side, the crevice is marked by the crescent-like free edge of the valve (Figure 2.7). Other than a few pits and crevices, the valve on the left atrial aspect is featureless and blends into the atrial wall.

Interventionists who utilize the patent foramen ovale to cross the septum instead of performing a septal puncture should take note that when the catheter emerges from the crescent-like free edge of the septum primum, its tip is pointing directly at the anterior wall of the left atrium. In this region, the atrial wall is very thin (Figure 2.7). McAlpine drew attention to this area, which is immediately inferior to the Bachmann's bundle, by describing it as "the unprotected area in the anterior wall of the left atrium."[23]

Atrial Septal Defect

Some defects commonly referred to as atrial septal defects (ASDs) are interatrial communications rather than deficiencies of the true atrial septum. Defects within the true septum, generally termed "secundum defects," are deficiencies of the valve covering the oval fossa. By contrast, sinus venosus defects, coronary sinus defects, and "ostium primum" defects are outside the confines of the true atrial septum, although, unequivocally, they permit interatrial shunting.[24]

Defects within the oval fossa (secundum defects) are located at the site of the embryonic "ostium secundum"; they are therefore not a deficiency of the "septum secundum," for the "septum secundum" is largely the infolded right atrial wall. Deficiencies, perforations, or a complete absence of the valve guarding the oval fossa are the most common types of interatrial communications, and they come in a variety of sizes and form.[25-27] The simplest form is that of the valve being too small to overlap the muscular rim, leaving an oval-shaped aperture between the rim and the edge of the valve. This form is most amenable to transcatheter repair, providing the muscular borders are adequate enough to not impinge on the orifices of the pulmonary veins, the

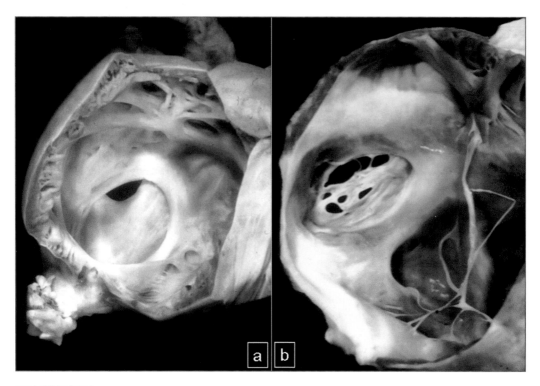

FIGURE 2.8   *Atrial Septal Defects*
These views of the right atrium show two examples of deficiency of the valve of the fossa ovale. **A.** There is an oval-shaped defect. **B.** The valve of the fossa is fenestrated, and the eustachian valve is comprised of thin strands.

atrioventricular valves, the caval veins, or the coronary sinus.[24-26] The valve itself may be perforated with single or multiple fenestrations (Figure 2.8). Sometimes, the valve appears like a net or is represented by a filigreed remnant. When associated with aneurysmal formation, the net may appear like a windsock. Although defects in the oval fossa do not alter the basic disposition of the sinus and atrioventricular nodes of the conduction system, very large or unusually located defects will reduce the distances between the margin of the defects and the atrioventricular node, the orifice of the coronary sinus, the right pulmonary veins, the aortic root, or the mitral valve.

The presence of a small defect in the oval fossa may facilitate passing the catheter through the atrial septum without having to make a perforation. However, the location of the aperture may or may not be ideal for subsequent maneuvers to reach the desired destinations in the left atrium. Crossing through an aperture in the anterosuperior margin of the fossa will be like crossing through a probe-patent foramen ovale. The angle of the catheter can make it more challenging to reach the area around the orifice of the right inferior pulmonary vein. Today, the major relevance of atrial septal defects to transseptal catheterization occurs when the interventionist encounters a device occluding the defect. Attempting to perforate an early generation device may be difficult, but trying to cross at the periphery of the septal occluder may run the risk of encroaching upon cardiac structures, as discussed above.

Conclusions

Structurally, the atrial septum is more complex than it seems at first glance. Differentiating the true atrial septum from its surroundings will help avoid complications when accessing the left atrium from the right atrium. Owing to its location and proximity to important structures like the aortic valve, the septum should be imaged from more than one perspective or from within the right atrium when selecting the best site to cross. Thickly fibrosed septum, patches, occluder devices, and aneurysmal valves of the oval fossa are particularly challenging for transseptal catheterization. Knowledge of normal anatomy, its variations, and abnormal anatomy is essential.

References

1. McAlpine WA. *Heart and Coronary Arteries.* Berlin: Springer, 1975:1.

2. Arráez-Aybar A, González-Lorrio F, Marantos-Gamarra DG, et al. Cardiac development onomatology: the real heart of the matter. *Ann Anat* 2003;185:525-533.

3. Whitmore I. Terminologia anatomica: new terminology for the new anatomist. *Anat Rec* 1999;257:50-53.

4. His W. Die area interposita, die Eustachische klappe und die spina vestibuli. *Anatomie Menschlicher Embryonen.* 1880;149-152.

5. Wessels A, Anderson RH, Markwald RR, et al. Atrial development in the human heart: an immunohistochemical study with emphasis on the role of mesenchymal tissues. *Anat Rec* 2000;259:288-300.

6. Arrechedera H, Alvarez M, Strauss M, et al. Origin of mesenchymal tissue in the septum primum: a structural and ultrastructural study. *J Mol Cell Cardiol* 1987;19:641-651.

7. Mommersteeg MTM, Soufan AT, de Lange FJ, et al. Two distinct pools of mesenchyme contribute to the development of the atrial septum. *Circ Res* 2006;99:351-353.

8. Webb S, Brown NA, Wessels A, et al. Development of the murine pulmonary vein and its relationship to the embryonic venous sinus. *Anat Rec* 1998;250:325-334.

9. Hutchins GM, Moore GW, Jones JF, et al. Postnatal endocardial fibroelastosis of the valve of the foramen ovale. *Am J Cardiol* 1981;47:90-94.

10. Marrouche NF, Natale A, Wazni OM, et al. Left septal atrial flutter: electrophysiology, anatomy and results of ablation. *Circulation* 2004;109:2440-2447.

11. Platonov PG, Mitrofanova L, Ivanov V, et al. Substrates for intra-atrial and interatrial conduction in the atrial septum: anatomical study on 84 human hearts. *Heart Rhythm* 2008;5:1189-1195.

12. Powell EDU, Mullaney JM. The Chiari network and the valve of the inferior vena cava. *Br Heart J* 1960;22:579-584.

13. Ho SY, Sánchez-Quintana D. The importance of atrial structure and fibers. *Clin Anat* 2009;22:52-63.

14. Schwinger ME, Gindea AJ, Freedberg RS, et al. The anatomy of the interatrial septum: a transesophageal echocardiographic study. *Am Heart J* 1990;119:1401-1405.

15. Shirani J, Zafari AM, Roberts WC. Morphologic features of fossa ovalis membrane aneurysm in the adult and its clinical significance. *J Am Coll Cardiol* 1995;26:466-471.

16. Hanaoka T, Suyama K, Taguchi A, et al. Shifting of puncture site in the fossa ovalis during radiofrequency catheter ablation: intracardiac echocardiography-guided transseptal left heart catheterization. *Jpn Heart J* 2003;44:673-680.

17. Shirani J, Roberts WC. Clinical, electrocardiographic and morphologic features of massive fatty deposits ("lipomatous hypertrophy") in the atrial septum. *J Am Coll Cardiol* 1993;22:226-238.

18. Ho SY, Anderson RH. How constant anatomically is the tendon of Todaro as a marker of the triangle of Koch? *J Cardiovasc Electrophysiol* 2000;11:83-89.

19. Ho SY, McComb JM, Scott CD, et al. Morphology of the cardiac conduction system in patients with electrophysiologically proven dual atrioventricular nodal pathways. *J Cardiovasc Electrophysiol* 1993;4:504-512.

20. Hagen PT, Scholz DG, Edwards WD. Incidence and size of patent foramen ovale during the first 10 decades of life: an autopsy study of 965 normal hearts. *Mayo Clin Proc* 1984; 59:7-20.

21. Ho SY, McCarthy KP, Rigby ML. Morphological features pertinent to interventional closure of patent foramen ovale. *J Interv Cardiol* 2003;16:1-6.

22. Marshall AC, Lock JE. Structural and compliant anatomy of the patent foramen ovale in patients undergoing transcatheter closure. *Am Heart J* 2000;140:303-307.

23. McAlpine WA. *Heart and Coronary Arteries.* Berlin: Springer, 1975:58.

24. Ho SY, McCarthy KP, Josen M, et al. Anatomic-echocardiographic correlates: an introduction to normal and congenitally malformed hearts. *Heart* 2001;86 (suppl 2):113-111.

25. Ferreira SM, Ho SY, Anderson RH. Morphological study of defects of the atrial septum within the oval fossa: implications for transcatheter closure of left-to-right shunt. *Br Heart J* 1992;67:316-320.

26. Chan KC, Godman MJ, Walsh K, et al. Transcatheter closure of atrial septal defect and interatrial communications with a new self-expanding nitinol double disc device (Amplatzer septal occluder): multicentre UK experience. *Heart* 1999;82:300-306.

27. Blom NA, Ottenkamp J, Jongeneel TH, et al. Morphogenetic differences of secundum atrial septal defects. *Pediatr Cardiol* 2005;26:338-343.

3

Radiographic Anatomy of the Atria for the Interventional Electrophysiologist

Isabelle Nault, Sébastien Knecht, Pierre Jaïs

Fluoroscopy has been used to help catheter navigation since the beginning of invasive cardiac electrophysiology (EP). It has several advantages, such as real-time dynamic visualization of the heart and catheters, availability in every EP laboratory, simplicity of use, instantaneous imaging without time-consuming data acquisition and manipulation, and well-known anatomical landmarks. It is not without limitations. With both the patient and the operator exposed to radiation, it gives only a 2-D image of a volume in which catheters have to be moved in all 3 axes, and at best gives only an indirect knowledge of the localization of most cardiac structures, which then have to be deduced by relative positioning to established landmarks, by examination under different views, and by the dynamic behavior of the catheters. Nonetheless, electrophysiologists rely widely on fluoroscopy for most invasive procedures, and other more modern imaging techniques, such as virtual navigating systems and intracardiac echocardiography, are used as an adjunct to fluoroscopy, without being sufficiently complete and reliable to replace it entirely. Fluoroscopy is also used to guide transeptal catheterization, frequently performed by electrophysiologists for catheter ablation of atrial fibrillation or other left-sided arrhythmias.

Knowledge of cardiac radiographic anatomy is therefore imperative for the invasive electrophysiologist in order to facilitate catheter manipulation and to avoid complications. This chapter outlines general cardiac anatomy, focussing on the atria and the interatrial septum.

Transseptal Catheterization and Interventions.
© 2010 Ranjan Thakur MD and Andrea Natale MD, eds.
Cardiotext Publishing, ISBN 978-0-9790164-1-7.

Fluoroscopic Views

To better appreciate catheter positioning within the heart volume using fluoroscopy, different projection angles can be used. In electrophysiology, the most useful views are posteroanterior (PA), left anterior oblique (LAO), and right anterior oblique (RAO). The lateral projection may also be useful during transseptal puncture and for pericardial access.

In the PA projection, the superior vena cava and the right atrium form the right cardiac border, while the aortic arch, the left main pulmonary artery, the left atrial appendage, and the left ventricle form the left cardiac border, respectively, from top to bottom (Figure 3.1). The catheter is seen moving from right to left and from high to low.

The RAO projection is useful to assess anterior and posterior positions as well as superior and inferior. In LAO, the superior, inferior, anterior, and posterior locations can be visualized. It is often used when mapping around the AV valve annulus or when attempting to engage the coronary sinus.

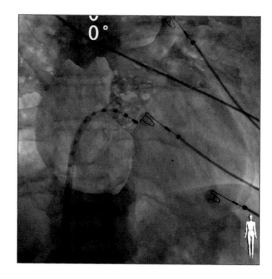

FIGURE 3.1   *Heart Anatomy over Fluoroscopy*

Computed tomography overlay of right atrium (yellow), left atrium (blue), and left ventricle (green). Posteroanterior (PA) projection. The right atrium forms the right cardiac border, and the left atrial appendage is seen at the superior part of the left cardiac border. The sheath and the catheter are through the transseptal puncture site. Reproduced with permission from Knecht et al, Europace, Computed tomography–fluoroscopy overlay evaluation during catheter ablation of left atrial arrhythmia, *Europace* (2008) 10, 931–938. Oxford University Press.

Dynamic Catheter Position Assessment

Dynamic evaluation of catheter position using fluoroscopy can prove very helpful. For example, a sheath or catheter pointing posteriorly, when given a clockwise torque, will be seen moving from right to left on the screen and the opposite observation can be made when it is oriented anteriorly. At the ostia of left pulmonary veins, clockwise torque moves the catheter tip to the posterior wall and counterclockwise torque to the anterior wall. However, at the level of the right pulmonary veins, the posterior wall can be reached by giving counterclockwise torque and clock-

wise motion will move the catheter posteriorly. The location of the venous ostia can be revealed by inserting a deflectable catheter inside the pulmonary vein, bending it and slowly withdrawing it: the catheter will "fall off" the vein at the ostium. Ablation should then be performed medial to the ostium to avoid pulmonary vein stenosis.

Right Atrium

The right atrium constitutes the right cardiac border in PA projection. It has a smooth posterior wall and a trabeculated anterior-lateral surface, separated by the crista terminalis. The sinus node is located at the superior cavoatrial junction and the atrioventricular node at the intersection of the interatrial septum with the atrioventricular junction. Several pathologic cardiac rhythms amenable to ablation arise from the right atrium and its contiguous structures, namely atrial tachycardias, right-sided accessory pathways, AVNRT, and right atrial flutter. Moreover, access to the left-sided atrium and ventricle is often obtained via transseptal catheterization throughout the fossa ovalis.

Superior Vena Cava

The superior vena cava (SVC) joins the right atrium at its superior and posterior aspect. It lies anterior to the right superior pulmonary vein (RSPV), and this has an implication for atrial fibrillation catheter ablation as far-field SVC venous potentials can sometimes be recorded in the RSPV. Another structure lying in the vicinity of the SVC is the right phrenic nerve. Ablation within the SVC should be performed cautiously with frequent monitoring of right diaphragmatic excursion. Pacing at maximal output prior to ablation is strongly advised to check for absence of phrenic nerve capture. The SVC can be easily catheterized using the PA projection.

Crista Terminalis

The terminal crest (crista terminalis) anatomically separates the anterior trabeculated right atrium from the posterior smooth wall. This C-shaped structure originates on the interatrial groove above the fossa ovalis, runs anteriorly to the junction between the right atrium and the SVC, and pursues its course downward along the lateral atrial wall, giving on its course the pectinate muscles forming the trabeculation of the anterolateral right

atrium. It ends by branching into several trabeculations at the inferior cavotricuspid isthmus, beneath the inferior vena cava.[1] The importance of the crista terminalis for electrophysiologists is reflected by 3 main findings: 1) Several atrial tachycardias are known to arise from this structure[2]; 2) It can be targeted for modification of the sinus node during ablation for inappropriate sinus tachycardia[3,4]; 3) During typical right atrial flutter, functional block along the crista terminalis delineates the macroentrant circuit.[5,6] The crista terminalis can be visualized in the frontal projection laterally along the right atrium, but it is best seen in LAO projection where it is parallel to the screen. Ablation along the lateral right atrium should give rise to caution about phrenic nerve injury, as the nerve courses laterally and anteriorly to the right atrium.[7] Previously mentioned precautions for avoiding phrenic nerve damage apply.

Sinus Node

The sinus node is located at the junction between the superior vena cava and the right atrial appendage, close to the epicardium. Its runs laterally and inferiorly through the crista terminalis to form a spindle-shaped structure that ends subendocardially, midway between the superior and inferior vena cava.[1] The sinus node is a well-protected structure due to the following: (1) It is deeply situated subendocardially, and is separated from the endocardium by the thick crista terminalis; (2) It is an elongated structure approximately 10 mm long and 3 mm thick; (3) The sinus node artery courses centrally and exerts a cooling effect on the surrounding nodal structure.[8]

Right Atrial Appendage

The right atrial appendage (RAA) is a broad structure that constitutes part of the anterolateral wall of the right atrium. It is approximately triangular in shape with a wide base, and a tip oriented superiorly and anteriorly. It has a trabeculated surface formed by the pectinate muscles arising from the crista terminalis, but catheters have to be manipulated with caution inside the appendage as the areas between the trabeculated muscular bundles consist of very thin atrial tissue, which can easily be perforated. As it is an anterior structure, a catheter placed inside the RAA will be oriented leftward on the fluoroscopy screen in LAO projection and rightward in RAO projection. In PA projection, the catheter will face the screen, more or less, and have a translational negation movement, from right to left and right again.

Inferior Vena Cava

The inferior vena cava (IVC) enters the right atrium inferiorly and posteriorly. The eustachian valve is a thin membrane spanning the anterior part of the IVC orifice in contiguity with the thicker eustachian ridge that separates the IVC from the coronary sinus inflows. It converges with the muscular area superior to the coronary sinus and inferior to the fossa ovalis. The IVC very rarely is the source of atrial tachycardia.

Cavotricuspid Isthmus

The cavotricuspid isthmus consists in the area of atrial myocardium lying between the tricuspid annulus and the inferior vena cava on the inferior part of the right atrium. It is the narrowest isthmus of atrial tissue along the right atrial flutter circuit, and is the ablation site for this common arrhythmia. A catheter dragged along this line will go from right to left in RAO projection, from the anterior tricuspid annulus to the posterior IVC. In LAO projection, the catheter will be perpendicular to the

screen, in the 6 o'clock position. The anatomy of the isthmus consists of 3 main zones: anteriorly, the vestibule of the tricuspid valve, which forms a rather smooth surface; the middle muscular trabeculations; and posteriorly, an area of fibrous and fatty tissue with scarce muscle fiber content adjacent to the inferior vena cava.[9] In more than half of patients, a pouch-like structure is present anterior to the IVC and the Thebesian valve, called the subeustachian sinus, or the sinus of Keith.[9] Power delivery inside such a pouch can be challenging as the cooling effect from the blood flow is reduced. In patients where conduction block is difficult to achieve, it can sometimes be useful to do an inferior right atrial angiography to locate and assess this area.

Tricuspid Annulus

The tricuspid valve annulus is mainly relevant to the electrophysiologist in cases of right-sided accessory pathways. It is best visualized in LAO, where the annulus is parallel to the screen.

Coronary Sinus Ostium

The coronary sinus (CS) flows into the inferior right atrium. The CS ostium lies inferior and anterior to the fossa ovalis. It is guarded by the Thebesian valve, which has a variable morphology in different individuals, usually a small valve, and sometimes a fenestrated membrane.[9] The coronary sinus can be entered using the frontal or, more typically, the LAO projection, where its course is parallel to the fluoro screen. In RAO, it is seen running perpendicular to the screen. The coronary sinus os is a useful landmark, as it marks the inferior part of the triangle of Koch (discussed below). The coronary sinus itself can be used to locate the mitral annulus in cases of left-sided accessory pathway mapping.

AV Node

The atrioventricular node is located at the top of the triangle of Koch. This anatomic area was first described by Koch in 1909.[10] The sides of the triangle are formed by the tendon of Todaro, posteriorly and laterally, and by the septal leaflet of the tricuspid valve anteriorly. The base of the triangle is a line at the level of the coronary sinus ostium. The compact AV node is located in most patients at the tip of the triangle. Transitional cells surround the compact node, with superficial and deeper extensions. The deep anterosuperior extensions penetrate further toward the left side of the atrial septum and bundle together to form the His bundle.[11] Unlike the sinus node, the compact AV node is very sensitive to radiofrequency injury. It is superficial and much smaller, measuring approximately 5.25 mm long, 2.5 mm to 3.5 mm wide, and 0.7 mm to 1.0 mm thick.[11] The inferior portion of the triangle of Koch, near the coronary sinus ostium, is of interest during ablation of the slow pathway for AVNRT. Even though there is no clear histopathological evidence of such a slow pathway, [11] "slow pathway potential," a signal typically recorded in patients with AVNRT, has been recorded in this lower area of the triangle of Koch, and ablation at these sites has resulted in successful cure of AVNRT.[12,13]

Interatrial Septum

Membranous Septum/Fossa Ovalis

The true interatrial septum is the area of the fossa ovalis, entirely covered and sealed in most patients by a membranous flap. However, up to one-quarter of the population has a probe-patent foramen ovale (PFO), allowing passage of the catheter through a weakness in the seal, often located in the anterosuperior part of the fossa ovalis. Although the antero-

superior location of the patency sometimes makes manipulation of the catheters in the left atrium more challenging, left-sided procedures, such as atrial fibrillation ablation, can be carried out using the PFO, and results are similar to those found if a transseptal puncture were used.[14]

In the posteroanterior projection, the area of the fossa ovalis seems to override the area where a His signal can be recorded. It is superior to the coronary sinus ostium (Figure 3.2). In RAO, the fossa ovalis is posterior to the His recording and superior to the coronary sinus.[15] It is usually located midway between the His recording anteriorly and the right

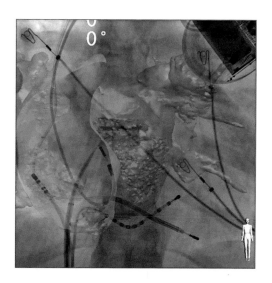

FIGURE 3.2   *Fossa Ovalis: Fluoroscopy and CT*

Computed tomography of the left atrium overlay on fluoroscopy. The endocardial surface of the right atrium is seen through the cut plan, and the fossa ovalis is visualized, guiding the transseptal puncture. In posteroanterior (PA) projection, the area of the fossa ovalis seems to override the area where a His signal can be recorded. It is superior to the coronary sinus ostium. Reproduced with permission from Knecht et al, Europace, Computed tomography–fluoroscopy overlay evaluation during catheter ablation of left atrial arrhythmia, *Europace* (2008) 10, 931–938. Oxford University Press.

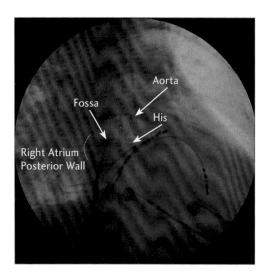

FIGURE 3.3   *Aorta and Fossa Ovalis*
Projection in RAO View

Right anterior oblique (RAO) projection. The fossa
ovalis is seen at the same horizontal level as the His
catheter, at equal distance from the posterior wall
of the right atrium and the His. A pigtail catheter
in the aorta illustrates the anterior position of the
ascending aorta relative to the fossa ovalis. Note
that the His catheter is approximately at the same
level as the pigtail in the aorta (it is, in fact, at the
level of the noncoronary cusp of the aortic valve).
Therefore, when the His is identified, a catheter
in the aorta is not required as a landmark for
transseptal catheterization. Courtesy of Dr. George
D. Veenhuyzen, Libin Cardiovascular Institute of
Alberta, Calgary, Alberta, Canada.

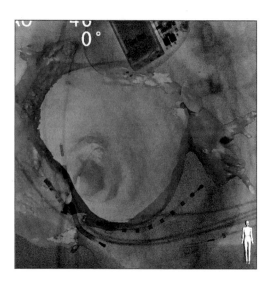

FIGURE 3.4   *Fossa Ovalis in LAO View:*
Endocardial View from CT

Left anterior oblique (LAO) projection. Computed
tomography of the left atrium overlay on fluoroscopy. The endocardial surface of the right atrium
is seen through the cut plan, and the fossa ovalis
is visualized, guiding the transseptal puncture. In
LAO, the puncture site is superior to the coronary
sinus, and is oriented approximately at the 2 o'clock
position.

atrial posterior wall posteriorly, at the same
horizontal level as the His (Figure 3.3). In
LAO, the puncture site is superior to the coronary sinus and is oriented approximately at the
2 o'clock position (Figure 3.4). The lateral projection can also be used to better visualize the
anteroposterior plan. With this incidence, the
needle should be oriented slightly posteriorly,
almost perpendicular to the screen (Figure
3.5). When preparing for a transseptal puncture, a long sheath should be advanced on a
guidewire positioned inside the superior vena
cava before the needle can be advanced inside

the sheath. The transeptal needle can be connected to a pressure monitor to visualize the
left atrial pressure curve upon LA entry. The
location of the fossa ovalis is confirmed by
pulling down the sheath and transseptal needle from the SVC into the right atrium with
a posteromedial orientation (sheath valve and
needle marker between the 4 and 6 o'clock
position), and as the transseptal apparatus
engages the fossa, a characteristic rightward
jump is seen on the fluoro screen, both in PA
and LAO projections. The position is further
confirmed if necessary by LAO, RAO, or lateral projections. Confirmation of correct positioning can also be done with radiocontrast
injection: The transseptal needle is advanced,
and contrast is injected. When at the fossa, the
contrast will stain with a characteristic round

shape, with a well-defined border, and will not wash out immediately (Figure 3.6). If the needle is oriented to the muscular septum or to the posterior wall, the contrast will spread diffusely in the myocardium with irregular and hazy borders (Figure 3.7). If staining and fluoroscopic position is consistent with the correct location, tenting of the interatrial septum can be visualized when pushing the needle forward with simultaneous injection contrast (Figure 3.6). Once the needle has crossed the septum and entered the left atrium, a small quantity of blood is withdrawn to ensure the absence of any air bubble; contrast is again injected and should be seen swirling around the left atrial cavity (Figure 3.8). When the left atrium is partially opacified, attention should be paid to its contours, notably the roof, to avoid trauma when advancing the transseptal apparatus. If contrast delineates the cardiac silhouette, the needle is in the pericardial space and should be withdrawn. If contrast flows superiorly in a pulsatile manner, aortic puncture should be suspected.

When left atrial access has been confirmed with contrast injection and pressure monitoring (Figure 3.9), the transseptal apparatus is slightly advanced so the tip of the dilator just protrudes into the left atrium, and the transseptal needle is withdrawn. A J guidewire is then advanced distally in one of the pulmonary veins (usually the left superior) until it is seen outside of the heart silhouette. In addition to further confirming that the left atrium has been correctly entered, this process allows advancement of the dilator and sheath without risk of injury to the left atrial walls or to the left atrial appendage.

Either intracardiac echocardiography or transoesophageal echocardiography can be

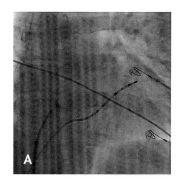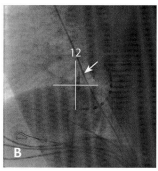

FIGURE 3.5 *Fossa Ovalis Staining with Dye and Position in Lateral View*

A. Transseptal with fossa ovalis staining.
B. Confirmation of the catheter's position with a lateral view. The transseptal apparatus is pointing slightly posterior, between the 12 o'clock and 1 o'clock positions.

used to guide transseptal punctures, but we do not consider these tools to be mandatory for standard transseptal catheterization. However, these imaging tools do allow the operator to directly visualize the transseptal needle, which can help in difficult cases.

Interatrial Groove

The interatrial groove is the area superior and posterior to the fossa ovalis. Although classically referred to as the muscular interatrial septum, it is actually formed by the apposition of the right and left atrial walls, separated by epicardial tissue and vascular structures, and therefore is more correctly called the interatrial groove.[8] A puncture at this site will not only be more difficult due to the thick tissue, but it also will also carry the risk of pericardial effusion, especially in heavily anticoagulated patients (Figures 3.10, 3.11).

Aorta

The atrial wall anterior and medial to the fossa ovalis is contiguous with the ascending aortic wall.[8] Hence; it is possible to puncture

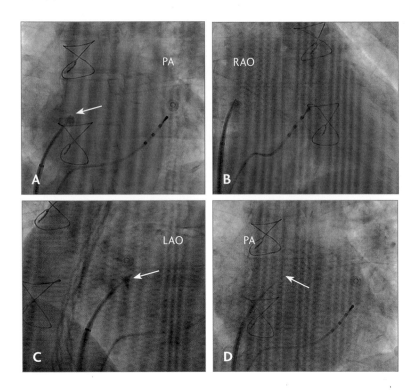

FIGURE 3.6   *Transseptal Position in All Views; Staining and Tenting of the Fossa Ovalis*
Septal staining with contrast. **A.** Note the smooth and round shape of the contrast media trapped inside the fossa ovalis. **B.** Right anterior oblique (RAO) view. Contrast is still seen, and the position of the fossa ovalis is between the 12 o'clock and 1 o'clock positions. **C.** Left anterior oblique (LAO) view. Contrast is still seen, and the position of the fossa ovalis is at the 2 o'clock position. Tenting of the fossa can also be seen before crossing into the left atrium. **D.** Left atrial access is confirmed by contrast infusion (white arrow). RAO = right anterior oblique; LAO = left anterior oblique; PA = posteroanterior.

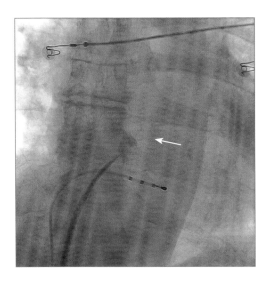

FIGURE 3.7   *Myocardial Puncture and Stain*
Contrast injected in the myocardium (arrow). When compared to staining of the fossa ovalis, intramyocardial staining has a hazy and asymmetrical distribution.

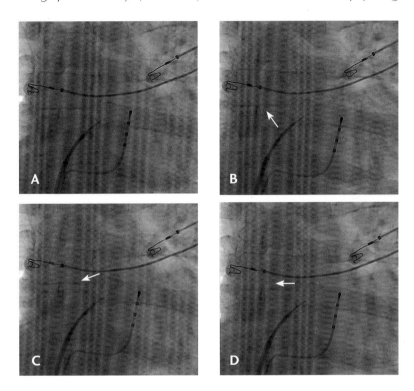

FIGURE 3.8   *Left Atrial Access Confirmation by Dye Injection*
Transseptal puncture in posteroanterior (PA) projection. Confirmation of left anterior (LA) access by contrast injection. The contrast can be seen injected through the transseptal needle and swirling around the left atrium (arrows).

the aorta accidentally if the transseptal needle is oriented anteriorly. Oblique fluoroscopy views are useful to assess the anteroposterior location. To help with anterior and posterior locations, a catheter can be placed on the AV node, recording a His signal, or a pigtail catheter can be introduced retrograde in the ascending aorta (Figure 3.3).

Left Atrium

When the fossa ovalis is crossed for transseptal access, the sheath enters the left atrium in its mid-anterior portion.

Pulmonary Veins

Typically, 4 pulmonary veins drain into the left atrium. However, anatomical variants are frequent, such as an additional middle pulmonary vein (typically on the right) or a common ostium for the ipsilateral pulmonary veins (more frequently on the left). All 4 venous ostia are found in the posterior part of the left atrium: Right-sided veins are, on average, 6 mm apart, and left-sided veins are approximately 8 mm apart.[16] The course of the upper veins is more superoposterolateral, and a catheter introduced deep inside an upper vein is seen outside the heart shadow in a PA view (Figures 3.12, 3.13). The lower veins have a more posterior course, more or less parallel to the x-ray beam in PA view. The LAO projection is the best to assess catheter position for the left-sided veins (the catheter points to the right when in the LIPV) (Figure 3.14) and RAO for the right-sided veins (the catheter

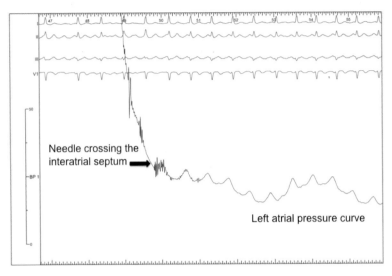

Needle crossing the
interatrial septum ➤

Left atrial pressure curve

FIGURE 3.9   *Left Atrial Access Confirmation*
by Pressure Monitoring
The transseptal needle is connected to a pressure manifold, and a left atrial
pressure curve is observed when the interatrial septum is crossed.

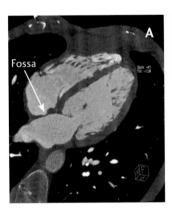
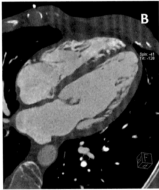

FIGURE 3.10   *Interatrial Septum*
Seen with CT Scan
Computerized tomography (CT) scan. **A.** The fossa
ovalis can be seen. It is surrounded by thicker tissue,
consisting of the interatrial groove superiorly and
the atrioventricular groove inferiorly. **B.** This slice
was taken anteriorly to the slice in A. The fossa is no
longer visible. Courtesy of Dr Michel Montaudon,
Hôpital Cardiologique Haut Leveque, Bordeaux-
Pessac, France.

points to the left when in the
RIPV) (Figure 3.15).

The key finding that
atrial ectopic beats arising
from muscular sleeves extending from the left atrium into
the pulmonary veins could
trigger atrial fibrillation
has prompted great interest
and innovation in catheter-
based ablation techniques.[17]

Although ablation was ini-
tially targeted at the ectopic foci, it was soon
realized that this could lead to pulmonary vein
stenosis, and a more proximal ablation within
the left atrium to isolate the pulmonary veins
has been adopted.[18] The true ostia of the pulmonary veins are difficult to visualize using
fluoroscopy due to the overlying left atrial
silhouette. However, the previously described
"catheter fall-off trick" in the section about

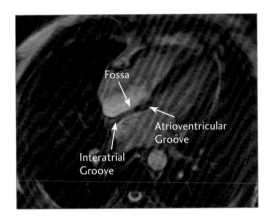

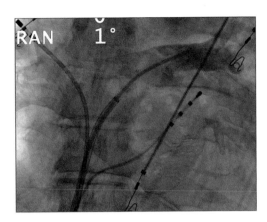

FIGURE 3.11   *Muscular and Membranous Parts of Interatrial Septum Show with MRI*

Magnetic resonance image (MRI) of the heart. The fossa ovalis can be seen. In addition, superiorly, the interatrial groove formed by the apposition of the atrial walls can be seen, separated by epicardial tissue and vascular structures in contiguity with the pericardial space. Inferiorly, the atrioventricular groove can also be seen, also contiguous with the pericardial space. Courtesy of Dr. Michel Montaudon, Hôpital Cardiologique Haut Leveque, Bordeaux-Pessac, France.

FIGURE 3.12   *CT Overlay on Fluoroscopy*

Computed tomography overlay on live fluoroscopy screen. Posteroanterior (PA) view, with ablation catheter inside the right superior pulmonary vein and a multipurpose catheter in the left superior pulmonary vein for angiographic confirmation of adequate overlay. Catheters inserted deeply inside the superior pulmonary veins are seen outside of the heart shadow on fluoroscopy. Reproduced with permission from Knecht et al, Europace, Computed tomography–fluoroscopy overlay evaluation during catheter ablation of left atrial arrhythmia, *Europace* (2008) 10, 931–938. Oxford University Press.

dynamic evaluation of catheter position can reproducibly delineate the venous ostia. Pulmonary venous angiography can also be performed, either by selective injection of each vein or by injecting the whole left atrium. If injecting the whole atrium, the lower veins are more difficult to distinguish. Adenosine can be used to achieve transient cardiac standstill and allow better opacification of the left atrial cavity and pulmonary veins.[19]

Left Atrial Appendage

The left atrial appendage is the only trabeculated structure in the left atrium. It is narrow and funnel shaped, and lies superiorly on the anterior surface of the left atrium. In PA view, it is often superimposed on the left superior pulmonary vein. In between the thicker trabeculation, the appendage tissue is very thin, and catheters should be moved with caution inside and around these fragile structures.

Bachmann Bundle

The Bachmann bundle arises from the terminal crest, at the junction between the superior vena cava and the right atrium. It then runs anteriorly and parallel to the AV groove to connect the left atrium, where it is joined by fibers oriented in different directions.[16] The Bachmann bundle is not the only electrical connection between the two atria, as other myocardial connections have been described.[16] With fluoroscopy, it is localized superiorly to the His recording and anteriorly, but posterior, to the right atrial appendage apex.[15]

Ligament of Marshall

The ligament of Marshall is the vestigial remnant of the left superior vena cava; it contains fibrous, vascular, and nervous tissue. It runs laterally to the left superior pulmonary vein and above the left atrial appendage. If part of it remains patent, the vein of Marshall, which drains into the coronary sinus, can be selectively opacified.[20] Ectopic atrial beats originating from the ligament of Marshall have been demonstrated both in atrial fibrillation and in atrial tachycardia in isolated cases.[21,22]

Mitral Annulus

Visualization of the mitral annulus is especially useful when mapping and ablating left-sided accessory pathways. The LAO projection is mostly used as the annulus is seen entirely facing the screen, and mapping can

be guided by a catheter inserted inside the coronary sinus delineating the inferior part of the annulus. In addition, ablation along the lateral mitral line (from the lateral mitral annulus to the left inferior pulmonary vein) has been proven to be necessary in the vast majority of patients with longstanding persistent atrial fibrillation.

Special Considerations

Recognizing Complications

Fluoroscopy can help with early recognition of certain complications of catheter ablation. During transseptal catheterization and during atrial fibrillation ablation, several maneuvers carry the risk of cardiac wall injury and subsequent pericardial effusion and tamponade. Tamponade can occur following traumatic transseptal puncture, if the puncture is performed in the posterior wall of the right atrium or in the interatrial groove where it enters the pericardial space, if the ascending aorta is punctured (too anterior) or if the needle is advanced too deep inside the left atria, injuring or crossing the roof or lateral wall of the left atrium. Cardiac perforation can also happen during catheter manipulation inside thin-walled areas, such as the atrial appendages, or as a consequence of a "steam pop" during radiofrequency delivery. One of the earliest signs of tamponade, even before a significant drop in blood pressure can be observed, is the sudden immobility or decreased excursion of the cardiac silhouette, best seen at the left superior cardiac border in PA projection. As fluid

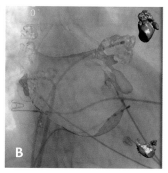

FIGURE 3.13   *Rotational Angiography Overlay on Fluoroscopy*

Posteroanterior (PA) view. **A.** Rotational angiography overlay on live fluoroscopy screen. It allows visualization of the pulmonary veins and their ostium, which is impossible with only fluoroscopy. The multipolar catheter is in the right inferior pulmonary vein and the ablation catheter is in the left superior pulmonary vein. **B.** The cut plan revealing the endocardial surface of the left atrium.

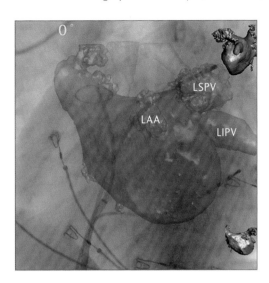

FIGURE 3.14   *Position and Orientation on Fluoroscopy of the Left Pulmonary Veins*

The left anterior oblique (LAO) projection is the best to assess catheter position for the left-sided veins. This figure shows the projection of the left veins in the LAO 30° view. The catheter is in the left superior pulmonary vein (LSPV) and is pointing rightward. The left atrial appendage (LAA) is not overlapping the veins and is seen anteriorly, in the central part of the fluoroscopic image. LIPV = left inferior pulmonary vein.

accumulates in the pericardial space, it is no longer possible to see the myocardial contraction on fluoroscopy. Prompt recognition of this sign can lead to early intervention.

Injury to the right phrenic nerve can occur while ablating near the ostium of the superior vena cava, inside the superior vena cava, on the lateral wall of the right atrium, or inside the right superior pulmonary vein. The left phrenic nerve can be injured by ablation deep inside the left atrial appendage. Phrenic nerve lesion results in ipsilateral hemidiaphragmatic paralysis, which is reversible if recognized early, but can be devastating if it goes unnoticed and causes permanent damage. Direct visualization of diaphragmatic excursion during inspiration confirms the integrity of the phrenic nerve and should be monitored during ablation of the aforementioned regions. Prior to ablation, pacing from the ablation catheter at maximal output should be performed to check the absence of phrenic capture. During radiofrequency delivery, coughing, phrenic stimulation, or absence of normal diaphragmatic movement should prompt immediate cessation of ablation.

Pulmonary vein stenosis is a known complication of pulmonary vein isolation, especially if ablation is performed inside the vein. In redo procedures, selective angiography of the pulmonary veins can detect asymptomatic stenosis and avoid further injury to the vein during reablation. However, if PV stenosis is suspected on the basis of clinical symptoms (exertional dyspnea, hemoptysis), computed tomography or magnetic resonance angiography should be performed.

Esophageal fistula to the mediastinum or to the left atrium is one of the most feared complications of atrial fibrillation catheter ablation.[23-25] In order to avoid esophageal injury, care should be taken when ablating in close proximity to the esophagus path posterior to the left atrium. To visualize the course of the esophagus, barium paste can be swallowed prior to the procedure, and the esophagus position can be monitored with fluoroscopy during the procedure.[26]

New Technologies Integrating Fluoroscopy for Imaging

To overcome some of the limitations of standard fluoroscopy, such as limited anatomical data, software has been developed that can overlay a high resolution 3-D image of the left atrium to the live fluoroscopy.[27] It allows

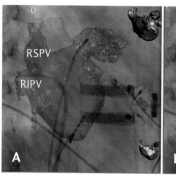
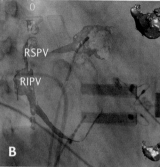

FIGURE 3.15   *Position and Orientation on Fluoroscopy of the Right Pulmonary Veins*

Right anterior oblique (RAO), 30°. This projection allows visualization of right-sided pulmonary veins. **A.** The entire left atrium. **B.** A cut plan of the left atrium. The second image allows visualization of the endocardial surface of the left atrium and the veins ostia. The multipolar catheter is in the right inferior pulmonary vein (RIPV) and is oriented leftward on the screen. The left superior vein and the left atrial appendage are overlapping in this projection (ablation catheter is in the left superior pulmonary vein) and the left inferior vein is seen parallel to the X-ray beam, penetrating the image. RSPV = right superior pulmonary vein.

visualization of precise details of the left atrial anatomy usually not seen with standard fluoroscopy, such as the pulmonary veins and their ostia. Different projections can be used, and the left atrial anatomy "moves along."

If using the CT overlay application, CT scanning can be done prior to the procedure and registered on the fluoroscopic image on the day of the procedure. This technique has the advantage of providing precise anatomic details of the heart (not only of the left atrium) (Figure 3.1). It can also be used to guide transseptal puncture (Figures 3.2, 3.4). However, the technique requires registration of the CT on live fluoroscopy, performed using pulmonary vein angiography with the help of catheter positioning. This registration

process can lead to erroneous superimposition of the images. Moreover, the CT is done prior to the procedure, in potentially different fluid load conditions, and thus may possibly differ from the real-time anatomy at the moment of the procedure.

The left atrial image can also be obtained by rotational angiography, performed just before the ablation, with the fluoroscopic equipment used for the procedure. It reflects the actual left atrial anatomy and is automatically registered on the fluoroscopy screen after automated segmentation. It has the advantage of being quick, simple, and reliable, offering a detailed left atrial anatomy and combining it with a tool commonly used and well-known to electrophysiologists (Figures 3.13, 3.14, and 3.15).

New Techniques for Transseptal Catheterization

In some patients, the fossa ovalis is unusually resistant to transseptal puncture. This resistance may prove especially true in patients who have undergone several procedures involving transseptal punctures and who may have developed fibrosis, which renders interatrial septum crossing difficult or sometimes impossible when using the standard technique. Excessive pushing and pressure on the needle and transseptal apparatus to overcome this resistance carry the risk of left atrial injury and perforation if the needle reaches the roof or lateral wall of the left atrium. Using radiofrequency current to help the needle cross the septum can overcome this resistance without having to apply force. First, the correct location of the needle at the fossa ovalis needs to be verified and confirmed by different fluoroscopic views and by contrast injection. Once it is certain that the needle is "tenting" the fossa without being able to cross it, radiofrequency unipolar current is delivered through the needle simply by touching the proximal end of the needle with the tip of the ablation catheter: The proximal end of the needle and the catheter are outside the patient, and the long plastic sheath prevents radiofrequency energy from being delivered to structures other than the fossa. Normally, 1 to 4 seconds of radiofrequency is enough for the needle to make its way through the interatrial septum, and no additional force is required than the usual tension put on the transseptal apparatus and needle.[28]

Radiation Awareness and Limitation

Malignancy risk and radiation injury risk to the patient, the operator, and staff are low to moderate with modern fluoroscopy equipment.[29-31] The operator should be constantly aware of radiation dose, and should try and keep it as low as possible. Do the following to minimize radiation dose[15,32-34]:

- Keep fluoroscopy time as short as possible.
- To minimize thyroid and breast exposure, use posteroanterior rather than anteroposterior X-ray beam direction.
- Use the PA or RAO projection instead of LAO whenever possible.
- Minimize the radiation field size to include only the area of interest.
- Use pulsed instead of continuous fluoroscopy, with low frame/second (ideally 7.5 f/s).

- Use low intensity resolution.
- Use digital fluorography instead of 35-mm film to store images
- Use adequate shielding for the staff and operator, and stay as far as possible from the fluoroscopy source.
- Avoid manipulation from jugular or subclavian approach when feasible.

Conclusion

Fluoroscopy is widely used as an imaging tool during electrophysiological interventions. It can be used alone or in combination with echocardiography for transseptal puncture and has the advantage of offering real-time imaging and being reliable and simple to use. Knowledge of fluoroscopic cardiac anatomy is necessary to perform safe and tailored procedures. Finally, awareness of the possible hazards of excessive exposure to radiation should result in strategies for limiting fluoroscopy doses in order to limit radiation exposition to the patient, the staff, and the operator.

Acknowledgments
The authors would like to thank Matthew Wright MD, PhD, Michel Montaudon MD, Georges Veenhuyzen MD, Seiichiro Matsuo MD, Shinsuke Miyazaki MD, Antoine Deplagne MD, Kang-Teng Lim MD, Frédéric Sacher MD, Rukshen Weerasooriya MD, Mélèze Hocini MD, François Laurent MD, and Michel Haïssaguerre MD for their assistance with this chapter.

References
1. Sanchez-Quintana D, Anderson RH, Cabrera JA, Climent V, Martin R, Farré J, Ho SY. The terminal crest: morphological features relevant to electrophysiology. *Heart* 2002;88:406-411.

2. Kalman JM, Olgin JE, Karch MR, Hamdan M, Lee RJ, Lesh MD. "Cristal Tachycardias": origin of right atrial tachycardias from the crista terminalis identified by intracardiac echocardiography. *J Am Coll Cardiol* 1998;31(2):451-459.

3. Lee RJ, Kalman JM, Fitzpatrick AP, Epstein LM, Fisher WG, Olgin JE, Lesh MD, Scheinman MM. Radiofrequency catheter modification of the sinus node for "inappropriate" sinus tachycardia. *Circulation* 1995;92(10):2919-2928.

4. Jayaprakash S, Sparks PB, Vohra J. Inappropriate sinus tachycardia (IST): management by radiofrequency modification of sinus node. *Aust N Z J Med* 1997;(4):391-397.

5. Tai CT, Chen SA, Chen YJ, Yu WC, Hsieh MH, Tsai CF, Ding YA, Chang MS. Conduction properties of the crista terminalis in patients with typical atrial flutter: basis for a line of block in the reentrant circuit. *J Cardiovasc Electrophysiol* 1998;9(8):811-819.

6. Yamaabe H, Misumi I, Fukushim H, Uneo K, Kimura V, Hokamura Y. Conduction properties of the crista terminalis and its influence on the right atrial activation sequence in patients with typical atrial flutter. *Pacing Clin Electrophysiol* 2002;25(2):132-141.

7. Vatasescu R, Shalganov T, Kardos A, Jalabadze K, Paprika D, Gyorgy M, Szili-Torok T. Right diaphragmatic paralysis following endocardial cryothermal ablation of inappropriate sinus tachycardia. *Europace* 2006;(10):904-906.

8. Ho SY, Anderson RH, Sanchez-Quintana D. Atrial structures and fibres: morphologic bases of atrial conduction. *Cardiovasc Res* 2002;54:325-336.

9. Cabrera JA, Sanchez-Quintana D, Ho SY, Medina A, Anderson RH. The architecture of the atrial musculature between the orifice of the inferior caval vein and the tricuspid valve: the anatomy of the isthmus. *Cardiovasc Electrophysiol* 1998;9:1186-1195.

10. Koch W. Weiter Mitteilungen über den Sinusknoten des Herzens. *Verh Dtsch Ges Pathol* 1909;13:85-92.

11. Sanchez-Quintana D, Davies DW, Ho SY, Oslizlok P, Anderson RH. Architecture of the atrial musculature in and around the triangle of Koch: its potential relevance to atrioventricular nodal reentry. *J Cardiovasc Electrophysiol* 1997;8:1396-1407.

12. Jackman WM, Beckman KJ, McClelland JH, Wang X, Friday KJ, Roman CA, Moulton KP, Twidale N, Hazlitt HA, Prior MI, et al. Treatment of supraventricular tachycardia due to atrioventricular nodal reentry, by radiofrequency catheter ablation of slow pathway conduction. *N Engl J Med* 1992;327(5):313-318.

13. Haïssaguerre M, Gaita F, Fischer B, Commenges D, Montserrat P, D'Ivernois C, Lemetayer P, Warin JF. Elimination of atrioventricular nodal reentrant tachycardia using discrete slow potentials to guide application of radiofrequency energy. *Circulation* 1992;85(6):2162-2175.

14. Knecht S, Wright M, Lellouche N, Nault I, Matsuo S, O'Neill M, Lomas O, Deplagne A, Bordachar P, Sacher F, Derval N, Hocini M, Jaïs P, Clémenty J, Haïssaguerre M. Impact of a patent foramen ovale on paroxysmal atrial fibrillation ablation. *J Cardiovasc Electrophysiol* 2008;19(12):1236-1241.

15. Farré J, Anderson RH, Cabrera JA, Sanchez-Quintana D, Rubio JM, Romero J, Cabestrero F. Fluoroscopic cardiac anatomy for catheter ablation of tachycardia. *Pacing Clin Electrophysiol* 2002;25:76-94.

16. Ho SY, Sanchez-Quitana D, Cabrera JA, Anderson RH. Anatomy of the left Atrium: implications for radiofrequency ablation of atrial fibrillation. *J Cardiovasc Electrophysiol* 1999;10(11):1525-1533.

17. Haïssaguerre M, Jaïs P, Shah DC, Takahashi A, Hocini M, Quiniou G, Garrigue S, LeMouroux A, LeMétayer P, Clémenty J.

Spontaneous initiation of atrial fibrillation by ectopic beats originating in the pulmonary veins. *N Engl J Med* 1998;339(10):659-666.

18. Robbins IM, Colvin EV, Doyle TP, Kemp WE, Loyd JE, McMahon WS, Kay GN. Pulmonary vein stenosis after catheter ablation of atrial fibrillation. *Circulation* 1998;98(17):1769-1775.

19. Tse HF, Lee KL, Lau CP. Adenosine tri-phosphate enhanced contrast pulmonary venogram to facilitate pulmonary vein ablation. *J Cardiovasc Electrophysiol* 2002;13(3):300.

20. Kim DT, Lai AC, Hwang C, Fan LT, Karagueuzian HS, Chen PS, Fishbein MC. The ligament of Marshall: a structural analysis in human hearts with implications for atrial arrhythmias. *J Am Coll Cardiol* 2000;36(4):1324-1327.

21. Polymeropoulos KP, Rodriguez LM, Timmermans C, Wellens HJ. Radiofrequency ablation of a focal atrial tachycardia originating from the Marshall ligament as a trigger for atrial fibrillation. *Circulation* 2002;105(17):2112-2113.

22. Hwang C, Karagueusian HS, Chen PS. Idiopathic paroxysmal atrial fibrillation induced by a focal discharge mechanism in the left superior pulmonary vein: possible roles of the ligament of Marshall. *J Cardiovasc Electrophysiol* 1999;10(5):636-648.

23. Scanavacca MI, D'Avila A, Parga J, Sosa E. Left atrial–oesophageal fistula following radiofrequency catheter ablation of atrial fibrillation. *J Cardiovasc Electrophysiol* 2004;15(8):960-962.

24. Pappone C, Oral H, Santinelli V, Vicedomini G, Lang CC, Manguso F, Torracca L, Benussi S, Alfieri O, Hong R, Lau W, Hirata K, Shikuma N, Hall B, Morady F. Atriooesophageal fistula as a complication of percutaneous transcatheter ablation of atrial fibrillation. *Circulation* 2004;109 (22):2724-2726.

25. Sonmez B, Demirsoy E, Yagan N, Unal M, Arbatli H, Sener D, Baran T, Ilkova F. A fatal complication due to radiofrequency ablation for atrial fibrillation: atriooesophageal fistula. *Ann Thorac Surg* 2003;76(1):281-283.

26. Good E, Oral H, Lemola K, Han J, Tamirisa K, Igic P, Elmouchi D, Tschopp D, Reich S, Chugh A, Bogun F, Pelosi F Jr, Morady F. Movement of the oesophagus during left atrial catheter ablation for atrial fibrillation. *J Am College Cardiol* 2005;46(11):2107-2110.

27. Knecht S, Skali H, O'Neill M, Wright M, Matsuo S, Chaudhry GM, Haffajee C, Nault I, Gijsbers GHM, Sacher F, Laurent F, Montaudon M, Corneloup O, Hocini M, Haïssaguerre M, Orlov MV, Jaïs P. Computed tomography–fluoroscopy overlay evaluation during catheter ablation of left atrial arrhythmia. *Europace* 2008;10:931-938.

28. Knecht S, Jaïs P, Nault I, Wright M, Matsuo S, Madaffari A, Lellouche N, O'Neill MD, Derval N, Deplagne A, Bordachar B, Sacher F, Hocini M, Clémenty J, Haïssaguerre M. Radiofrequency puncture of the fossa ovalis for resistant transseptal access. *Circ Arrhythm Electrophysiol* 2008;1:169-174.

29. Efstathopoulos EP, Katritsis DG, Kottou S, Kalivas N, Tzanalaridou E, Giazitzoglou E, Korovesis S, Faulkner K. Patient and staff radiation dosimetry during cardiac electrophysiology studies and catheter ablation procedures: a comprehensive analysis. *Europace* 2006;8(6):443-448.

30. McFadden SL, Mooney RB, Shepherd PH. X-ray dose and associated risks from radiofrequency catheter ablation procedures. *Br J Radiol* 2002;75(891):253-265.

31. Theocharopoulos N, Damilakis J, Perisinakis K, Manios E, Vardas P, Gourtsoyiannis N. Occupational exposure in the electrophysiology laboratory: quantifying and minimizing radiation burden. *Br J Radiol* 2006;79(944):644-651.

32. Perisinakis K, Damilakis J, Theocharopoulos N, Manios E, Vardas P, Gourtsoyiannis N. Accurate assessment of patient effective radiation dose and associated detriment risk from radiofrequency catheter ablation procedures. *Circulation* 2001;104(1):58-62.

33. Lickfett L, Mahesh M, Vasamreddy C, Bradley D, Jayam V, Eldadah Z, Dickfeld T, Kearney D, Dalal D, Lüderitz B, Berger R, Calkins H. Radiation exposure during catheter ablation of atrial fibrillation. *Circulation* 2004;110(19):3003-3010.

34. Wittkampf FHM, Wever EFD, Vos K, Geleijns J, Schalij MJ, Van der Tol J, Robles de Medina EO. Reduction of radiation exposure in the cardiac electrophysiology laboratory. *Pacing Clin Electrophysiol* 2000;23(11):1638-1644.

Indications and Contraindications of Transseptal Catheterization

Michael Kühne, Hakan Oral

Transseptal catheterization describes the passage of a cardiac catheter from the right atrium through the interatrial septum into the left atrium. Unless a patent foramen ovale is present, as is the case in 20% to 25% of the population, a transseptal needle is used to create a primary puncture of the interatrial septum.[1,2] The primary puncture is followed by advancing a dilator and a sheath into the left atrium, allowing access to the left atrium with the mapping or ablation catheter. If more than one catheter is used simultaneously in the left atrium, two separate punctures of the septum can be performed ("double transseptal") or two catheters are advanced through the same primary puncture. This chapter provides an overview of the current indications and contraindications of transseptal catheterization in electrophysiology.

Transseptal Catheterization and Interventions.
© 2010 Ranjan Thakur MD and Andrea Natale MD, eds.
Cardiotext Publishing, ISBN 978-0-9790164-1-7.

Background

The technique of accessing the left atrium via the transseptal route was first described 50 years ago.[3] Previously, the left atrium was accessed using several other methods that carried considerable procedural risks, such as the suprasternal approach through the great vessels, the posterior transthoracic technique (puncture of the left atrium lateral to the spine), the transbronchial approach, and the subxiphoid approach.[4,5] Transseptal catheterization has been employed to provide access to the left atrium and left ventricle since the 1960s, but with the development of coronary angiography in the late 1960s and the 1970s, the retrograde aortic approach has been more frequently used to access the left ventricle. Therefore, until recently, invasive cardiologists only rarely had sufficient experience performing transseptal catheterization unless they were trained in high-volume centers where balloon mitral valvuloplasty was performed.[6] In his textbook on cardiac catheterization, William Grossman once wrote that "the infrequency with which the procedure is currently needed has made it difficult for most laboratories to maintain operator expertise and to train cardiovascular fellows in transseptal puncture, and has given the procedure an aura of danger and intrigue."[7] However, over the last few years, there has been a resurgence of transseptal catheterization due to a dramatic increase in left atrial procedures for catheter ablation.

A number of clinical scenarios exist in which it may be useful to gain access to the left atrium for diagnostic or therapeutic indications. Since the introduction of transseptal catheterization, when the technique was primarily used to measure left atrial pressure, the indications for transseptal catheterization have changed markedly over the last 5 decades. A recent study from 33 centers reported that among 5520 transseptal catheterizations for catheter ablation of arrhythmias, 78% was performed to target atrial fibrillation, and transseptal catheterization was successfully performed in 99%. The primary reason for inability to perform transseptal catheterization was abnormal anatomy of the interatrial septum.[8]

Indications

More than 10 years have passed since a landmark study described a technique targeting ectopic beats arising from the pulmonary veins to eliminate triggers for atrial fibrillation using radiofrequency catheter ablation.[9] After refinements of this technique in many clinical studies in recent years, catheter ablation of atrial fibrillation has become widely available. Left atrial ablations targeting atrial fibrillation are now the most frequent indica-

tion for transseptal catheterization. However, a number of other clinical situations in the management of patients with cardiac arrhythmias require access to the left atrium, and this is most frequently achieved via the transseptal route. Table 4.1 summarizes current indications for transseptal catheterization in cardiac electrophysiology.

TABLE 4.1

Indications for Transseptal Catheterization

Atrial fibrillation

Atypical/Left atrial flutter

Left atrial tachycardia (focal/reentry)

Left-sided accessory pathways

Ventricular tachycardia

Rare indications (eg, "left atrial" atrioventricular nodal reentry tachycardia)

Atrial Fibrillation

There are different approaches to managing patients with atrial fibrillation non-pharmacologically. However, unless a patient undergoes surgical treatment of atrial fibrillation (Maze procedure) or a surgical technique such as epicardial radiofrequency ablation (AtriCure Inc, West Chester, OH),[10] the arrhythmia is targeted endocardially with an ablation catheter for energy delivery, currently radiofrequency energy in most cases. Although some ablation strategies applied in the 1990s were limited to the right atrium, the significance of the left atrium and the pulmonary veins was soon recognized.[11] Therefore catheter-based treatment strategies targeting atrial fibrillation all have in common that they require access to the left atrium. This is achieved by transseptal catheterization.

If more than 1 catheter is used in the left atrium at the same time, 2 separate punctures of the interatrial septum can be performed (double transseptal). Alternatively, 2 catheters can be passed through the same primary puncture of the septum. There are no specific recommendations to use single or double transseptal technique, but some operators prefer a single puncture in case the first puncture is difficult.

Repeat procedures to treat recurrences of atrial fibrillation or occurrences of other arrhythmias, such as left atrial flutters, may be necessary in some patients.[12] When performing these procedures, the interatrial septum can be distorted, thickened, or fibrotic due to the development of scar tissue in the area of the previous puncture. The changes in the architecture of the interatrial septum can be quite significant in some patients, making repeat transseptal catheterization more challenging. More pressure may be required to puncture the septum due to the fibrotic changes; the typical drop of the catheter into the fossa ovalis may be more difficult to appreciate; and tenting of the interatrial septum may be absent. In these cases, intracardiac ultrasound may be particularly helpful. Data on the safety and efficacy of repeat transseptal catheterization is relatively scarce. Transseptal puncture for repeat transseptal catheterization may be necessary in some patients in whom the first left atrial procedure had been performed through a patent foramen ovale.[13]

When transseptal catheterization appears difficult due to fibrotic changes, novel approaches such as radiofrequency energy delivery via the transseptal needle or a dedicated radiofrequency transseptal system (Baylis Medical, Montreal, Ontario, Canada) may be indicated to successfully puncture the interatrial septum.[14,15]

Left Atrial Tachycardia and Flutter

Primary atrial tachycardias may be observed in approximately 10% of patients presenting with paroxysmal supraventricular tachycardia (and no previous left atrial procedures). Some of these atrial tachycardias may originate from the left atrium, and transseptal access may be necessary to map and ablate them.

Left atrial tachycardia or flutter may also develop after left atrial ablation of atrial fibrillation.[16] Approximately half of these arrhythmias may be transient and not require any interventional therapy. However, in the remaining patients repeat transseptal catheterization often is necessary to eliminate these tachycardias.

Relatively few data exist on transseptal catheterization and ablation of left atrial arrhythmias in patients with mechanical valve prostheses. The major concern of left atrial ablation in these patients is catheter entrapment in the prosthetic valve. One study concluded that transseptal catheterization and ablation of atrial fibrillation in patients with mitral valve prosthesis is feasible. However, the complication rate was higher, with a greater radiation exposure and a higher incidence of post-ablation atrial tachycardias.[17] In a series of 227 transseptal catheterizations for left atrial procedures, 9 patients (4%) had valve prostheses, and transseptal puncture was successfully performed in all of them.[18] If a decision is made to proceed with transseptal catheterization in patients with valve prostheses, experienced operators are required, and using an additional imaging modality may be helpful.

Left-sided Accessory Pathways and AV Nodal Reentry Tachycardia

Approximately 60% of all accessory pathways are left-sided. Catheter ablation can be performed using a transseptal or a retrograde aortic approach. Traditionally, left-sided accessory pathways have been ablated using the retrograde aortic approach. The disadvantage of this technique is the fact that it requires arterial access resulting in longer vascular recovery. Furthermore, catheter maneuverability can be impaired by parts of the mitral valve apparatus, making the mapping procedure more difficult. However, catheter stability is excellent during application of energy. Using transseptal catheterization, mapping of the mitral annulus can be performed with great ease compared to the retrograde aortic approach where the subvalvular structures can adversely affect catheter maneuverability. However, catheter stability may be less favorable with the antegrade approach through a transseptal puncture than with the retrograde approach. Arterial access may not be necessary during transseptal access, and duration of vascular recovery is shorter compared to the retrograde approach (Table 4.2). One study found that the retrograde and transseptal approaches may be complementary and that the two have similar complication rates.[19]

Atrioventricular nodal reentry tachycardia (AVNRT) utilizing a slow pathway more readily accessible from the left side may constitute <1% of patients with typical (slow/fast) AVNRT. In some of these patients, successful treatment of the arrhythmia can be achieved by performing transseptal catheterization and ablation of a slow pathway component close to the inferolateral mitral annulus.[20] Left septal ablation of the fast pathway in AVNRT has also been reported.[21]

TABLE 4.2

Transseptal Versus Retrograde Aortic Approach for Catheter Ablation of Left-sided Accessory Pathways

	Transseptal Approach	Retrograde Approach
Catheter stability	Difficult	Good
Catheter maneuverability	Excellent	Difficult
Heating	Good	May be difficult
Access	No arterial access necessary	Longer vascular recovery
Costs	Higher if intracardiac echocardiography is used	Lower compared to transseptal with intracardiac echocardiography

TABLE 4.3

Contraindications of Transseptal Catheterization in Electrophysiology

Left atrial thrombus

Left atrial tumor

Severe bleeding diathesis

Significant extracardiac anatomical abnormalities (eg, deformity of the chest or spine)

Inability to lie flat

PFO or ASD closure device

PFO = patent foramen ovale
ASD = atrial septal defect

Ventricular Tachycardia

Transseptal catheterization is rarely necessary when attempting catheter ablation of ventricular tachycardia. Mapping of the left ventricle, particularly the left ventricular outflow tract, aortic cusps, and mitral annulus through transseptal catheterization can be more difficult. However, it may be easier to map the papillary muscles. A transseptal approach is preferred in patients with severe atherosclerotic disease of the aorta, with major aortic malformations or dissection, or in patients with severe aortic stenosis or with mechanical aortic valve prosthesis. With the advent of magnetic navigation (Stereotaxis), catheter maneuverability in the left ventricle may also be easier using a transseptal approach.

Contraindications

Although, with the use of intracardiac echocardiography, transeptal puncture can be safely performed even in patients with sig-nificant anatomical variations, in certain conditions the risks of performing a transseptal puncture may outweigh the benefits. The electrophysiologist should be well aware of these conditions and carefully consider the risks before proceeding with a transseptal puncture (Table 4.3).

Left Atrial Thrombus and Tumor

Thrombus in the left atrium (mostly left atrial appendage) may occur in patients with atrial fibrillation.[22-24] A left atrial thrombus may be identified by transesophageal echocardiography, intracardiac echocardiography, or a CT scan of the left atrium. However, transesophageal echocardiography has been considered the gold standard. Because a thrombus, particularly a fresh thrombus, can be dislocated during catheter manipulation in the left atrium, and because the risk of thromboembolic events is higher after restoration of sinus rhythm, transseptal puncture may be best avoided for catheter ablation of atrial fibrillation or left atrial flutter in patients with a left atrial thrombus or tumor.

Presence of a Percutaneous PFO or ASD Closure Device

Most operators would not perform transseptal catheterization in a patient with a history of either a percutaneous closure of a patent foramen ovale or an atrial septal defect with a closure device, particularly after a recent implant. The procedure presents the potential risk of dislodgement of the device and the risk of systemic embolization due to coagulum or fibrous material that may have formed around the closure device. However, successful transseptal catheterization in the presence of a percutaneously implanted closure device has recently been reported.[25-27]

Severe Bleeding Diathesis

The concern in patients with severe bleeding diathesis is that there may be uncontrollable bleeding if inadvertent puncture of the adjacent structures, such as the aorta or free wall of the atrium, occurs. However, transseptal access can be considered in these patients if effective and rapid reversal of the bleeding diathesis is possible or if the coagulation abnormality is corrected prior to the procedure. More recently, transseptal puncture in the presence of continuing systemic anticoagulation with warfarin has been routinely performed to minimize the risk of thromboembolic complications, particularly during the discontinuation and reinitiation of anticoagulant therapy before and after the procedure.[28] In these patients, anticoagulant activity can be reversed by infusion of fresh frozen plasma and/or factor VII complex.

Anatomical Variations and Abnormalities

Severe anatomical abnormalities of the spine (eg, kyphoscoliosis) or chest deformities (eg, prior pneumonectomy, pectus excavatum) are not absolute contraindications to transseptal catheterization, but may present as a challenge. Due to rotation and repositioning of the heart in the chest, standard maneuvers to position the transseptal needle in the fossa ovalis may not be helpful. In these patients, intracardiac echocardiography can be particularly helpful.

For example, a persistent left inferior vena cava draining into the azygous system may pose a particular challenge as the left atrium cannot be accessed through a femoral venous approach and access through a jugular vein and superior vena cava may be considered (Figure 4.1). However, the superior approach to access the left atrium can be challenging and requires operator experience. Additional imaging modalities such as intracardiac echocardiography may be helpful.

Special Considerations in Patients with Congenital Heart Disease

The presence of baffles, conduits, and other intraatrial patches poses a unique challenge. Transseptal puncture should be performed by experienced operators familiar with both the underlying congenital abnormality and the corrective surgery. In a prior study, transseptal catheterization was performed in 39 patients with intraatrial baffles or patches. These patients had a history of patch repair of atrial septal defect or atrioventricular canal, D-transposition of the great arteries treated with the Mustard or Senning procedure, single ventricle variant with Fontan operation, or total anomalous pulmonary venous return repair. The materials used for the patch repairs included pericardium, native atrial tissue, Dacron, GORE-TEX, and Teflon. Transseptal catheterization was successfully performed in 97.4% of patients. The authors concluded that transseptal catheterization through intraatrial patches can be performed safely and successfully in the early and late postoperative period, independent of the material used to create the patch, and that there were no residual shunts after the transseptal catheterization.[29]

Conclusions

Transseptal catheterization is routinely and safely performed in electrophysiology laboratories around the world and is necessary for catheter ablation in the left atrium targeting

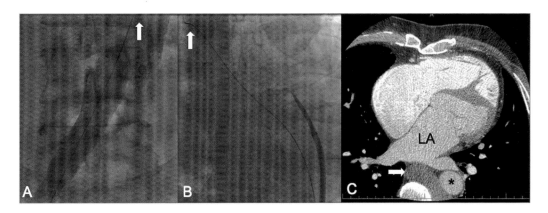

FIGURE 4.1   *Inability to Access the Left Atrium with a Femoral Vein Approach*
Due to a Persistent Left Inferior Vena Cava Draining into the Azygous System
A. Anteroposterior view: Venous access from the right groin. The guidewire and the intravenous contrast are in the right iliac vein and the left-sided inferior vena cava (arrow). **B.** Anteroposterior view at the level of the left atrium: The tip of the dilator is in the azygous vein. The guidewire is in the azygous vein close to the entry into the superior vena cava (arrow). **C.** Computed tomography of the chest (axial view) shows the connection (arrow) from the left to the azygous vein on the right. The connection is posterior to the left atrium (LA). The asterisk denotes the descending aorta.

a variety of arrhythmias, particularly atrial fibrillation.

As left atrial procedures are being performed routinely, there has been substantial improvement in operator experience, and trainees now have ample opportunity to acquire the skills to perform transseptal puncture. Furthermore, additional imaging modalities, particularly intracardiac echocardiography, has been very helpful for the safe execution of the procedure, even in the most challenging patients. Nevertheless, in each patient the risks and benefits of transseptal catheterization should be carefully considered, as inadvertent complications may result in catastrophic outcomes.

References

1. Bloomfield DA, Sinclair-Smith BC. The limbic ledge: a landmark for transseptal catheterization. *Circulation* 1965;31:103-107.
2. Sweeney LJ, Rosenquist GC. The normal anatomy of the atrial septum in the human heart. *Am Heart J* 1979;98:194-199.
3. Ross J Jr, Braunwald E, Morrow AG. Transseptal left atrial puncture: a new technique for the measurement of left atrial pressure in man. *Am J Cardiol* 1959;3:653-655.
4. Morrow AG, Braunwald E, Ross J Jr. Left heart catheterization: an appraisal of techniques and their application in cardiovascular diagnosis. *Arch Intern Med* 1960;105:645-655.
5. Ross J Jr. Transseptal left heart catheterization. A 50-year odyssey. *J Am Coll Cardiol* 2008;51:2107-2115.
6. Babaliaros VC, Green JT, Lerakis S, Lloyd M, Block PC. Emerging applications for transseptal left heart catheterization: old techniques for new procedures. *J Am Coll Cardiol* 2008;51:2116-2122.
7. Baim DS, Grossman W. Percutaneous approach, including transseptal catheterization and apical left ventricular puncture. In: Grossman W, Baim DS, eds. *Cardiac*

Catheterization, Angiography, and Intervention. 6th ed. Philadelphia: Lippincott, Williams & Wilkins, 2000.

8. De Ponti R, Cappato R, Curnis A, et al. Trans-septal catheterization in the electrophysiology laboratory: data from a multicenter survey spanning 12 years. *J Am Coll Cardiol* 2006;47:1037-1042.

9. Haïssaguerre M, Jaïs P, Shah DC, et al. Spontaneous initiation of atrial fibrillation by ectopic beats originating in the pulmonary veins. *N Engl J Med* 1998;339:659-666.

10. Gillinov AM, McCarthy PM, Marrouche N, et al. Contemporary surgical treatment for atrial fibrillation. *Pacing Clin Electrophysiol* 2003;26:1641-1644.

11. Jaïs P, Shah DC, Takahashi A, et al. Long-term follow-up after right atrial radiofrequency catheter treatment of paroxysmal atrial fibrillation. *Pacing Clin Electrophysiol* 1998;21:2533-2538.

12. Callans DJ, Gerstenfeld EP, Dixit S, et al. Efficacy of repeat pulmonary vein isolation procedures in patients with recurrent atrial fibrillation. *J Cardiovasc Electrophysiol* 2004;15:150-155.

13. Marcus GM, Ren X, Tseng ZH, et al. Repeat transseptal catheterization after ablation for atrial fibrillation. *J Cardiovasc Electrophysiol* 2007;18:55-59.

14. Bidart C, Vaseghi M, Cesario DA, et al. Radiofrequency current delivery via transseptal needle to facilitate septal puncture. *Heart Rhythm* 2007;4:1573-1576.

15. Sakata Y, Feldman T. Transcatheter creation of atrial septal perforation using a radiofrequency transseptal system: novel approach as an alternative to transseptal needle puncture. *Catheter Cardiovasc Interv* 2005;64:327-332.

16. Chugh A, Oral H, Lemola K, et al. Prevalence, mechanisms, and clinical significance of macroreentrant atrial tachycardia during and following left atrial ablation for atrial fibrillation. *Heart Rhythm* 2005;2:464-471.

17. Lang CC, Santinelli V, Augello G, et al. Transcatheter radiofrequency ablation of atrial fibrillation in patients with mitral valve prostheses and enlarged atria: safety, feasibility, and efficacy. *J Am Coll Cardiol* 2005;45:868-872.

18. Barbato G, Pergolini F, Carinci V, Di Pasquale G. Transseptal approach for left atrial arrhythmia ablation in patients with valve prostheses. *J Cardiovasc Med* (Hagerstown) 2008;9:273-276.

19. Lesh MD, Van Hare GF, Scheinman MM, et al. Comparison of the retrograde and transseptal methods for left free wall accessory pathways. *J Am Coll Cardiol* 1993;22:542-549.

20. Chen SA, Tai CT, Lee SH, Chang MA. AV nodal reentrant tachycardia with unusual characteristics: lessons from radiofrequency catheter ablation. *J Cardiovasc Electrophysiol* 1998;9:321-323.

21. Kobza R, Hindricks G, Tanner H, Kottkamp H. Left-septal ablation of the fast pathway in AV nodal reentrant tachycardia refractory to right septal ablation. *Europace* 2005;7: 149-153.

22. Corrado G, Beretta S, Sormani L, et al. Prevalence of atrial thrombi in patients with atrial fibrillation/flutter and subtherapeutic anticoagulation prior to cardioversion. *Eur J Echocardiogr* 2004;5:57-61.

23. Manning WJ, Silverman DI, Keighley CS, Oettgen P, Douglas PS. Transesophageal echocardiographically facilitated early cardioversion from atrial fibrillation using short-term anticoagulation: final results of a prospective 4.5-year study. *J Am Coll Cardiol* 1995;25:1354-1361.

24. Stoddard MF, Dawkins PR, Prince CR, Ammash NM. Left atrial thrombus is not uncommon in patients with acute atrial fibrillation and a recent embolic event: transesophageal echocardiographic study. *J Am Coll Cardiol* 1995;25:452-459.

25. Lakkireddy D, Rangisetty U, Prasad S, et al.

Intracardiac echo-guided radiofrequency catheter ablation of atrial fibrillation in patients with atrial septal defect or patent foramen ovale repair: a feasibility, safety, and efficacy study. *J Cardiovasc Electrophysiol* 2008;19:1137-1142.

26. Cook S, Meier B, Windecker S. Transseptal TandemHeart implantation through an Amplatzer atrial septal occluder. *J Invasive Cardiol* 2007;19:198-199.

27. Zaker-Shahrak R, Fuhrer J, Meier B. Transseptal puncture for catheter ablation of atrial fibrillation after device closure of patent foramen ovale. *Catheter Cardiovasc Interv* 2008;71:551-552.

28. Wazni OM, Beheiry S, Fahmy T, et al. Atrial fibrillation ablation in patients with therapeutic international normalized ration: comparison of strategies of anticoagulation management in the periprocedural period. *Circulation* 2007;116:2531-2534.

29. El-Said HG, Ing FF, Grifka RG, et al. 18-year experience with transseptal procedures through baffles, conduits, and other intra-atrial patches. *Catheter Cardiovasc Interv* 2000;50:434-439.

5

EQUIPMENT FOR TRANSSEPTAL PUNCTURES

PETER LEONG-SIT, DAVID CALLANS

The transseptal puncture was originally described in the late 1950s by Drs. John Ross, Edwin Brockenbrough, and Eugene Braunwald.[1,2] Over several years, with experiments on canines, human cadavers, and then patients, they developed the most basic equipment required for a percutaneous transseptal puncture. Although the initial reported series of 450 transseptal punctures in 1962 gave rise to relatively low complication rates,[3] major complications occurred, such as aortic puncture, pericardial tamponade, systemic arterial embolism, and inferior vena cava perforation.[4] Expectedly, there have been many advances in technology and in the equipment used over the last 5 decades. These improvements allow the clinician to perform a safer transseptal puncture and more frequently avoid the many possible complications. More recent publications would suggest that the procedure still has tangible risks: a 2.7% risk of pericardial effusion, a 1.0% risk of pericardial tamponade, and a 0.4% risk of a neurologic event.[5]

The basic set of tools required for the procedure includes a wire to guide the insertion of sheaths into the heart, a long needle to puncture the interatrial septum, and a long sheath to traverse the septum. Optional auxiliary tools to assist in a safer procedure include air filters, X-ray contrast dye, pressure lines, various forms of echocardiography, and catheters placed for anatomic reference. Emerging tools include laser or radiofrequency assistance to puncture the interatrial septum, needle systems with additional safety features, and equipment designed for use with internal jugular vein access.

Transseptal Catheterization and Interventions.
© 2010 Ranjan Thakur MD and Andrea Natale MD, eds.
Cardiotext Publishing, ISBN 978-0-9790164-1-7.

Needles

Arguably, the most critical advance in the percutaneous transseptal puncture was the invention and modification of the transseptal needle. Most of this work was originally done by Ross, who invented the transseptal needle, and by Brockenbrough, who modified it to a version not dissimilar to the modern needle. Since that time, several manufacturers have devised versions of the transseptal puncture needle. All versions of the needle are long, curved, and stainless steel, and designed to be introduced via the right femoral vein. The needles have an arrow-shaped handle that indicates the direction of the needle tip and that allows for steerable control of the rotational direction of the needle tip (Figure 5.1). The needles are 18-gauge in adult-sized sheaths (19-gauge in pediatric needles) and taper to a size of 21-gauge. The curve of the needle between the shaft and the needle tip varies with different size options. For example, St. Jude Medical has a series of transseptal needles. The Brockenbrough (BRK) is a small-curved needle with a shaft-to-needle-tip angle of approximately 19°, whereas the BRK-1 is a large-curved needle with an angle of approximately 55°. Pediatric options also include the BRK-2 with an intermediate curve. The length of the needle also varies depending on the length of the sheath being used. The majority of sheaths require a standard-length needle of 71 cm (pediatric needles are 56 cm). Longer sheaths with steerable mechanisms, such as the Agilis NxT Steerable Introducer sheath (St. Jude Medical Inc, St. Paul, MN), require a longer needle of 98 cm. All needles come with a stylet that fills the lumen of the needle and extends beyond the needle tip. The stylet is used when introducing the needle into a sheath; it prevents the needle tip from scraping the inner lumen of the sheath.

Introducers and Sheaths

Many sheaths are available for use with the transseptal puncture needle. The shape and curve of the sheath are designed to first assist in providing support to the transseptal needle during the transseptal puncture and, more importantly, to give support and stability to the mapping or ablation catheter to reach various parts of the left atrium and ventricle. Manufacturers have designed several different sheaths to serve this purpose.

General design features of these sheaths include a side port with a hemostasis valve. All come with a dilator that fits within the lumen of the sheath and extends beyond the sheath tip to add structural support during cannulation of the vein as well as during transseptal puncture.

Generally, sheaths can be categorized as steerable or fixed. An example of a basic multi-purpose fixed sheath would be the Mullins-style sheath manufactured by several companies. The sheath is approximately 60 cm long with a large distal curve of 180° and a diameter of 6 cm. It is generally softer and more pliable than newer sheaths and provides less structural support to the catheter. St. Jude Medical, Inc, C. R. Bard, Inc, and Boston Scientific, Inc have each developed a series of sheaths with varying curves (Figure 5.2). St. Jude Medical, Inc has several Swartz transseptal guiding introducers, such as the LAMP series of 63-cm-length sheaths with curves of 45°, 90°, or 135°. The Swartz SL series of sheaths come in 63-cm or 81-cm lengths and in both size 8 F and 8.5 F. This series was designed to assist in stabilizing the catheter on the mitral annulus at various sites, initially for left-sided accessory pathway ablation. With the exception of the SL4, the sheaths all have a primary curve of 50° followed by a secondary curve of 0° (SL0), 45° (SL1), 90° (SL2), 135° (SL3), and 180° (SL4).

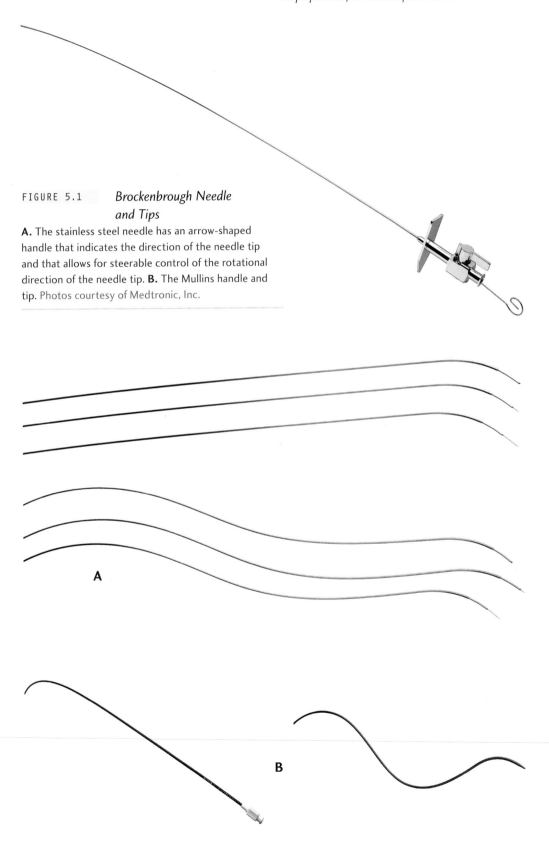

FIGURE 5.1   *Brockenbrough Needle and Tips*

A. The stainless steel needle has an arrow-shaped handle that indicates the direction of the needle tip and that allows for steerable control of the rotational direction of the needle tip. **B.** The Mullins handle and tip. Photos courtesy of Medtronic, Inc.

A

B

The SL4 has a lesser primary curve of 35°. C. R. Bard, Inc has a series of transseptal sheath kits called the Channel FX with a sheath length of 61 cm and a size of 8 F. The series has three curves available: 55°, 90°, and 120°. Boston Scientific Corporation has the Convoy Advanced Delivery Sheath Kit series with curves ranging from 15° to 150°.*

Another innovation in sheath design is a steerable mechanism to assist in catheter stability and placement at various locations in the heart. An example would be the Agilis NxT Steerable Introducer (St. Jude Medical,

---

*Boston Scientific has discontinued the Convoy sheath.

FIGURE 5.2   *Sheaths with Varying Curves*
A. The Swartz LAMP series of LAMP sheaths from St. Jude Medical, Inc. **B.** The Swartz SL series of SL sheaths, also from St. Jude Medical, Inc. Permission to reproduce these images granted by St. Jude Medical, Inc. **C.** The Convoy series of sheaths from Boston Scientific Corporation. Courtesy of Boston Scientific.

Inc, St. Paul, MN) (Figure 5.3). The sheath is designed with a handle that can control the sheath tip with bi-directional deflection. The sheaths have small-curl and medium-curl options; are 91 cm in length, including the steering handle mechanism (71 cm usable length); and require the longer transseptal needle (98 cm). The steerable and stiffer composition of the sheath gives additional structural and directional support to the catheter and allows for additional control of the catheter tip location. C. R. Bard, Inc also has the Channel steerable sheath, which has 67 cm usable length and is available in 8 F or 9 F sizes. It has a unidirectional steering mechanism, which can vary from 0° to 180°. It is compatible with an 89-cm transseptal needle.

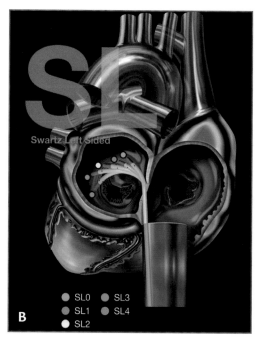

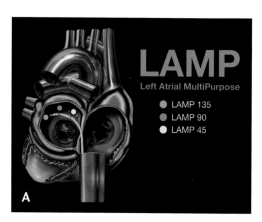

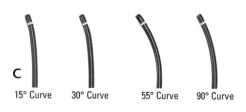

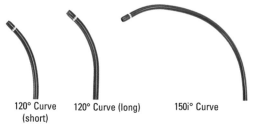

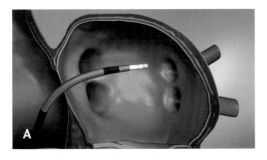

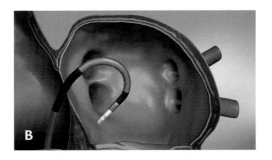

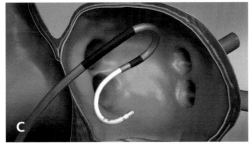

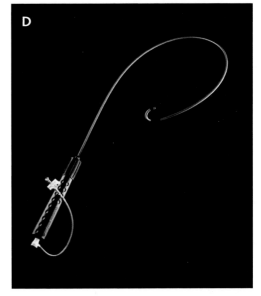

FIGURE 5.3   *Steerable Sheath*
The Agilis NxT Steerable Intro-
ducer from St. Jude Medical, Inc in the straightened
position (**A**) and flexed (**B**). A steerable sheath
allows for dual curves when used in conjunction with
a steerable catheter (**C**). The handle controls the
amount of flex on the sheath by rotating the handle
clockwise or counterclockwise (**D**). Permission to
reproduce these images granted by St. Jude Medical, Inc.

Guidewires

Guidewires are required for safe advancement
of sheaths and/or dilators through the vascular anatomy. Most introducer and sheath kits
come with a standard wire. Many wires are
available and generally have a J-tipped curve
to reduce the risk of vascular injury during
advancement of the wire. The maximum
guidewire diameter that will fit into most
sheaths and dilator system is 0.032 inches, but
varies depending on the sheath. The J curve
has a standard curve radius of 3 mm, and
some are finger-straightenable while others do
not have a straightening mechanism. Other
wire options are available for difficult venous
anatomy, such as stenosed or tortuous vessels.

An example would be the Glidewire (Terumo
Medical Corporation, Somerset, NJ). The
wire's hydrophilic polymer-coated surface
allows for a frictionless advancement when
the coating is in contact with saline solution,
and it's made with a superelastic alloy core
that helps eliminate kinking. These design
features assist in wire advancement when the
vascular anatomy proves challenging.

Additionally, guidewires that fit through
the hub of the transseptal needle can also be
used. Some techniques involve the confirmation of left atrial positioning as well as left
atrial wall protection by advancing a guidewire through the needle hub and out through
a left-sided pulmonary vein. These wires are
once again J-tipped, but at 0.014 inches are
smaller in diameter to allow the wire to fit
through the needle tip.

Auxiliary Tools

While a transseptal puncture can be performed with only the equipment described above (a transseptal needle, a sheath and introducer system, and a guidewire), there are many other auxiliary tools available for the clinician to assist in minimizing complications: pressure transducers, radiopaque contrast agents, catheters placed for anatomic landmarks, and echocardiographic tools.

Pressure Transducer

First, there is the pressure transducer, which can be attached to the needle hub. This device allows a measurement of mean right and left atrial pressures. The pressure transducer can be attached to the needle hub either during the transseptal puncture or following the puncture to confirm left atrial pressures. Using the former technique, a mean right atrial pres-

sure can be measured, followed by a blunting of the pressure signal during needle contact with the septum. Following puncture through the septum into the left atrium, a mean left atrial pressure confirms correct positioning of the needle and excludes the possibility of transaortic puncture (Figure 5.4).

Fluoroscopic Contrast Medium

Radiopaque contrast can also be used to assist in confirmation of needle position. The contrast agent can be used at full strength or diluted 1:1 with normal saline. When used, the contrast agent is drawn into a hand-held syringe and attached to the transseptal needle hub. Once the needle is positioned at the fossa ovalis, a small hand injection of the contrast agent stains the adjacent tissue and allows for visualization of the intraatrial septum (Figure 5.5). After the needle is advanced through the septum and into the left atrium, injection of

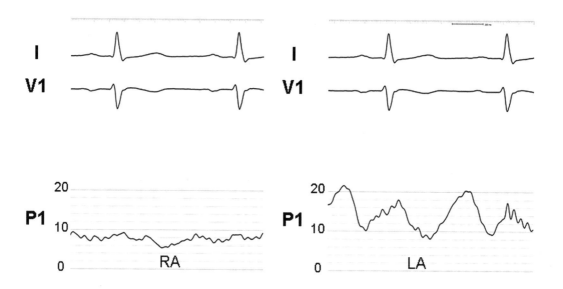

FIGURE 5.4   *Pressure Transduction During a Transseptal Puncture*
Pressure transduction demonstrates normal right atrial pressures and waveform (RA) and normal left atrial pressures (LA) after a successful transseptal puncture. P1 = transduced pressure in mmHg; I and V1 = surface electrocardiographic leads.

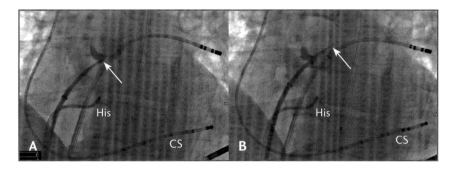

FIGURE 5.5   *Use of Contrast Medium*
A. Staining of the interatrial septum at the tip of the transseptal needle (arrow) can be seen prior to transseptal puncture. **B.** The needle tip and the dilator (arrow) can be seen past the stained septum following successful transseptal puncture. CS = coronary sinus catheter; His = His catheter.

contrast medium confirms needle tip positioning with contrast flow from the left atrium into the left ventricle or, conversely, with brisk flow in a cranial direction, which would indicate inadvertent transaortic cannulation.

Catheters for Anatomic Landmarks

Standard diagnostic electrophysiology catheters can be used to obtain fluoroscopic landmarks when other imaging modalities, such as echocardiography, are not employed. Standard quadripolar diagnostic catheters can be positioned at the His position, and decapolar diagnostic catheters in the coronary sinus.[6] Additionally, or alternatively, a pigtail catheter can be positioned arterially to the aortic root, but it would, of course, require arterial access. A catheter positioned at the His can be of great value.[7] The fossa ovalis is generally at the level of the His catheter, and the needle tip should generally be posterior to the His catheter. A coronary sinus catheter is also useful, as the needle tip should generally be pointing in a path parallel to the coronary sinus. It also approximates the left atrial free wall in the left anterior oblique projection.

The pigtail catheter positioned in the aortic root provides an anterior landmark to avoid.

Echocardiography

Direct echocardiographic visualization of the intraatrial septum and of the site of transseptal puncture have assisted in the safety of the procedure. Transthoracic echocardiography has little role given the limited resolution and inadequate view of the intraatrial septum. However, transesophageal echocardiography provides adequate views of the intraatrial septum to assist in the procedure. Two other intracardiac options are also available. First, there is the intravenous ultrasound (IVUS) catheter, which provides a 360° lateral cross-sectional view. It is an 8 F probe, and can be introduced through an 8 F sheath into the right atrium. The newest form of intracardiac echocardiography, such as the ACUSON AcuNav (Siemens Medical Solutions USA, Inc, Malvern, PA), provides a standard echocardiographic format view from inside the heart. It is an 8-F, 110-cm-long probe, and has a frequency range from 5.0 MHz to 10.0 MHz. The imaging plane is steerable 160° in both an anterior-posterior plane and in the left-right plane. In addition to 2-D imaging, it has the capability of pulsed-wave, continuous-wave, color, and tissue Doppler. It provides an intracardiac echocardiographic format recognizable to those who are already familiar with transthoracic and transesophageal echocardiography. These modalities can be invaluable as they provide direct visualization of the intraatrial septum and give rise to important information, such as the level of the intended transseptal puncture, the thickness of the septum at that point, and the degree of the anterior-posterior direction of the intended puncture. During the puncture, the tenting of the stretched septum can be seen, as well as the needle as it traverses the septum (Figure 5.6). Visualization of bubbles in the left atrium during flushing of the sheath further confirms correct localization. Furthermore, the intracardiac echocardiography probe can be useful during the ablation itself; it provides visualization of the pulmonary veins during atrial fibrillation ablation, of the mitral annulus during accessory pathway ablation, and of the left ventricle and outflow tract during ventricular tachycardia or premature ventricular contraction (PVC) ablation.

Emerging Tools

There are many emerging tools to assist with a safe transseptal puncture. Several manufacturers have sheath/dilator/needle combination systems, such as the ACross Transseptal Access System (St. Jude Medical, Inc, St. Paul, MN). This interlocking and integrated system combines the sheath, dilator, and transseptal needle to assist with directional orientation of the sheath with the needle and to improve control of needle deployment. The system comes with the option of an 8.5 F Swartz SL1 or LAMP 90 sheath in 63- or 81-cm lengths. St. Jude Medical, Inc has also designed the LA-Crosse system (not approved in the United States), which allows for transseptal puncture from the right internal jugular vein. This system provides a second option in case the lower extremity venous anatomy precludes the usual approach. A thickened or fibrous septum, the presence of a septal aneurysm, or a small left atrium can make transseptal punctures more difficult. Scarring of the intraatrial septum may become more common as the number of repeat procedures grow, for scarring often occurs following an

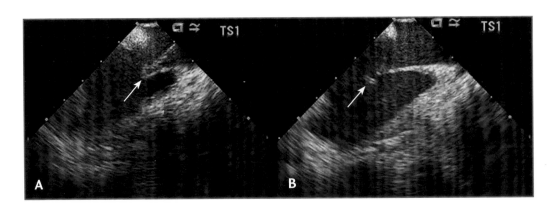

FIGURE 5.6   *Intracardiac Echocardiography*
          A. Tenting of the interatrial septum due to forward pressure from the sheath (arrow) prior to transseptal puncture. **B.** The needle tip (arrow) can be seen in the left atrium following successful transseptal puncture. IAS = interatrial septum; LA = left atrium; RA = right atrium.

initial transseptal puncture. Auxiliary tools such as J-curve needles, laser assistance, and radiofrequency assistance are being designed to assist with such situations. The SafeSept Transseptal Guidewire (Pressure Products, Inc, San Pedro, CA) is a flexible J-curve needle with a 0.014-inch diameter and a length of 120 cm; its design enhances the needle's safety in the left atrium during needle advancement (Figure 5.7). The CLiRpath X-80 (Spectranetics Corporation, Colorado Springs, CO) provides laser assistance at the tip of the needle in order to traverse thickened septums. The Toronto Transseptal Catheter (Baylis Medical Company, Inc, Montreal, Canada) is a radiofrequency transseptal system. In place of the traditional transseptal needle, this system incorporates a sheath with a catheter that delivers radiofrequency energy at the tip, which enables it to cross the septum with less mechanical force.

Summary

Advances in percutaneous ablation techniques for left-sided atrial and ventricular arrhythmias have led to the reemergence and growth of the transseptal puncture. Many technological advances now assist in making the procedure easier and safer. Innovative tools and auxiliary equipment need to be continually designed to help minimize complications and optimize the safety of such procedures.

References

1. Brockenbrough EC, Braunwald E. A new technique for left ventriculography and transseptal left heart catheterization. *Am J Cardiol* 1960;6:1062-1064.

2. Ross J Jr. Transseptal left heart catheterization: a 50-year odyssey. *J Am Coll Cardiol* 2008;51:2107-2115.

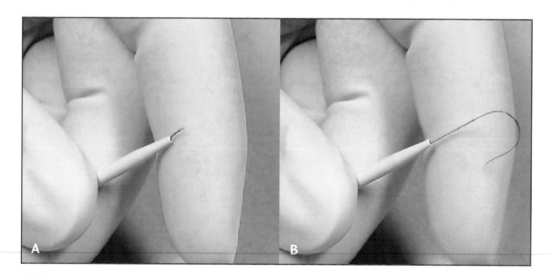

FIGURE 5.7   *J-Curve Transseptal Needle*
A. The needle tip is straight as it emerges from the sheath. **B.** Following deployment of the transseptal needle, the flexible tip conforms to its J shape. Courtesy of Pressure Products Inc.

3. Brockenbrough EC, Braunwald E, Ross J Jr. Transseptal left heart catheterization: a review of 450 studies and description of an improved technic. *Circulation* 1962;25: 15-21.

4. Lundqvist C, Olsson SB, Varnauskas E. Transseptal left heart catheterization: a review of 278 studies. *Clin Cardiol* 1986;9: 21-26.

5. Fagundes RL, Mantica M, De Luca L, et al. Safety of single transseptal puncture for ablation of atrial fibrillation: retrospective study from a large cohort of patients. *J Cardiovasc Electrophysiol* 2007;18:1277-1281.

6. Gonzalez MD, Otomo K, Shah N, et al. Transseptal left heart catheterization for cardiac ablation procedures. *J Interv Card Electrophysiol* 2001;5:89-95.

7. Cheng A, Calkins H. A conservative approach to performing transseptal punctures without the use of intracardiac echocardiography: stepwise approach with real-time video clips. *J Cardiovasc Electrophysiol* 2007;18:686-689.

6

Fluoroscopy-Guided Transseptal Catheterization

Michael M. Shehata, Kalyanam Shivkumar

Transseptal left heart catheterization has reemerged as an important tool in the field of interventional electrophysiology. The technique was originally introduced in 1959 as a strategy to directly measure left atrial (LA) pressure and left ventricular (LV) pressure.[1] It emerged as an alternative to previous techniques for direct LA access, which included the suprasternal approach (a long needle passed retrosternally through the great vessels into the LA), the posterior transthoracic method (a needle passed lateral to the vertebral column into the LA), the transbronchial approach, and the direct puncture of the left ventricle by the subxiphoid (apical approach).[2] The transseptal approach was subsequently modified by Brockenbrough and colleagues,[3] by Gorlin and colleagues,[4] and by Mullins and colleagues.[5]

Today, transseptal left heart puncture is rarely performed for diagnostic purposes, but a rapidly emerging use for catheter-based ablation procedures involving the left atrium and ventricle has made the technique increasingly relevant. The field of interventional electrophysiology currently accounts for the most common context in which transseptal puncture is being performed. This dramatic rise in transseptal procedures has been driven by ablative procedures for atrial fibrillation. Additionally, transseptal puncture is utilized for the ablation of left mitral annular accessory pathway connections, left atrial tachycardias and macro-reentrant flutters, as well as ablation for ventricular tachyarrhythmias involving the left ventricle or left ventricular outflow tract. Transseptal access to the left atrium and ventricle helps to avoid complications inherent to the retrograde transaortic approach, including dislodgment of atheromatous material, dissection of the aortic wall, and potential damage to the aortic valve.

Transseptal Catheterization and Interventions.
© 2010 Ranjan Thakur MD and Andrea Natale MD, eds.
Cardiotext Publishing, ISBN 978-0-9790164-1-7.

While multiple imaging modalities have emerged to assist in safely performing transseptal puncture, a biplanar fluoroscopic-guided technique remains the mainstay of this procedure. The operator must have a detailed familiarity with the regional anatomy of the interatrial septum and the fluoroscopic landmarks that help to define the anatomy. Additionally the operator must have a thorough understanding of the technical aspects of the procedure. (This is aided in the field of electrophysiology by the use of diagnostic electrode catheters that are placed in standard anatomic positions.)

The following material is presented for both the basic and advanced operator in providing guidance for a fluoroscopic approach to transseptal catheterization. Data on cardiac anatomy, the functional anatomy of the heart, fluoroscopic correlations, and imaging studies will be incorporated to provide a framework for the safe performance of this procedure.

Anatomy

The interatrial septum is anatomically complex with several important structures within its immediate vicinity. The left atrium, the aorta, the pericardium, and the ostium of the coronary sinus are structures that are closely related to the medial wall of the right atrium. The fossa ovalis represents the true interatrial portion of the septum. It is bounded anteriorly by the aortic sinus of Valsalva and posteriorly by the pericardium (Figure 6.1). The fossa ovalis also represents the thinnest portion of the interatrial septum.

The plane of the interatrial and interventricular septum can be well appreciated using a left anterior oblique (LAO) view at 30° to 40° via fluoroscopy (Figure 6.2a). The use of the right anterior oblique (RAO) view allows the operator to view the anterior to posterior extent of the fossa ovalis (Figure 6.2b). These standard views provide the optimal orthogonal views of the interatrial septum. While interventional cardiologists typically use an anteroposterior (AP) and lateral fluoroscopic view (Figures 6.3a and 6.3b) with a pigtail catheter placed in the aortic root for imaging during transseptal procedures, the use of orthogonal LAO and RAO views is more anatomic, provides more careful consideration of the boundaries of the fossa ovalis, and can be accomplished without the use of a pigtail catheter placed in the aorta, thus eliminating the need for arterial access.

In the field of cardiac electrophysiology, the positioning of electrode catheters can be used as anatomical landmarks to help define the fossa ovalis. Multipolar electrode catheters are placed from a femoral vein and right internal jugular approach and positioned under fluoroscopic guidance into the right atrial appendage, the His-bundle region, the distal coronary sinus, and the right ventricle. The fluoroscopic angles of the RAO and LAO projections should be selected based on the orientation of the interventricular septum, as determined by the direction of the electrode catheter recording His-bundle activation. The angle of the LAO projection is chosen such that the tip of the His-bundle catheter (and therefore the basal portion of the interventricular septum) is oriented perpendicular to this plane (Figure 6.4). The angle of the RAO projection is then set perpendicular to the LAO plane.[6]

In the RAO projection, the location of the posterior wall of the right atrium can be determined by both the radiopaque border of the atrial wall overlying the radiolucent lung field as well as by the body (proximal portion) of the coronary sinus catheter entering from the right internal jugular or left subclavian approach. The aortic root is indicated by the

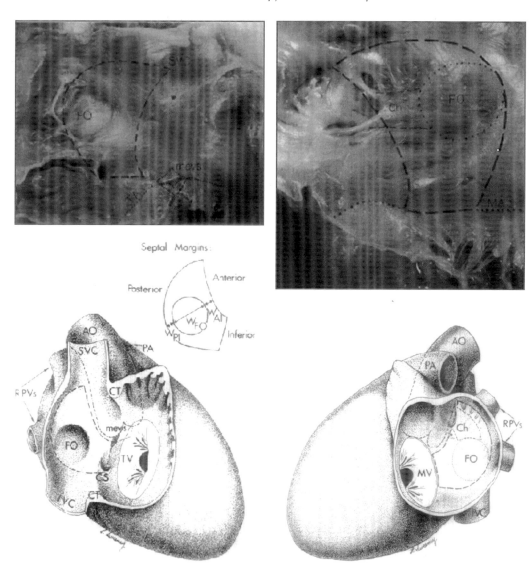

FIGURE 6.1   *Anatomy of the Interatrial Septum*

Anatomic views of the interatrial septum and fossa ovalis from the right and left atrial aspects. Dashed lines in the upper panels demarcate the inferior, anterior, and posterior margins of the fossa ovalis. Sweeney LJ, Rosenquist GC. The normal anatomy of the atrial septum in the human heart. *Am Heart J* Aug 1979;98(2):194-199.

position of the electrodes recording the proximal His-bundle activation (Figure 6.5a). In the LAO projection, the right margin of the aortic root is also indicated by the position of the catheter recording His-bundle activation. The margins of the left atrial free wall are best delineated by the position of the distal poles of the coronary sinus electrode catheter, and the roof of the left atrium by the inferior border of the left main bronchus (Figure 6.5b).

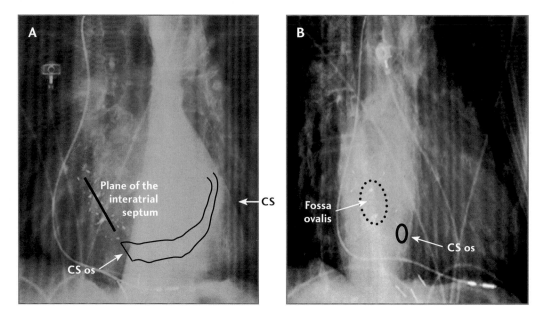

FIGURE 6.2   *Anatomy of the Interatrial Septum, LAO and RAO Fluoroscopic Views*
A. Left anterior oblique (LAO) fluoroscopic view of the interatrial septum. Solid line denotes the plane of the atrial septum overlying a septal occluder device that had been placed in this patient. LAO = 30° **B.** Right anterior oblique (RAO) fluoroscopic view of the interatrial septum. Dashed circle represents the fossa ovalis overlying a septal occluder device. This view helps to define the anterior and posterior extent of the fossa ovalis. CS = coronary sinus.

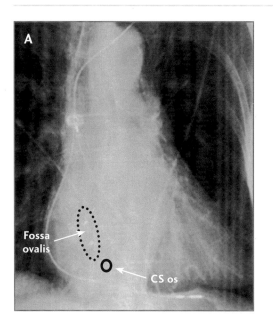
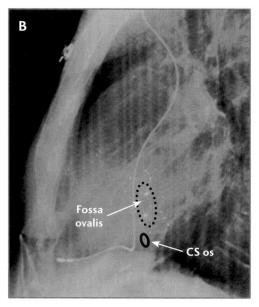

FIGURE 6.3   *Anatomy of the Interatrial Septum, AP and Lateral Views*
A. Anteroposterior fluoroscopic view of the interatrial septum. Dashed oval line demarcates the fossa ovalis. **B.** Lateral fluoroscopic view of the interatrial septum. Dashed oval line demarcates the fossa ovalis. CS = coronary sinus.

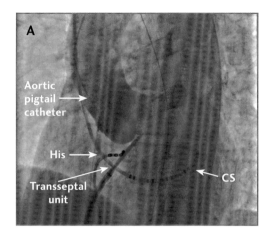

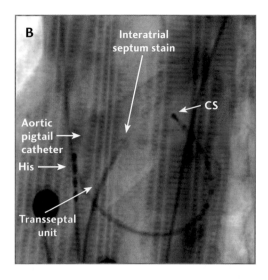

FIGURE 6.4   *Steep LAO and LAO/Lateral Views with Catheters*
A. Left anterior oblique (LAO) fluoroscopic view with aortography outlining the contour of the aortic sinuses. An electrode catheter at the His-bundle position delineates the anterior aspect of the interatrial septum. **B.** Steep LAO fluoroscopic view with aortic pigtail catheter placed in the aortic root. An electrode catheter at the His-bundle position delineates the anterior aspect of the interatrial septum. The transseptal unit is placed at the fossa ovalis with contrast injected to stain the septum. CS = coronary sinus, His = His bundle.

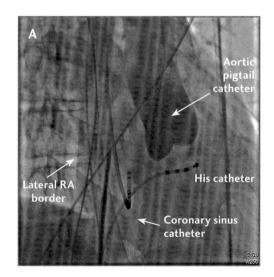

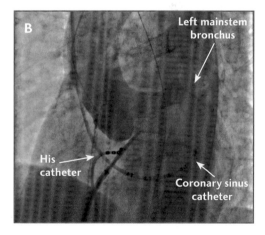

FIGURE 6.5   *RAO and LAO View of Transseptal with Catheters*
A. Right anterior oblique (RAO) fluoroscopic view with aortography to delineate the aortic root. The lateral right atrial wall is seen as a shadow overlying the spine. The right sinus of Valsalva delineates the anterior border of the interatrial septum. **B.** Left anterior oblique (LAO) fluoroscopic view outlining the terminal left main bronchus, which represents the superior border of the left atrium. The electrode catheter at the His-bundle location marks the right anterior aspect of the interatrial septum. CS = coronary sinus, His = His bundle.

Procedure

The optimal fluoroscopic guidance for the transseptal procedure requires the use of biplanar imaging with an AP and lateral tube that allow rotation and iso-centering for a simultaneous RAO and LAO projections. Single plane fluoroscopy can also be used with rotation between the two views during the procedure. For accurate visualization of all anatomic structures, the use of high-resolution fluoroscopy with frame rates of 15 frames per second is recommended over pulsed fluoroscopy during this procedure.

The fluoroscopy tube is first positioned in AP view for introduction of the transseptal sheath system. Under fluoroscopic guidance, an 8 F or 8.5 F transseptal sheath, 62 cm length of varying shape (SL0-SL4 for access to the left atrium or Mullins type for left ventricular access) with a dilator is introduced over a 0.032-inch guidewire to the superior vena cava (SVC) with the tip pointed medially. (The guidewire can then be positioned into the left subclavian vein, and the sheath and dilator advanced over the wire in this location). The patient should be heparinized before starting the transseptal procedure. The guidewire should then be removed, and the dilator aspirated and then flushed with heparinized saline solution.

Next, a Brockenbrough (BRK) transseptal needle with the stylet in a locked position is inserted into the dilator and slowly advanced, allowing free rotation of the needle to accommodate the curvatures of the sheath and dilator system. For the majority of adult cases, a standard BRK or BRK-1 curve-type needle is appropriate. The BRK needle has a pointer on the hub, which orients the operator to the direction of the needle. The use of fluoroscopy as the needle and stylet are advanced toward the distal portion of the dilator allows direct visualization of the needle tip and proper positioning of the tip just inside the distal end of the dilator. Once the needle is in this position, the stylet is then removed from the needle. The needle is then flushed with heparinized saline and attached to a three-way, high-pressure stopcock and pressure transducer. A right atrial pressure waveform should be recorded. Using a high-pressure stopcock allows the stopcock to move freely without rotating the needle. Next, a 10-cc Leur lock syringe filled with radiopaque contrast is then attached to the perpendicular port on the stopcock and any visible air bubbles are carefully aspirated back into the syringe. The needle is then forward filled with a small amount of contrast solution (1-2 cc) under fluoroscopy.

At this time, the pointer hub of the transseptal needle will be directed anteriorly at 12 o'clock, pointing toward the sternum. Using the LAO fluoroscopic view with an angle that has been previously set according to a septal location via the His-bundle electrode catheter, the sheath, dilator, and needle are then slowly withdrawn caudally as a single unit with clockwise rotation as continuous right atrial pressure monitoring is performed. The proper orientation of the pointer hub can vary substantially among patients based on variations in septal anatomy; however, a position from 2 o'clock through 5 o'clock is generally required to maintain the needle perpendicular to the fossa ovalis. Positioning based on fluoroscopic anatomical landmarks and the location of electrode catheters is considered most accurate. During the transseptal drag, one hand should be used to hold the sheath and dilator and the other to hold the needle in a fixed relationship to avoid inadvertent advancement of the needle. The contrast syringe can be allowed to rest on the hypothenar eminence of the right thumb.

Care must be taken to observe the levels of the left main bronchus, the His-bundle catheter, and the coronary sinus catheter. As the unit is dragged toward the junction of the SVC and right atrium, it is in contact with the ascending aorta. As the unit is pulled further caudally and moves posteriorly away from the aorta, the tip will demonstrate a pronounced jump leftward (medially) in the LAO projection (Figure 6.6). With slightly more withdrawal of the unit, a second jump may be notable further leftward as the tip of the unit falls below the superior limbus and engages in the fossa ovalis. In the LAO projection, the dilator tip, which is properly engaged in the fossa ovalis, will be located at or below the level of the His-bundle catheter and leftward behind the aorta, superior to the coronary sinus catheter and well below the left bronchus.

In the RAO projection, the tip of the dilator should be positioned approximately midway between the lateral right atrial border silhouette and the proximal electrodes of the His-bundle catheter (Figure 6.7). There should be no exaggerated curve of the dilator tip in this view, and the tip should appear to be moving into the screen. The coronary sinus catheter will appear foreshortened in this view, and the transseptal assembly should parallel the electrodes of this catheter, which also delineates the atrioventricular groove. The level of the dilator tip should be at the same level or slightly higher than the electrodes recording proximal His-bundle activation and well superior to the coronary sinus ostium. If one chooses to use a pigtail catheter placed within the aortic root as a landmark, ensure that the needle tip is below and rightward of the aorta between the pigtail and the vertebral column.

At this point, with the dilator tip properly engaged in the fossa ovalis, attention is turned toward crossing the interatrial septum with the transseptal needle. With the needle just inside the dilator tip, contrast media from

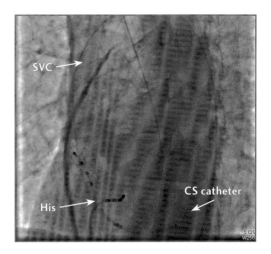

FIGURE 6.6   *LAO View with Sheath in SVC*

The transseptal sheath unit being dragged inferiorly demonstrates a "jump" medially in the left anterior oblique (LAO) projection as it moves posteriorly away from the ascending aorta. (CS = coronary sinus; His = His bundle; SVC = superior vena cava.

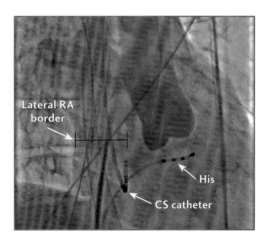

FIGURE 6.7   *RAO View with Aortogram (50% Distance Between CS and Lateral RA Border)*

The transseptal sheath unit is positioned at the fossa ovalis approximately midway between the lateral right atrial (RA) border and the coronary sinus (CS) catheter. Aortography demonstrates that the sheath is directed relatively posteriorly towards the fossa ovalis and away from the aortic root. His = His bundle.

the attached syringe can be injected in order to stain the septum. Care must be taken not to lose the orientation of the assembly during this time. Next, observe the movement of the structure that has been stained, as the interatrial septum will move in the transverse plane in the LAO projection and appear tented. The aorta will move in the long axis, perpendicular to the interatrial septum. However, anatomic distortions, the body habitus of the patient, and the imaging capabilities of the fluoroscopy system may preclude these interpretations.

Once the proper position of the needle tip within the fossa ovalis has been confirmed, the needle should be advanced across the septum and into the left atrium under continuous pressure monitoring and continuous fluoroscopy in the LAO projection. If there is any resistance to needle advancement, reevaluate all landmarks, as the needle may be positioned at the limbus. It is crucial to remember that the fossa ovalis is the only true interatrial portion of the septum. If the needle is positioned anterior to the limbus, it may cross into the aorta; if positioned posterior to the fossa, it may enter into the pericardial space. Entrance into the left atrium is confirmed when the pressure tracing shows a left atrial waveform with accentuated X and Y dips. Confirmation of entry into the left atrium can be aided by injection of a small amount of radiopaque contrast medium to opacify the left atrial cavity. If contrast medium enters into the pericardial space instead of into the left atrium it will create a thin outline of the heart and enter the transverse sinus. If the contrast enters the aorta, contrast will be seen briskly flowing from an inferior to a superior direction. If pericardial exit or aortic entry occurs with the needle, do not advance the dilator over the needle. The needle should be immediately withdrawn, and the patient should be

monitored closely to assess for any hemodynamic consequences.

Difficulty in attempting to cross the interatrial septum with the needle can be encountered in certain cases. These include patients undergoing repeat transseptal access, patients with cardiac surgical repair involving the interatrial septum, or patients with anatomic variants, including lipomatous or aneurysmal interatrial septal aneurysms. To overcome these challenges, a technique using radiofrequency energy, via an electrocautery needle, applied directly to the needle hub, can assist with needle delivery.[7]

The next major step is to advance the sheath-dilator assembly across the interatrial septum over the fixed needle. Once the proper needle entry into the left atrium has been confirmed, and with the needle in a fixed position, gently advance the sheath-dilator assembly. Remember that the interatrial atrial septum is moving back on the dilator while the dilator is advancing. The tenting depth is already the distance the dilator has moved into the left atrium. Therefore, all that is required is a small movement to advance the dilator across the septum (Figure 6.8). The interatrial septum will move inferiorly and to the patient's right side as the dilator passes into the left atrium. When the interatrial septum stops moving, the dilator is approximately in the midpoint of the left atrium.

The next major step in the transseptal procedure is to advance the sheath over the fixed dilator and needle into the left atrium. The needle should be withdrawn back into the dilator so that it is just within the tip. At this point the needle and dilator should still be across the septum. With the dilator now in a fixed position, the sheath should be advanced over the dilator and needle into the left atrium. The transseptal assembly should not get close to the posterior wall or to the superior portion of the left atrium as delineated by the terminal portion of the left main bronchus.

The last major step is the removal of the transseptal needle and dilator from the sheath. First, the needle should be withdrawn from the dilator; then a syringe should be immediately attached to the hub of the dilator, and blood should be withdrawn. The aspirated blood should appear bright red, as it is arterial blood. Continuous aspiration of blood back into the syringe as the dilator is being withdrawn from the sheath is an important step to avoid entrapment of air into the sheath and potential air embolism. Next, aspirate blood through the side arm of the sheath, and then flush it with care using heparinized saline to avoid air bubbles. Once successful transseptal catheterization is con-

firmed and the patient's vital signs are stable, anticoagulation can be initiated with intravenous heparin to maintain activated clotting times in the desirable range. The sidearm of the sheath should be attached to continuous flush at a low flow rate with heparinized saline throughout the procedure.

If a second transseptal sheath is required for the procedure, such as may be necessary in pulmonary vein isolation procedures, a separate transseptal puncture can be performed with the same steps as outlined. An alternative approach to avoid damaging the existing transseptal sheath can also be performed. Through the existing transseptal sheath, advance a Toray wire length (Toray Industries, Inc, Tokyo, Japan) under fluoroscopic guidance into the left atrium (Figure 6.9), and

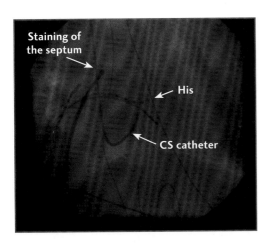

FIGURE 6.8   *Staining of the Interatrial Septum Prior to Needle Deployment (RAO View)*

Right anterior oblique (RAO) view of the transseptal unit with contrast administered through the needle to stain the interatrial septum prior to deployment of the needle. The stained septum can appear tented as the needle crosses into the left atrium. CS = coronary sinus; His = His bundle.

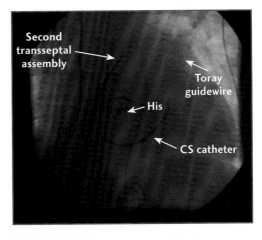

FIGURE 6.9   *LAO View with Toray Wire in Place for Second Transseptal Puncture*

A Toray guidewire has been placed in the left atrium through an initial transseptal puncture. A second transseptal assembly is positioned at the interatrial septum, and the needle is shown crossing into the left atrium in a left anterior oblique (LAO) fluoroscopic view. Use of the Toray guidewire may help minimize any trauma to the left atrium and/or the first transseptal sheath assembly as the second puncture is performed. CS = coronary sinus; His = His bundle.

retain it as a guidewire. Because of its shape, this wire minimizes any potential trauma to the left atrium. The sheath is then brought back into the right atrium, and a second transseptal puncture is performed with the same previous steps. Once the second transseptal sheath has been placed into the left atrium, the first sheath can be advanced over the retained Toray guidewire and the transseptal dilator under fluoroscopic guidance.

Conclusions

Knowledge of fluoroscopic transseptal catheterization is essential for safe transseptal catheterization. This is even more relevant as overreliance on imaging alone can sometimes be detrimental and also leaves the operator at a significant disadvantage when dealing with situations where there is no echo imaging support, such as due to equipment failure or lack of venous access. Fluoroscopic transseptal catheterization can be performed safely, and it nicely complements other strategies that are used for transseptal access.

References

1. Ross J Jr, Braunwald E, Morrow AG. Transseptal left atrial puncture: a new technique for the measurement of left atrial pressure in man. *Am J Cardiol* 1959;3(5):653-655.

2. Morrow AG, Braunwald E, Ross J Jr. Left heart catheterization: an appraisal of techniques and their applications in cardiovascular diagnosis. *Arch Intern Med* 1960;105:645-655.

3. Braunwald E, Brockenbrough EC, Talbert JL, et al. Selective left heart angiocardiography by the transseptal route. *Am J Med* 1962;33:213-222.

4. Gorlin R, Krasnow N, Levine HJ, et al. A modification of the technic of transseptal left heart catheterization. *Am J Cardiol* 1961;7:580.

5. Mullins CE. Transseptal left heart catheterization: experience with a new technique in 520 pediatric and adult patients. *Pediatr Cardiol* 1983;4(3):239-245.

6. Gonzalez MD, Otomo K, Shah N, et al. Transseptal left heart catheterization for cardiac ablation procedures. *J Interv Card Electrophysiol* 2001;5(1):89-95.

7. Bidart C, Vaseghi M, Cesario DA, et al. Radiofrequency current delivery via transseptal needle to facilitate septal puncture. *Heart Rhythm* 2007;4(12):1573-1576.

7

Transseptal Catheterization Guided by Transthoracic and Transesophageal Echocardiography

Matthew P. Smelley, Bradley P. Knight

Since the introduction of transseptal puncture and catheterization (TSP) in 1959,[1-7] the technique has evolved from a means of directly measuring left-sided cardiac pressures to a means of providing therapy for left-sided arrhythmias and mitral valve disease. Transseptal catheterization, however, is associated with a small risk of complications, and is not successful in every case. One review of 1279 transseptal punctures at a single center documented a success rate of 90% with a major complication rate of 1.3%, including cardiac tamponade (1.2%), systemic embolization (0.08%), and aortic perforation (0.08%).[8] A second single-center experience of 278 procedures listed an overall success rate of 91% with a complication rate of 1.1% for aortic perforation, 3.2% for systemic embolization, and 0.7% for tamponade.[9] In terms of short- and long-term outcomes up to 18 months, there was no difference among transseptal procedures performed for the diagnosis of valvular heart disease, catheter ablation of arrhythmias, and mitral valvuloplasty. Patients undergoing valvuloplasty had a higher chance of a residual atrial septal defect, but this occurrence did not affect long-term prognosis.[10] These three studies used fluoroscopic landmarks alone and not echocardiography to perform the transseptal puncture.

In skilled hands, TSP can be performed successfully using only fluoroscopic landmarks for guidance. However, congenital and acquired anatomic variations and the potential for life-threatening complications has led to a demand for methods of directly visualizing the interatrial septum to improve the success rate in all cases and to avoid the chance of an unwanted event. Transthoracic (TTE), transesophageal (TEE), and intracardiac echocardiography (ICE) have been used to provide additional imaging during TSP.

Transseptal Catheterization and Interventions.
© 2010 Ranjan Thakur MD and Andrea Natale MD, eds.
Cardiotext Publishing, ISBN 978-0-9790164-1-7.

ICE catheterization provides direct visualization of the interatrial septum during TSP,[11-14] but the universal use of an ICE catheter is problematic due to the high cost of the equipment and the need for technical training. With these limitations in mind, there remains a role for TTE and TEE guidance. This chapter will focus on the use of TTE and TEE for transseptal puncture. Specific references to 3-D TEE imaging will be made. The use of ICE is discussed in chapter 8.

Anatomy Pertinent to Transseptal Catheterization

The safest place to gain access to the left atrium (LA) from the right atrium (RA) is through the fossa ovalis (FO). The FO is found in the posterior interatrial septum, and is surrounded by a muscular limbus. The anatomy of the FO and the immediate surrounding cardiac structures can vary based on congenital and acquired heart disease.

A patent foramen ovale (PFO) (Figure 7.1) can be found in the range of 25% to 30% of patients and allows direct access to the left atrium.[15-17] During an autopsy study of 965 normal hearts, a PFO was found in 27% of patients. The incidence and size of the PFO did not vary significantly between genders. However, the incidence progressively declined with age, while the size of the PFO increased with age from a mean of 3.4 mm in the first decade of life to 5.8 mm in the tenth decade of life.[15]

Atrial septal aneurysms are typically defined as an oscillating aneurysmal dilatation of the septum with at least 10 mm to 15 mm of movement into either atrium during the cardiorespiratory cycle.[16,17] The prevalence of these aneurysms varies depending upon the study technique, from 1% at autopsy,[18] 0.22% to 4.0% with echocardiography,[16,17,19,20] and 4.9% during cardiac surgery.[21] The presence of an aneurysm increases the risk of LA wall perforation during TSP,[22] and, therefore, should be noted when using echocardiography at the beginning of the procedure. In diseased hearts, the normal anatomy can be distorted, potentially leading to an increased rate of complications if fluoroscopic landmarks are used alone. Patients with a dilated aortic root, an enlarged atria, prior cardiac surgery, or kyphoscoliosis may have a dysmorphic FO.

Echocardiography has the advantage over radiographic imaging by being able to image the soft tissue variations described for both congenital and acquired heart disease. Direct visualization of the FO provides reassurance to the operator, and may be associated with a reduction in the risk of complications, especially in patients with altered atrial anatomy.

Technique for Transseptal Puncture Using Supplemental Echocardiographic Guidance

In our laboratory, the majority of transseptal catheterizations are for LA ablation procedures, usually atrial fibrillation. These procedures are typically performed using intravenous sedation. For this reason, in our lab ICE is used more often than TEE to guide the procedure. However, endotracheal intubation and general anesthesia is occasionally necessary for patients who are obese, have a high-risk airway for sedation, have a history of being difficult to sedate, or request complete amnesia for the procedure. When gen-

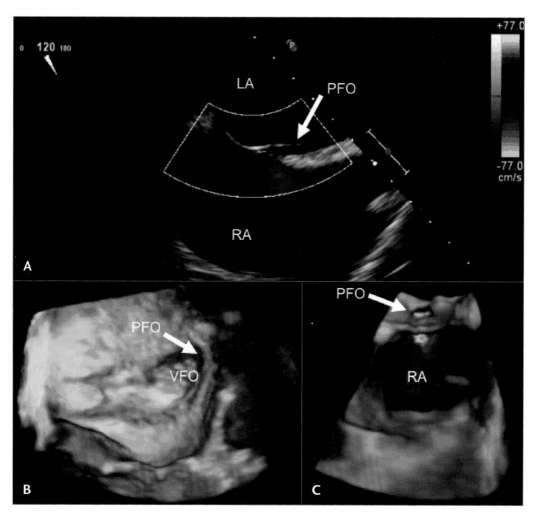

FIGURE 7.1   *TEE Views of a PFO*

In panel **A**, the transesophageal echocardiography (TEE) probe is positioned behind the left atrium and adjusted to obtain a bicaval view. A patent foramen ovale (PFO) can often be visualized using 2-D imaging alone with color Doppler, but sometimes it requires the injection of agitated saline timed with a Valsalva maneuver to open the PFO and demonstrate the interatrial communication. In this case, using color Doppler alone (arrow), flow can be seen crossing the PFO. Panel **B** shows a 3-D TEE image of a PFO demonstrating a communication between the left and right atria (arrow). The muscular limbus surrounds the flap-like valve of the fossa ovalis (VFO). In panel **C**, color Doppler during a 3-D TEE shows flow across the PFO into the right atrium. LA = left atrium; PFO = patent foramen ovale; RA = right atrium; VFO = valve of fossa ovalis.

eral anesthesia is used, the procedure can be guided easily by TEE. With TEE guidance, the esophagus is intubated after anesthesia is induced, and the TEE probe is advanced into position behind the LA.

Ultrasound techniques supplement, but do not substitute for, standard fluoroscopic techniques. It is recommended that the physician follow standard methods and use ultrasound to confirm that the transseptal apparatus is properly positioned before puncturing the septum. Also, a survey of the cardiac anatomy should be performed using echocardiography to confirm the orientation of the septum in relationship to the aorta and posterior wall of the atria.

When the TSP is performed during an electrophysiology procedure, a His-bundle and coronary sinus (CS) catheter can be used to provide additional fluoroscopic landmarks and help make adjustments to the angulation of the left anterior oblique (LAO) and right anterior oblique (RAO) cameras. A quadripolar catheter positioned correctly over the His bundle can also approximate the noncoronary cusp of the aortic valve. It is this cusp of the aorta that is adjacent to the interatrial septum (Figure 7.2). A CS catheter can help define on fluoroscopy where the atrioventricular groove is located and mark the posterior-inferior border of the atrium. If the atrial and ventricular electrograms on the CS catheter are of similar size, then the catheter is within the body of the CS and not in a ventricular branch. The CS catheter then approximates the posterior left atrium and mitral valve.

In the LAO view, the His-bundle catheter should be pointed directly at the image intensifier along the septum. In the RAO view, the CS catheter is perpendicular to the image. In one study, the use of this RAO technique with a pigtail catheter in the aorta demonstrated a transseptal puncture success rate of 99% with a nonfatal complication rate of 2.8%.[23] This success rate is considerably higher than the 90% to 91% success rates previously described using fluoroscopic landmarks alone.[8,9] However, when using ultrasound to guide TSP, placement of a catheter in the aorta as a landmark is probably not necessary, and is not done in our laboratory.

The physician should be familiar with the transseptal apparatus. Various transseptal introducers combine different sheath lengths with their dilators. The typical Brockenbrough needle is 71 cm in length with an arrow at the hub that points in the direction of the curve of the needle tip. Before starting the case, this relationship should be confirmed, and the needle should be advanced into the dilator. The needle flange and sidearm of the sheath should always have the same orientation. When the needle tip is withdrawn just into the dilator tip, there is usually a space between the dilator hub and needle flange of roughly 2 cm, or 2 fingerbreadths.

Many transseptal sheaths and dilators are available. The choice depends on the clinical circumstances, the desire to have or not to have a soft tip at the end of the sheath, and the operator's familiarity with the system. After right femoral venous access is obtained, a 0.032-inch J wire should be positioned in the superior vena cava under fluoroscopic guidance. Over the J wire, the sheath and dilator should be advanced into the superior vena cava or left innominate vein. Care must be taken to always advance the apparatus over the wire to avoid perforation.[24-26] Once in the superior vena cava, the J wire is removed, and the needle and stylet are advanced within 1 cm to 2 cm of the tip of the dilator. Next, the stylet is removed and the needle is flushed. In most patients, the transseptal punctures can be performed with a standard Brockenbrough needle. In patients with an enlarged RA, the needle can be bent to increase the radius of the curve to reach the atrial septum, or a different needle type with an increased curve radius can be used (ie, BRK-1 and BRK-2).

A manifold system can be useful during TSP. It typically has 4 ports: the pressure transducer, contrast reservoir, saline reservoir, and waste. The pressure waveform should be calibrated and scrutinized for accuracy. Through the needle, contrast can be injected to confirm the location of the dilator within the SVC. Using TEE or TTE, a stable probe

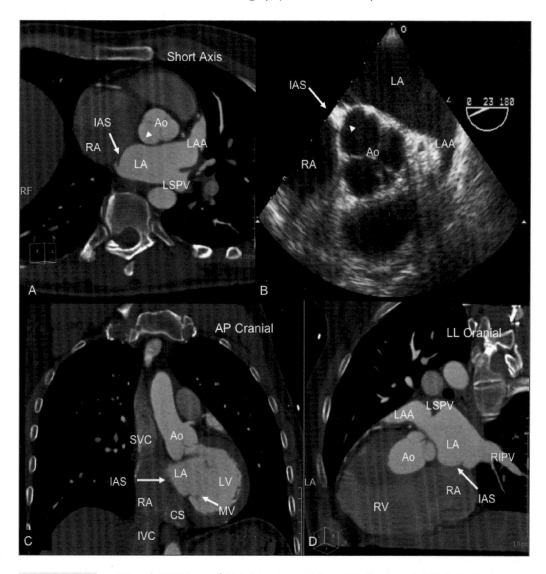

FIGURE 7.2   *CT and TEE Views of Atrial Anatomy Relevant to Transseptal Catheterization*

In panel **A**, a short axis computed tomography (CT) scan shows the relationship between the interatrial septum and the aorta and posterior pericardium. Notice the anterior location of the left atrial appendage. The arrowhead in this picture and in panel B points to the location of the noncoronary cusp of the aorta that is adjacent to the interatrial septum. A catheter in the His-bundle position approximates this location. In panel **B**, a short axis transesophageal echocardiography (TEE) image displays the proximity of the aorta to the left atrial appendage and interatrial septum. In panel **C**, an anterior-posterior and cranial CT scan demonstrates the anterior location of the aorta and the inferior location of the coronary sinus. In panel **D**, a left lateral CT scan shows the relationship between the interatrial septum, left atrial appendage, aorta, and pulmonary veins. Ao = aorta; CS = coronary sinus; IAS = interatrial septum; IVC = inferior vena cava; LA = left atrium; LAA = left atrial appendage; LSPV = left superior pulmonary vein; MV = mitral valve; RA = right atrium; RIPV = right inferior pulmonary vein; SVC = superior vena cava.

position should be obtained where imaging of the interatrial septum is optimal. When using TEE, a bicaval view is typically used during the transseptal puncture. When using surface echocardiography, an apical four chamber or subcostal view may provide the best images.

The transseptal apparatus should be withdrawn from the SVC into the RA as a single unit with care taken not to change the distance between the flange and dilator hub. Inadvertent punctures can occur if the needle is exposed. The curve of the needle should be oriented between the 3 o'clock to 5 o'clock position as viewed from the patient's feet, so that the tip is pointed leftward and slightly posterior. This orientation should allow the apparatus to fall into the FO and avoid the aorta. As the apparatus is withdrawn, the assembly will move slightly leftward in the LAO view as the tip crosses from the SVC into the RA. A second leftward hop may occur as the tip crosses the aortic knob, followed by a third leftward movement as the tip crosses the superior limbus into the FO (Figure 7.3). In the RAO view, the position of the tip of the apparatus should be posterior, well away from the aorta. The tip should also be pointed parallel to the CS catheter, a position that helps ensure the catheter is not pointed too posteriorly, which could result in inadvertent perforation of the posterior LA. Rotating the arrow of the transseptal needle between 3 o'clock and 5 o'clock will move the catheter from an anterior to posterior position.

At this stage, the TEE or TTE probe should be used to confirm proper positioning of the assembly and to optimize the location of the dilator tip just before puncturing the septum. When the tip of the dilator is properly positioned, it can be visualized within the FO tenting the membrane (Figure 7.4). The echocardiography probe can be manipulated to confirm the location of the tip relative to the aorta and the posterior wall of the left atrium.

The transseptal needle is then slowly advanced out of the sheath against the septum (Figure 7.4 and 7.5). Care should be taken during this step to avoid advancing the assembly superior to the fossa. Echocardiography can be used as the needle is advanced to confirm that it is embedded in the fossa rather than riding up the right side of the septum. This may not be detectable radiographically. The needle is then advanced beyond the dilator tip. If the needle does not puncture the septum, the entire transseptal apparatus should be advanced to add increased stiffness to the assembly and to help push the needle through the membrane. Successful puncture of the fossa can usually be felt through the hub of the needle as a pop or release of pressure.

Several methods can be used to confirm that the tip of the needle has entered the LA. Pressure measurements should be consistent with LA hemodynamics, and injection of contrast through the needle tip will result in opacification of the LA on fluoroscopy. Although not always a reliable indicator, the aspiration of fluid from the left atrium should have the appearance of bright red, oxygenated arterial blood. Before the dilator is advanced over the needle, echocardiography can be used to demonstrate that the needle is within the body of the LA, that the tenting of the fossa has resolved, and that contrast injection results in the appearance of microbubbles in the LA. After the dilator is advanced over the needle, echocardiography can be used to reconfirm that the dilator tip is freely moving within the body of the LA. At this stage, the sheath can be advanced over the dilator, or the needle can be replaced with a guidewire positioned in the LA or pulmonary vein to provide a rail over which the sheath can be safely advanced over the dilator. The guidewire can usually be seen on echocardiography

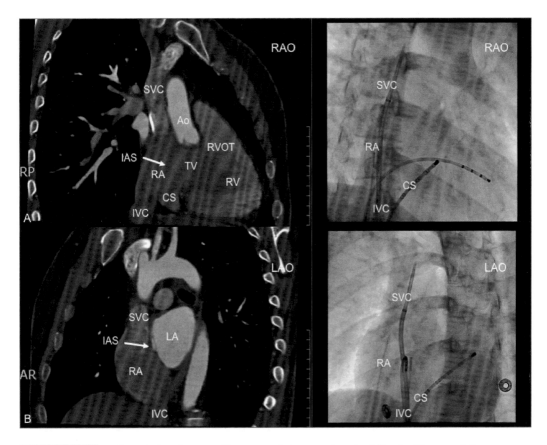

FIGURE 7.3   *Correlation Between Fluoroscopic Images Acquired During Transseptal Catheterization and CT Images to Demonstrate Atrial Anatomy Pertinent to Transseptal Catheterization*

Panel **A** shows a computed tomography (CT) and right anterior oblique (RAO) fluoroscopic view of the heart. In this fluoroscopic view, notice the position of the transseptal sheath in the superior vena cava (SVC). As the sheath is pulled down into the right atrium, there are typically 3 separate locations where the tip of the apparatus will move leftward. The first transition is from the SVC to the right atrium, the second is at the level of the aortic knob, and the third is into the fossa ovalis. In this view, the apparatus should be directed posteriorly toward the left atrium away from the anteriorly located aorta. Panel **B** shows a CT and left anterior oblique (LAO) fluoroscopic view of the heart. In this view, the transseptal apparatus should be directed to the patient's left in the direction of the left atrium. Ao = Aorta; AP = anterior posterior; CS = coronary sinus; IAS = interatrial septum; IVC = inferior vena cava; LA = left atrium; LAO = left anterior oblique, RA = right atrium; RAO = right anterior oblique; RV = right ventricle; RVOT = right ventricular outflow tract; SVC = superior vena cava; TV = tricuspid valve.

to confirm that, as the sheath is advanced into the LA, the wire remains in a stable position. The sheath should be aspirated to remove any bubbles and flushed with heparinized saline.

Occasionally, as the tip of the needle is advanced, the pressure will dampen. If contrast is injected at this point, there may be staining of the interatrial septum. This staining is a sign that the needle should be advanced further, provided that the location of the needle is still within the FO as seen on echocardiography. If the needle cannot

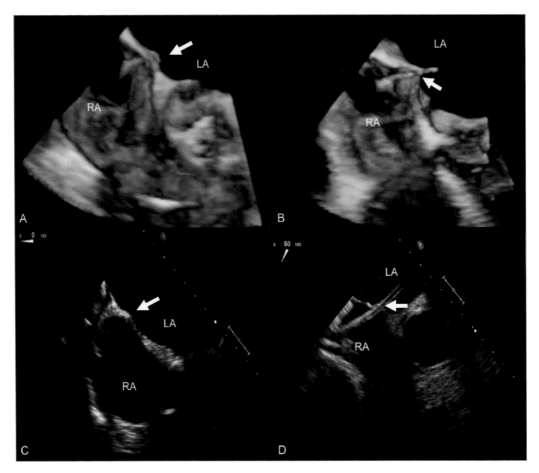

FIGURE 7.4   *2-D and 3-D TEE Images Acquired During Transseptal Catheterization*
        Panel **A** shows a 3-D TEE view of the interatrial septum showing tenting (arrow) of the
fossa ovalis from the transseptal apparatus. Panel **B** shows a 3-D TEE view after puncture of the interatrial
septum within the fossa ovalis (arrow). In panel **C**, using 2-D TEE imaging, the transseptal apparatus is shown
tenting the muscular portion of the interatrial septum. The apparatus was gradually moved more inferiorly into
the foramen ovale before puncture. In panel **D**, a 2-D TEE image from the same patient as panel C shows the
transseptal apparatus crossing the interatrial septum at the level of the fossa ovalis. LA = left atrium;
RA = right atrium.

be advanced into the LA, then the needle should be retracted, and the process should be repeated. The needle should be removed, and the guidewire should be repositioned through the sheath and dilator into the SVC for a second attempt. If an aortic pressure is transduced, or if there is staining of the aorta or pericardium, the needle should be promptly removed and the patient evaluated for hemodynamic compromise. The dilator

should never be advanced in this circumstance. It is rare for the needle to cause significant cardiac damage alone, but if the dilator is advanced over a needle that is not in proper position, then severe trauma can occur.

After successful TSP, the TEE or surface echo probe can continue to be used to guide the remainder of the procedure, if desired. When using TEE to guide an ablation procedure for atrial fibrillation, an

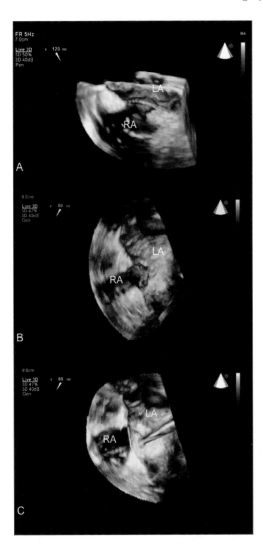

important consideration is to avoid movement of the esophagus with the TEE probe to a location near the ablation catheter. Radiofrequency ablation of the LA in close proximity to the esophagus can result in a LA-esophageal fistula.

Experience Using Surface Echocardiography to Guide Transseptal Puncture

Transthoracic echocardiography has been used to visualize the FO to guide TSP. In a series of 13 patients, the investigators showed that on the short-axis and four-chamber views, the interatrial septum could be demarcated from the ascending aorta. They described tenting of the septum when the apparatus was in the FO, and injected saline to document the location of the needle tip in the left and right atrium. The authors suggested that TTE was additive to fluoroscopic imaging alone, and they felt it may reduce complications and improve efficacy.[27]

In a prospective study of 56 patients, the utility of TTE as an aid to TSP was evaluated. In 720 transseptal cases without echocardiography guidance, the authors reported 5 inadvertent punctures of the aorta or atrial wall resulting in 2 deaths and 2 cases of cardiac tamponade. The transseptal apparatus

FIGURE 7.5   *3-D TEE Images Acquired During Double Transseptal Catheterization*

Panels **A**, **B** and **C** show 3 transesophageal echocardiography (TEE) images acquired sequentially in the same patient. Panel A shows the fossa ovalis separating the left (LA) and right atrium (RA) before manipulation. Panel **B** shows successful puncture of the intraatrial septum at the level of the fossa ovalis. After the dilator was advanced slightly across the septum, the needle was replaced by a guidewire, and the septum was dilated. The transseptal apparatus was pulled back into the right atrium, leaving only the guidewire across the septum. A steerable electrophysiology ablation catheter was then guided through the transseptal puncture site next to the wire. The transseptal sheath was then advanced over the wire so that both the transseptal sheath and the ablation catheter were positioned in the LA across a single puncture site. The shaft of the ablation catheter and the body of the sheath can both be seen crossing the septum next to each other in panel **C**.

was positioned under fluoroscopic guidance in the FO, and with gentle pressure if the dilator crossed into the LA, then the patient most likely had a PFO. This type of crossing occurred in 43% of patients, and in all of these cases, TTE showed that the catheter was in the region of the FO. If any difficulty was met with advancing the dilator, then TTE was used to guide the puncture. The interesting finding was that in 48% of these patients, the transseptal apparatus was not within the FO and required repositioning.[28]

Another study of 75 patients with symptomatic rheumatic mitral stenosis in India showed that balloon mitral valvuloplasty was safe and feasible using TTE guidance alone in most cases. The puncture was performed by using firm pressure, noting entry into the LA by injecting saline contrast, and then observing the change in pressure waveform. TEE was required in 3 patients, and fluoroscopy was required to complete the procedure in 4 cases. The study's authors stated that TTE was helpful in reducing the risk of entry into the LA transpericardially through the RA wall. They also felt that TEE helped to correctly position the needle within the FO, resulting in easier manipulation of the catheters in the LA.[29] Using TEE guidance alone, the same group has also published a case report of performing a mitral commissurotomy in a critically ill patient.[30] They have also successfully performed TSPs for percutaneous mitral valve commissurotomy in pregnant patients.[29]

TTE is limited by occasional suboptimal visualization of the atrial septum and FO, superimposition of catheter and TEE probe images on fluoroscopy, the problem of acquiring images in a sterile environment, and inadequate acoustic windows.[31] TTE has largely been supplanted by TEE and ICE, but is an option when only a surface probe is available.

Experience Using TEE to Guide Transseptal Puncture

The potential for TEE to guide TSP was demonstrated in the early 1990s. The rationale for using TEE rather than TTE, was to more reliably visualize the interatrial septum secondary to better acoustic windows[31] and to obtain images without disrupting the surgical field. In a series of 4 patients presenting for mitral balloon commissurotomy, the investigators demonstrated that TEE could be used to visualize the FO and the transseptal apparatus and to help ensure that the needle puncture was performed within the FO. In patients with an enlarged LA, TEE was able to reproducibly identify the FO, whereas fluoroscopy was less reliable. Another advantage of using TEE during these cases was the immediate assessment of valvular function during the procedure.[31] Two other studies from the same year demonstrated similar benefits of TEE over TTE. The main advantages were the proper positioning of catheters, early recognition of complications, and the assessment of LA clot and mitral regurgitation.[32,33]

A second, larger study evaluating the utility of TEE in percutaneous mitral valvuloplasty in 35 consecutive patients demonstrated that TEE was helpful in guiding the transseptal puncture, aided in balloon localization, and tended to decrease the frequency of significant mitral regurgitation. In a subsequent study of 46 transseptal catheterizations guided by TEE for ablation of left-sided pathways in patients with normal-sized atria, the investigators had only 1 complication of cardiac perforation and tamponade (2.2%).[34] With these early studies, the efficacy and safety of TEE to guide transseptal catheterization was established. TEE not only facilitates TSP, but can also be used to exclude LA thrombus, to guide the intervention, and to monitor for complications during the procedure.

Three-dimensional techniques have recently been incorporated into TEE imaging. A TEE probe that is currently available commercially is capable of both 2-D and 3-D imaging (X7-2t TEE probe, Philips Healthcare, Andover, MA). The use of 3-D TEE during transseptal puncture is still in the investigational stages, and whether or not the 3-D images improve safety or efficacy is unknown. However, the 3-D TEE probe does create images that are useful and easy to interpret. The images lack the resolution of cardiac CT or MRI, but they do give an impression of depth and perspective, which adds another dimension to localizing the transseptal apparatus in more than one plane (Figures 7.1, 7.4, 7.5). Case reports have been published that demonstrate the effectiveness of performing transseptal catheterization with 3-D TEE imaging.[35-37]

Summary

The goal of transseptal catheterization is to safely gain access to the left atrium to address the clinical issue confronting the patient while minimizing or negating the risk of any unwanted complications. Although complications are relatively uncommon, it is the potential for a life-threatening incident that has led to the incorporation of echocardiography as a routine component of this procedure. This imaging modality allows for the direct visualization of the transseptal needle within the FO in relation to the immediate surrounding cardiac structures, particularly the aorta and posterior wall of the LA. Although each has its limitations, TTE, TEE, and 3-D TEE can all be successfully implemented to guide TSP. Using echocardiography to define the patient's anatomy, especially in patients with congenital or acquired heart disease, is a powerful adjunct to fluoroscopic guidance alone.

References

1. Ross J, Braunwald E, Morrow AG. Transseptal left atrial puncture: a new technique for the measurement of left atrial pressure in man. *Am J Cardiol* 1959;3:653-655.

2. Cope C. Technique for the transseptal catheterization of the left atrium: preliminary report. *J Thorac Surg* 1959;37:482-486.

3. Brockenbrough E, Braunwald E. A new technique for left ventricular angiography and transseptal left heart catheterization. *Am J Cardiol* 1960;6:219-231.

4. Brockenbrough EC, Braunwald E, Ross J Jr. Transseptal left heart catheterization: a review of 450 studies and description of an improved technique. *Circulation* 1962; 25:15-21.

5. Braunwald E. Transseptal left heart catheterization. *Circulation* 1968;37(suppl 3):74-79.

6. Mullins CE. Transseptal left heart catheterization: experience with a new technique in 520 pediatric and adult patients. *Pediatr Cardiol* 1983;4:239-245.

7. Inoue K, Owaki T, Nakamura T, et al. Clinical application of transvenous mitral commissurotomy by a new balloon catheter. *J Thorac Cardiovasc Surg* 1984;87:394-402.

8. Roelke M, Smith AJ, Palacios IF. The technique and safety of transseptal left heart catheterization: the Massachusetts General Hospital experience with 1,279 procedures. *Cathet Cardiovasc Diagn* 1994;32:332-339.

9. Blomstrom-Lundqvist C, Olsson S, Varnauskas E. Transseptal left heart catheterization: a review of 278 studies. *Clin Cardiol* 1986; 9:21-26.

10. Liu TJ, Lai HC, Lee WL, et al. Immediate and late outcomes of patients undergoing

transseptal left-sided heart catheterization for symptomatic valvular and arrhythmic diseases. *Am Heart J* 2006;151:235-241.

11. Szili-Torok T, Kimman G, Theuns D, et al. Transseptal left heart catheterisation guided by intracardiac echocardiography. *Heart* 2001;86:E11.

12. Hung JS. Atrial septal puncture technique in percutaneous transvenous mitral commissurotomy: mitral valvuloplasty using the Inoue balloon catheter technique. *Cathet Cardiovasc Diagn* 1992;26:275-284.

13. Hung JS, Fu M, Yeh KH, et al. Usefulness of intracardiac echocardiography in transseptal puncture during percutaneous transvenous mitral commissurotomy. *Am J Cardiol* 1993;72:853-854.

14. Epstein LM, Smith T, TenHoff H. Nonfluoroscopic transseptal catheterization: safety and efficacy of intracardiac echocardiographic guidance. *J Cardiovasc Electrophysiol* 1998;9:625-630.

15. Hagen PT, Scholz DG, Edwards WD. Incidence and size of patent foramen ovale during the first 10 decades of life: an autopsy study of 965 normal hearts. *Mayo Clin Proc* 1984;59(1):17-20.

16. Pinto FJ. When and how to diagnose patent foramen ovale. *Heart* 2005;91:438-440.

17. Hara H, Virmani R, Ladich E, et al. Patent foramen ovale: current pathology, pathophysiology, and clinical status. *J Am Coll Cardiol* 2005;1;46:1768-1776.

16. Hanley PC, Tajik AJ, Hynes JK, Edwards WD, Reeder GS, Hagler DJ, Seward JB. Diagnosis and classification of atrial septal aneurysm by two-dimensional echocardiography: report of 80 consecutive cases. *J Am Coll Cardiol* 1985;6:1370-1382.

17. Olivares-Reyes A, Chan S, Lazar EJ, Bandlamudi K, Narla V, Ong K. Atrial septal aneurysm: a new classification in two hundred five adults. *J Am Soc Echocardiogr* 1997;10: 644-656.

18. Silver MD, Dorsey JS. Aneurysms of the septum primum in adults. *Arch Pathol Lab Med* 1978;102:62-65.

19. Agmon Y, Khandheria BK, Meissner I, Gentile F, Whisnant JP, Sicks JD, O'Fallon WM, Covalt JL, Wiebers DO, Seward JB. Frequency of atrial septal aneurysms in patients with cerebral ischemic events. *Circulation* 1999;99:1942-1944.

20. Pearson AC, Nagelhout D, Castello R, Gomez CR, Labovitz AJ. Atrial septal aneurysm and stroke: a transesophageal echocardiographic study. *J Am Coll Cardiol* 1991;18:1223-1229.

21. Burger AJ, Sherman HB, Charlamb MJ. Low incidence of embolic strokes with atrial septal aneurysms: A prospective, long-term study. *Am Heart J* 2000;139:149-152.

22. Ren JF, Marchlinski FE. Utility of intracardiac echocardiography in left heart ablation for tachyarrhythmias. *Echocardiography* 2007;24:533-540.

23. Croft CH, Lipscomb K. Modified technique of transseptal left heart catheterization. *J Am Coll Cardiol* 1985;5:904-910.

24. Androuny AZ, Sutherland DW, Griswold HE, Ritzman LW. Complications with transseptal left heart catheterization. *Am Heart J* 1963;65:327-333.

25. Braunwald E: Transseptal left heart catheterization. *Circulation* 1968;37 suppl III:74-79.

26. Arora R, Kalra GS, Murty GS, Trehan V, Jolly N, Mohan JC, Sethi KK, Nigam M, Khalilullah M. Percutaneous transatrial mitral commissurotomy: immediate and intermediate results. *J Am Coll Cardiol* 1994;23:1327-1332.

27. Kronzon I, Glassman E, Cohen M, Winer H. Use of two-dimensional echocardiography during transseptal cardiac catheterization. *J Am Coll Cardiol* 1984;4:425-428.

28. Hurrell DG, Nishimura RA, Symanski JD, Holmes DR Jr. Echocardiography in the invasive laboratory: Utility of two-dimensional

echocardiography in performing transseptal catheterization. *Mayo Clin Proc* 1998;73: 126-131.

29. Trehan V, Mukhopadhyay S, Nigam A, Yusuf J, Mehta V, Gupta MD, Girish MP, Tyagi S. Mitral valvuloplasty in Inoue balloon under transthoracic echocardiographic guidance. *J Am Soc Echocardiogr* 2005;18:964-969.

30. Trehan VK, Nigam A, Mukhopadhyay S, Yusuf J, UmaMahesh CR, Gupta MD, Girish MP, Sharma M. Bedside percutaneous trans-septal mitral commissurotomy under sole transthoracic echocardiographic guidance in a critically ill patient. *Echocardiography* 2006;23:312-314.

31. Ballal RS, Mahan EF, Nanda NC, Dean LS. Utility of transesophageal echocardiography in interatrial septal puncture during percuta-neous mitral balloon commissurotomy. *Am J Cardiol* 1990;66:230-232.

32. Chan K, Marquis J, Ascah C, Morton B, Baird M. Role of transesophageal echocar-diography in percutaneous balloon mitral val-vuloplasty. *Echocardiography* 1990;7:115-123.

33. Jaarsma W, Visser CA, Suttorp MJ, Haagen FD, Ernst SM. Transesophageal echocar-diography during percutaneous balloon mitral valvuloplasty. *J Am Soc Echocardiogr* 1990;3:384-391.

34. Hahn K, Gal R, Sarnoski J, Kubota J, Schmidt DH, Bajwa TK. Transesophageal echocardiographically guided left atrial transseptal catheterization in patients with normal-sized atria: incidence of complica-tions. *Clin Cardiol* 1995;18:217-220.

35. Lim KK, Sugeng L, Lang R, Knight BP. Double transseptal catheterization guided by real-time 3-dimensional transesophageal echocardiography. *Heart Rhythm* 2008;5: 324-325.

36. Baker GH, Shirali GS, Bandisode V. Trans-septal left heart catheterization for a patient with a prosthetic mitral valve using live three-dimensional transesophageal echocar-diography. *Pediatr Cardiol* 2008;29:690-691.

37. Chierchia GB, Van Camp G, Sarkozy A, de Asmundis C, Brugada P. Double transseptal puncture guided by real-time three-dimen-sional transesophageal echocardiography during atrial fibrillation ablation. *Europace* 2008;10:705-706.

8

Intracardiac Echocardiography to Guide Transseptal Puncture

Conor D. Barrett, Luigi Di Biase,
J. David Burkhardt, Rodney P. Horton,
Sheldon M. Singh, Moussa Mansour,
Andrea Natale

For many interventionalists who are training in left atrial mapping and ablation, gaining access to the left atrium (LA) is perceived as a stressful and challenging portion of the procedure. In expert hands, transseptal punctures can be safely performed with the utilization of fluoroscopy alone, but there are many instances where the additional information obtained by intracardiac echocardiography (ICE) is invaluable.[1,2] This is more so when patients are therapeutically anticoagulated for the procedure, when the inherent risks are higher. To reduce the periprocedural risk of stroke and access complications, many centers now routinely perform atrial fibrillation (AF) ablation procedures while the patient is therapeutically anticoagulated with warfarin and administer heparin *prior* to the transseptal puncture.[3-5]

Although for some procedures (eg, mapping of accessory pathways), a retrograde aortic approach may be undertaken, this obviously requires arterial access and increases the risk of access complications. A transseptal approach frequently is easier and necessary for left-sided pathway ablations, and is obligatory in some patients (eg, those with severe aortic stenosis or with an artificial aortic valve). For other procedures, in particular ablation for AF, transseptal catheterization is obligatory.[6] The usual location of transseptal puncture for AF ablation procedures is shown in Figure 8.1.

Because of the inherent risks associated with transseptal puncture, it makes sense that all necessary precautions are undertaken to ensure the safety of the procedure. In an analogous situation, it has been previously observed that central venous access complications (including the reduction of attempts for success) can be reduced by direct, real-time visualization with ultrasound.[7] Moreover, as

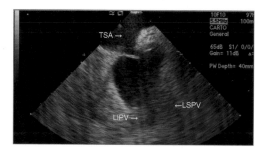

FIGURE 8.1   This is the usual level of approach for transseptal puncture in patients undergoing AF ablation. In the near field, the thin portion of the fossa is tented by the transseptal apparatus (the dilator). This approach provides the best orientation, with the left-sided pulmonary veins in view in the far field. LIPV = left inferior pulmonary vein; LSPV = left superior pulmonary vein; TSA = transseptal apparatus.

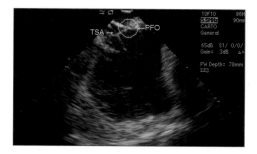

FIGURE 8.2   A patent foramen ovale (PFO) is circled in this diagram. The dilator of a second sheath is at this region; if the sheath is placed across such a patent foramen, the sheath tends to be directed more anteriorly. A transseptal sheath (TSA) has already been placed in the LA as indicated.

those familiar with AF ablation will testify, the appropriate approach to the transseptal and subsequent orientation of the sheaths in the left atrium is of extreme importance in increasing the ease of mapping and ablation of the posterior wall and the pulmonary venous antra. If a patent foramen ovale exists, passage through it is possible; such a course directs the transseptal apparatus in a more anterior direction, which is a suboptimal orientation for AF ablation procedures. The appearance of a second transseptal dilator at the level of a patent foramen ovale (PFO) is shown in Figure 8.2. It therefore makes sense to employ a real-time imaging modality that will increase the safety of transseptal puncture and, through correct orientation, decrease subsequent procedural time. Intracardiac echocardiography (ICE) is such a modality.

Procedural Considerations

Two forms of intracardiac echocardiography transducers are available: (1) a rotational (radial/mechanical) crystal transducer providing a circumferential view of the area of interest and (2) a phased array transducer providing sector visualization of the area of interest. Both catheters are available with imaging frequencies between 5 MHz to 10 MHz. The rotational catheters provide good quality near-field images and are employed in coronary interventions most frequently. It is our practice to utilize a phased-array catheter (available in 8 F and 10 F diameters), as these catheters provide better real-time definition of the anatomy in both the near- and far-field perspectives.

Transseptal punctures are routinely performed via right femoral venous access. The ICE catheter is advanced from the left femoral vein. It is advisable to advance the catheter into the inferior vena cava (IVC) under fluoroscopic guidance, which can be achieved by gentle flexion of the catheter at the level of the iliac vein. The catheter is then advanced into the right atrium. It is our general practice to position the ICE catheter in the mid-right atrium for the purpose of transseptal puncture (Figure 8.3). Gentle clockwise rotation

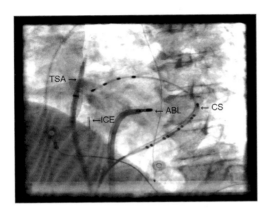

FIGURE 8.3   The usual position of the intracardiac echocardiography (ICE) catheter in the mid-right atrium, as viewed on fluoroscopy. ABL = ablation catheter; CS = coronary sinus; TSA = transseptal apparatus.

of the ICE catheter moves the plane of imaging posteriorly, such that the anterior (aortic root) and subsequently more posterior structures (anterior left atrium, mitral valve, and left atrial appendage) are sequentially viewed (Figures 8.4, 8.5). Further clockwise rotation of the catheter moves the plane of imaging more posteriorly, such that the left-sided pulmonary veins come into view in the far field

(Figure 8.6). At this orientation, in the near field, the interatrial septum (IAS) is clearly visualized. On occasion, if the ICE catheter is located too close to the septum, gentle retroflexion of the catheter provides for better imaging of the IAS. Further clockwise rotation brings the right-sided pulmonary veins into the field of view. The IAS remains in view in the near field throughout such posterior rotation. It is easily seen that the more posterior the orientation, the shorter the distance from the IAS to the opposing LA wall and roof (Figure 8.7). A puncture at this site, particularly without ICE guidance, may result in cardiac perforation and tamponade. Transseptal puncture should not be attempted in the more anterior plane with the aortic valve in view; an attempt at left atrial access at this level may result in damage or perforation of the aortic root.

The basic methodology employed for the transseptal puncture is the same as when utilizing fluoroscopy alone. A long 0.032-inch guidewire is advance to the superior vena cava (SVC) under fluoroscopic guidance. It is good practice to visualize the J tip of the guidewire outside the heart (to at least the

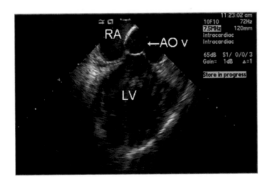

FIGURE 8.4   The more anterior structures as viewed on intracardiac echocardiography (ICE). Transseptal puncture is not attempted at this level. AOv = aortic valve; LV = left ventricle; RA = right atrium.

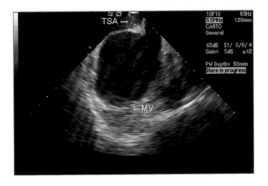

FIGURE 8.5   More posterior structures than those observed in Figure 8.4 are seen (with clockwise rotation of the probe). This orientation is still, nonetheless, anterior. MV = mitral valve TSA = transseptal apparatus.

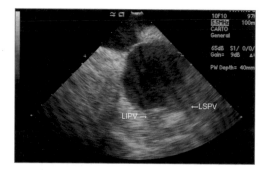

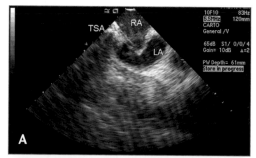

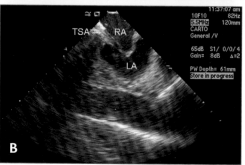

FIGURE 8.6 Further clockwise rotation of the probe brings the left-sided pulmonary veins into view in the far field. The thin portion of the fossa ovalis is readily appreciated in this view. Transseptal puncture for atrial fibrillation (AF) ablation is frequently performed with this view, for it allows easier access to the pulmonary veins and posterior left atrial wall. LIPV = left inferior pulmonary vein; LSPV = left superior pulmonary vein.

FIGURE 8.7 **A-B.** Yet further clockwise rotation brings the more posterior aspect of the intraatrial septum (IAS) into view. As can be easily appreciated, the opposing wall may be damaged by the transseptal needle or dilator with such an approach. Occasionally, this approach is necessary, and it is obvious that intracardiac echocardiography (ICE) provides for additional safety in such circumstances. LA = left atrium; RA = right atrium; TSA = transseptal apparatus.

level of the tracheal carina) to ensure that the long sheath is not inadvertently placed in the right atrial appendage. The long transseptal sheath of choice is advanced over the long J wire. The guidewire is removed, and the dilator aspirated and flushed with heparinized saline. Next, a flushed transseptal needle is advanced (with its stylet in place) to within 2 cm to 4 cm of the tip of the dilator. The stylet is withdrawn, and the needle is again aspirated and flushed with heparinized saline and then with radiopaque contrast. The whole apparatus is gently withdrawn into the right atrium in the left anterior oblique (LAO) view, with the guiding orientation (marker on the transseptal needle) usually oriented at between 4 o'clock and 6 o'clock so as to avoid the aortic root. A "jump" to the septum is usually clearly visualized on fluoroscopy, and the exact positioning of the tip of the apparatus is then confirmed on the ICE image (Figure 8.1). While it is possible to advance the ICE probe into the SVC and follow the transseptal apparatus as it is pulled

back into the RA, it is not our practice to do so. We find it easiest to accurately position the ICE probe before the transseptal portion of the procedure is commenced, such that the IAS is clearly visualized. Once the apparatus "jumps" to the septum (as viewed in the LAO perspective), the precise location and orientation of the transseptal apparatus can be determined. The goal is to position the dilator at the thinnest portion of the septum in the correct plane (Figure 8.1). From this point, ICE and fluoroscopy can be utilized to cross into the LA, and the ICE image can be invaluable.

The optimal anteroposterior orientation of the transseptal apparatus will depend on the reason for entering the LA. For interventional procedures aiming at mapping the more anterior or anterolateral LA structures (eg, in ablation of frequently observed accessory pathways), it makes sense to cross the IAS with a more anterior trajectory. This is achieved with the IAS clearly in view in the near field with the mitral valve and LAA in view in the far field. An anterior approach is shown in Figure 8.5. This is also the optimal approach for LAA occlusion device procedures. For procedures targeting more posteriorly placed structures (the pulmonary venous antra and the posterior wall of the LA for AF ablation) the transseptal puncture is best performed with the left-sided pulmonary veins in the far-field view. Further clockwise rotation brings the right-sided veins into view in the far field. Crossing the septum with such a posterior orientation is possible, but it is readily appreciated that this provides for less room, and the posterior wall of the LA may be more easily inadvertently damaged. A posterior approach is shown in Figure 8.7. We recommend crossing the IAS with the left-sided veins in view for AF ablation cases (Figure 8.8).

Once the correct trajectory is decided on and confirmed on ICE, the IAS at the level of the fossa ovalis is tented with the dilator of the transseptal apparatus. While tenting of the fossa generally reflects stable contact between the transseptal apparatus and the fossa, it is not unusual for the transseptal apparatus to advance superiorly with gentle pressure.[8] This vertical displacement can be visualized with ICE and can alert the operator to the need for repositioning. Once correctly positioned and the fossa tented, the needle is then advanced to the tip of the dilator, and a small amount of contrast may be injected if the operator wishes to observe

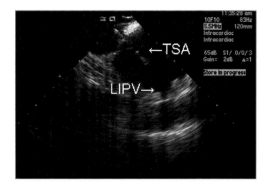

FIGURE 8.8　The transseptal needle has crossed the septum, with the left-sided pulmonary veins in view. LIPV = left inferior pulmonary vein; TSA = transseptal apparatus.

fluoroscopic confirmation of septal staining. With the IAS and the site of maximum tenting clearly in view, the needle is advanced beyond the dilator to further tent the septum. It is expected that with gentle pressure the transseptal needle will pass through the IAS into the LA (Figure 8.8). A small injection of contrast (<1 mL is sufficient) will reveal a reassuring appearance of contrast in the

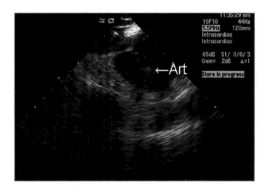

FIGURE 8.9　A small volume of contrast is injected through the transseptal needle, with the subsequent appearance of artifact (appearing as bubbles) in the left atrium. Art = artifact from contrast in the left atrium.

LA on ICE imaging. Such an appearance is shown in Figure 8.9. The whole apparatus is then rotated counterclockwise (if a posterior approach was used) to move the needle away from the posterior LA wall. The needle is fixed and the dilator advanced slowly over the needle. Once the dilator is visualized in the LA, the sheath is advanced gently over the dilator into the chamber. ICE is used at each stage to visualize the sequential process. The needle and dilator are removed, and the sheath is aspirated and flushed and then infused with heparinized saline.

Special Situations

The above description of the transseptal puncture is, fortunately, an accurate reflection of how the procedure is generally performed. Unfortunately, however, it is not that unusual for some degree of difficulty to be encountered at some stage during the puncture. This is increasingly the case as repeat procedures are more commonly performed and as procedures are more frequently performed in those with prior atrial septal defect (ASD) or PFO repair and with abnormal cardiac chamber orientation. In such situations, ICE is an invaluable tool. While foreknowledge of such potential issues may be available, in some cases abnormal IAS morphologies and rotation may only become evident at the time of the procedure. The routine use of ICE removes this uncertainty for the procedure.

(1) The Post-surgical, Thickened or "Lipomatous Hypertrophied" IAS

Patients may have a hypertrophied (often referred to as "lipomatous hypertrophy") septum, which can make transseptal puncture

challenging as the thickened septum may require a degree of pressure in excess of that normally employed in order to cross into the LA. Too much force applied to the apparatus may result in the needle jumping across the septum and piercing the posterior wall or roof. The use of ICE in such situations may help to define the thinnest region of the sep-

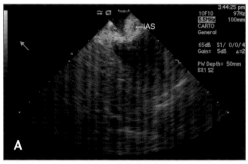

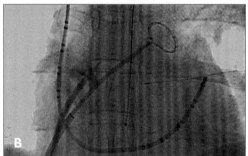

FIGURE 8.10   **A.** "Lipomatous hypertrophy" of the interatrial septum. In this case there is no identifiable fossa ovalis, and the septum is unfortunately quite thick. The septum is being tented with the dilator. **B.** Fluoroscopic image of the transseptal puncture in the same patient. IAS = thickened interatrial septum.

tum, thereby increasing the likelihood of safe and successful puncture. In the absence of an identifiable thin region, ICE gives further information regarding the trajectory of the needle and increases the safety of the puncture. An example of a hypertrophied septum is shown in Figure 8.10.

A similar situation is observed in patients who have had prior patch closure of an ASD and in those who have other surgical closures of the septum. Similarly, post-surgical patients (eg, those who have undergone mitral valve surgery) frequently have some degree of chamber rotation. In such patients, we have found that the approach to the transseptal puncture is frequently in a more posterior position than usual (with the transseptal needle oriented beyond the usual 6 o'clock position). The familiar appearance of a thin fossa ovalis may not be present in such patients (Figure 8.11). Thus, the septum may prove difficult to tent and puncture. ICE gives further information regarding the site of the closure and the degree of tenting of the septum. Increasingly,

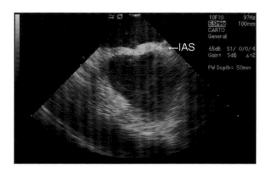

FIGURE 8.11   The appearance of the inter-atrial septum in a patient who had undergone a prior mitral valve repair. The septum is uniformly thickened, and no identifiable thin fossa was identifiable. IAS = interatrial septum.

as more repeat left atrium instrumentation procedures are performed, a thickened septum may be encountered at the time of the repeat procedure.

Recently, the possibility of applying radiofrequency (RF) energy to the external aspect of the needle as it initially tents the septum in order to cross into the LA has been reported.[9] A dedicated RF transseptal needle for transseptal puncture is commercially available (Baylis Medical Company, Montreal, Canada). This proprietary transseptal needle has a distal atraumatic flexible tip, which makes perforation most unlikely without the application of RF energy through the needle. As we do not routinely employ RF energy to perform the transseptal puncture, we prefer to continue to use a Brockenbrough needle for our procedures. When difficulty crossing the septum is encountered, we then employ RF assistance to cross into the LA. This is accomplished by the usual tenting of the septum at the desired location with the dilator of the transseptal apparatus. Radiofrequency energy is applied to the transseptal needle as the needle is just advanced out of the dilator to puncture the septum. This can be accomplished by placing a radiofrequency ablation catheter on the external aspect of the needle at the hub or by the use of a unipolar electrocautery pen (Bovie Medical Corporation, St. Petersburg, FL). We use an electrocautery pen in the "pure cut" mode, and have found that 20 W to 40 W, delivered near the hub of the needle, is sufficient to cross the septum in most cases. Radiofrequency energy application is generally needed for about 1 second in order to cross the septum; once artifact is visualized in the LA on ICE, the radiofrequency energy is immediately withdrawn. We have found this to be a useful method of crossing into the LA in refractory cases. However, it should be noted that the initial aperture created by an RF-mediated puncture is unlikely to close acutely. Therefore, if the aortic root were to be inadvertently entered while employing RF energy, it may lead to a serious complication. ICE imaging is the ideal method to avoid such an issue. Also, to prevent inadvertent damage to the LA walls, it is imperative that RF is immediately withdrawn once the needle has crossed into the LA. The precise moment of the transsep-

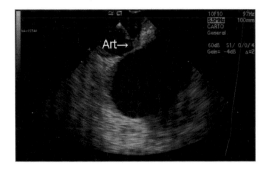

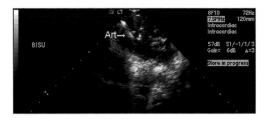

FIGURE 8.12   The use of radiofrequency energy to assist in transseptal puncture. Heating artifact appears at the tip of the needle at the level of the interatrial septum (Art).

FIGURE 8.13   The use of radiofrequency energy to assist in transseptal puncture. In this case the septum was highly mobile and can be seen tenting well into the left atrium. Heating artifact appears at the tip of the needle at the level of the interatrial septum (Art).

tal needle entering the LA is easily identified with ICE imaging. We feel that if RF energy is used as an adjunct to transseptal puncture, ICE imaging should be routinely employed. Examples of radiofrequency energy-assisted transseptal puncture are shown in Figures 8.12 and 8.13.

(2) *The Aneurysmal or Multiseptated IAS*

The opposite of a rigid septum is the highly mobile or aneurysmal IAS, which may be encountered. If ICE is not employed in such cases, the degree of mobility of the septum may not be readily appreciated. In such cases, the septum can occasionally be seen to tent all the way across to the opposing LA wall. Examples of aneurysmal and highly mobile septums are shown in Figures 8.14, 8.15, and 8.16. It is obvious that if one were to continue to push without ICE guidance in such cases, the lateral or posterior LA wall could be easily punctured. In some cases of aneurysmal septums, application of RF to the needle may facilitate entry into the LA. In such circumstances, real-time imaging with ICE is invaluable. A similar situation may be encountered with a multiseptated septum, which is most frequently a "double septum." If the presence of 2 septa is not appreciated (in the absence of ICE imaging), the reason for difficulty in crossing into the LA may not be realized. The reason for such "double-staining" as observed on fluoroscopy with contrast is readily observed on ICE (Figure 8.17).

(3) *The Septum with a "Closure Device" in Place*

Transseptal puncture may be necessary in patients who have previously undergone closure of an atrial septal defect or a patent foramen ovale with a closure device. It is obvious that such transseptal access is more challenging in such situations. ICE imaging provides excellent real-time localization of the device as well as information as to the best site and approach to transseptal puncture. It is often best to approach such punctures from below the device; frequently the anteroposterior direction has to be modified based on how the device has been placed on the septum. The use of ICE makes this easier and safer. Small movements of the transseptal apparatus in the anteroposterior plane (with gentle

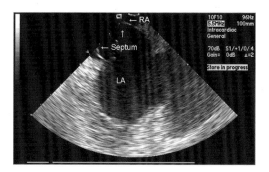

FIGURE 8.14   An aneurysmal septum, in this frame seen bowing into the right atrium (RA). LA = left atrium.

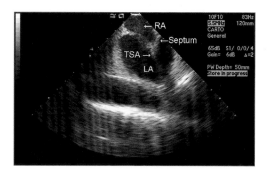

FIGURE 8.16   Another patient with a highly mobile septum. LA = left atrium; RA = right atrium; TSA = transseptal apparatus.

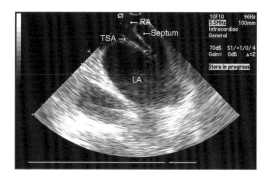

FIGURE 8.15   Subsequent tenting of the septum, just prior to transseptal puncture, in the same patient as in Figure 8.14. It is readily appreciated that significant mobility of such a septum may result in inadvertent damage to the opposing left atrial wall. Intracardiac echocardiography (ICE) in such situations increases the safety of transseptal puncture. LA = left atrium; RA = right atrium; TSA = transseptal apparatus.

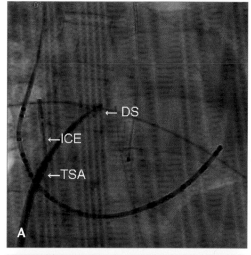

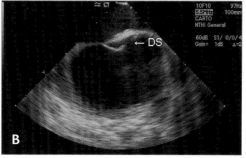

FIGURE 8.17   **A.** Fluoroscopic image of double staining of the interatrial septum (DS). **B.** The corresponding intracardiac echocardiography (ICE) image. The reason for the apparent double staining on fluoroscopy is readily identified as a double septum (DS). TSA = transseptal apparatus.

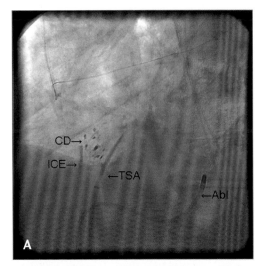

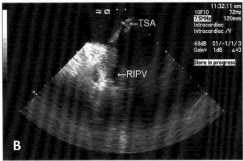

FIGURE 8.18   **A-B.** Successful transseptal puncture in a patient with a previously placed atrial septal defect (ASD) closure device (CD). The orientation of the transseptal apparatus (TSA) frequently has to be altered to avoid the closure device. Abl = ablation catheter in the coronary sinus; ICE = intracardiac echocardiography probe; RIPV = right inferior pulmonary vein.

counterclockwise or clockwise torque) is frequently necessary to approach the septum away from the device, such that transseptal puncture may be performed. Examples of ICE and corresponding fluoroscopic images of patients with septal closure devices undergoing transseptal puncture are shown in Figures 8.18 and 8.19.

Recognition of Complications

The use of ICE imaging during transseptal puncture is also invaluable for monitoring potential complications associated with the procedures, including pericardial tamponade associated with inadvertent cardiac perforation. Moreover, the development of thrombus on the transseptal apparatus or septum may easily be identified prior to and subsequent to transseptal perforation (Figure 8.20). When observed, thrombus removal by aspiration should be attempted.

Conclusion

ICE has gained widespread use during the performance of transseptal puncture. The addition of this imaging modality makes the procedure safer and increases the ease of access to the left atrium. In other situations, with atypical anatomy and in those who have undergone prior procedures, ICE can be an invaluable tool.

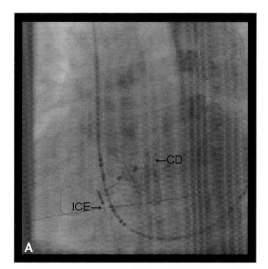

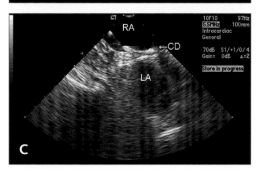

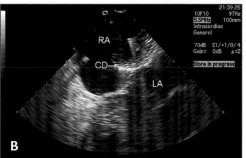

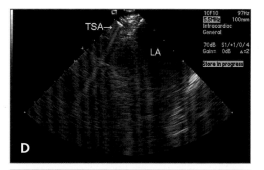

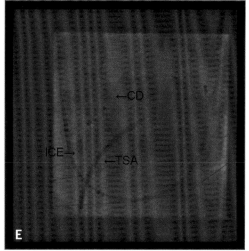

FIGURE 8.19 **A-E.** Successful transseptal puncture in a patient with another form of atrial septal defect (ASD) closure device (CS) present. Sequentially more posterior images reveal that a suitable site exists, away from the device, through which the transseptal apparatus could successfully be passed. CD = closure device; ICE = intracardiac echocardiography probe; LA = left atrium; RA = right atrium; TSA = transseptal apparatus.

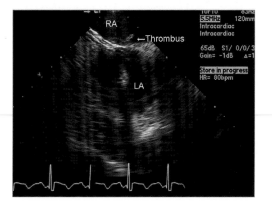

FIGURE 8.20 The appearance of thrombus formed on the right side of the interatrial septum. Transseptal puncture has already been performed. Such thrombi may be aspirated into a long sheet with the aid of intracardiac echocardiography (ICE) guidance. LA = left atrium; RA = right atrium.

References

1. Daoud EG, Kalbfleisch SJ, Hummel JD. Intracardiac echocardiography to guide transseptal left heart catheterization for radio-frequency catheter ablation. *J Cardiovasc Electrophysiol* 1999;10:358-363.

2. Epstein LM, Smith T, TenHoff H. Nonfluo-roscopic transseptal catheterization: safety and efficacy of intracardiac echocardio-graphic guidance. *J Cardiovasc Electrophysiol* 1998;9:625-630.

3. Kanj MH, Wazni OM, Natale A. How to do circular mapping catheter-guided pulmonary vein antrum isolation: the Cleveland Clinic approach. *Heart Rhythm* 2006;3:866-869.

4. Wazni OM, Rossillo A, Marrouche NF, et al. Embolic events and char formation during pulmonary vein isolation in patients with atrial fibrillation: impact of different anticoagulation regimens and importance of intracardiac echo imaging. *J Cardiovasc Electrophysiol* 2005;16:576-581.

5. Wazni OM, Beheiry S, Fahmy T, et al. Atrial fibrillation ablation in patients with therapeutic international normalized ratio: comparison of strategies of anticoagulation management in the periprocedural period. *Circulation* 2007;116:2531-2534.

6. Ren JF, Marchlinski FE, Callans DJ, et al. Clinical use of AcuNav diagnostic ultra-sound catheter imaging during left heart radiofrequency ablation and transcatheter closure procedures. *J Am Soc Echocardiogr* 2002;15:1301-1308.

7. Hind D, Calvert N, McWilliams R, et al. Ultrasonic locating devices for central venous cannulation: meta-analysis. *BMJ* 2003;327:361.

8. Hanoka T, Suyama K, Taguchi A, et al. Shift-ing of puncture site in the fossa ovalis during radiofrequency catheter ablation. *Jpn Heart J* 2003;44;673-680.

9. Knecht S, Jaïs P, Nault I, et al. Radiofre-quency puncture of the fossa ovalis for resistant transseptal access. *Circ Arrhythm Electrophysiol* 2008;1:169-174.

9

Transseptal Catheterization for Electrophysiology Procedures in Children and Patients with Congenital Heart Disease

Edward P. Walsh, Richard J. Czosek, John K. Triedman

Transseptal puncture was already a familiar maneuver in pediatric catheterization laboratories long before the launch of interventional electrophysiologic (EP) procedures. The technique had been employed routinely since the 1970s for accessing left heart structures for hemodynamic data and for angiography in patients with congenital heart disease (CHD) whenever a retrograde arterial approach was deemed inappropriate for anatomic reasons.[1,2] Thus, when radiofrequency (RF) ablation burst upon the scene some 2 decades ago, the transseptal approach was adopted early at many pediatric centers as a very natural and comfortable method to address left-sided arrhythmia targets.[3-5] Experience with transseptal EP procedures in children and in patients with CHD accumulated rather rapidly as a consequence. The fact that this entire textbook is now being dedicated to the topic clearly reflects how indispensable the tool has become for invasive electrophysiologists dealing with patients of all ages.

This chapter will review transseptal EP procedures in children with a focus on techniques needed to maximize safety in a small heart. Additionally, we will attempt to address some of the unique challenges encountered in patients with complex CHD where atrial anatomy is grossly distorted and/or the intraatrial septum has been modified by a surgical patch or occlusion device that can thwart conventional needle puncture. It should be emphasized that the information contained herein reflects our institutional experience and bias, but that many technical alternatives exist that may be equally effective in experienced hands. We offer our approach as a starting point for electrophysiologists involved with children and patients with CHD, but recognize that technology is changing constantly and that each operator

Transseptal Catheterization and Interventions.
© 2010 Ranjan Thakur MD and Andrea Natale MD, eds.
Cardiotext Publishing, ISBN 978-0-9790164-1-7.

must build upon their own clinical experience to arrive at a methodology that best suits their patients' needs.

Anatomic Features in Small Children and Patients with Congenital Heart Defects

The Normal Pediatric Heart

Safe transseptal catheterization in a child obviously demands strict attention to small chamber size and reduced wall thickness that could increase the risk of needle perforation. On a bright note, the atrial septum in children can often be traversed easily without exposure to the risks of needle puncture owing to a relatively high incidence of a patent foramen ovale (PFO) at younger ages. Pathologic studies have documented that fusion of the septal components (septum primum and septum secundum) is a gradual and imperfect postnatal process, such that the foramen will remain patent to a thin metal probe at autopsy in about 90% of infant hearts, 60% of young children, 40% of adolescents, and about 25% of adults.[6] This does not necessarily translate to patency for a catheter or sheath in the EP laboratory since the channel may be narrow and torturous. In practice, a deflectable EP catheter can only be coaxed unaided through the foramen in under half this number of cases, but it's a sizable percentage nonetheless, and nothing is ever lost by trying. We therefore insist on a routine check for foramen patency with a mapping catheter in all young patients before reaching for a Brockenbrough needle.

Small atrial chamber size will influence the equipment chosen for transseptal catheterization. For patients with a body weight less than about 30 kg (roughly, age <10 years),

the radius of curvature and shaft length on standard adult-sized sheaths and transseptal needles are excessive. It is recommended that special pediatric-sized sheaths and needles be selected for this purpose. Such equipment is available commercially in sizes 6 F and 7 F, with lengths and curve designs that better conform to the geometry of a small heart (Table 9.1, Figure 9.1). At body weights from about 30 kg to 40 kg, the operator can choose either a pediatric-sized or adult-sized apparatus depending upon the individual patient's body habitus. Selecting the pediatric-sized device in a thin but tall child could result in the 44-cm sheath being too short to reach into the left atrium. If uncertainty ever exists about this choice, one can simply position a pediatric sheath over the surface of the patient's body between the femoral puncture site and the mid-chest area while looking briefly with fluoroscopy to be assured the sheath tip extends well over the silhouette of the LA. Patients with body weights of more than 40 kg can usually accept standard adult transseptal equipment without difficulty.

A fundamental caveat regarding pediatric catheterization is that subtle hand motions by the operator can result in surprisingly dramatic catheter (or needle) motions relative to the small cardiac chambers of young children. Clinical experience and a rather "gentle touch" are mandatory to perform transseptal EP procedures safely in this population.

Special Atrial Features in Patients with Congenital Heart Disease

In both children and adults with CHD, transseptal EP procedures demand that the operator have clear understanding of the underlying anatomic defect as well as details of all surgical interventions. Those CHD

TABLE 9.1

Technical Specifications for Pediatric-sized and Adult-sized Transseptal Equipment

	Pediatric	Adult
Standard Sheath Sizes*	6 F or 7 F	7 F, 8 F, or 9 F
Sheath Length	44 cm	59 cm
Dilator Length	52 cm	67 cm
Guidewire Size	0.025 in	0.032 in
Needle Length	56 cm	71 cm
Needle Gauge	22 tip / 19 shaft	21 tip / 18 shaft

* Larger sizes available as a custom product for special interventions

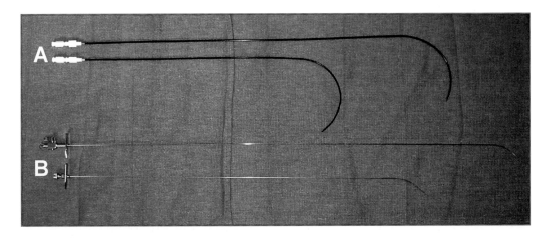

FIGURE 9.1   Comparison of pediatric-sized and adult-sized transseptal systems. **A.** Adult and pediatric sheath/dilator. **B.** Adult and pediatric Brockenbrough needles.

lesions that impact most significantly on gross atrial anatomy and status of the intraatrial septum are listed in Table 9.2.

On the simple end of this spectrum is the phenomenon of a left superior vena cava (LSVC) draining into the coronary sinus (CS). This normal variant can seriously distort landmark recognition during transseptal puncture in patients of all ages. The diagnosis might be overlooked on a preablation transthoracic echocardiogram in patients with poor acoustic windows, but should be nearly impossible to miss as soon as an EP catheter is advanced toward the CS at the beginning of a study (Figure 9.2). The CS (including its orifice) will be enlarged to many times normal

TABLE 9.2

Congenital Heart Defects That Affect Transseptal Catheterization

Left superior vena cava draining to coronary sinus

Repaired atrial septal defect (alone or in combination with other defects)
- Suture closure
- Patch closure
- Transcatheter device closure (Amplatzer, CardioSEAL, STARFlex)

Atrial baffles for transposition of the great arteries
- Mustard procedure
- Senning procedure

Fontan operation for single ventricle
- Atrial-pulmonary connection (various forms)
- Lateral tunnel
- Extracardiac conduit

Other defects causing severe atrial enlargement (eg, Ebstein's anomaly)

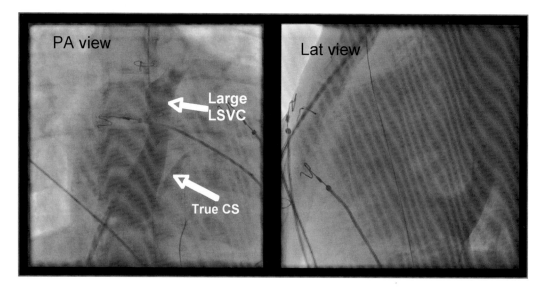

FIGURE 9.2   Left superior vena cava (LSVC) draining in a widely dilated proximal coronary sinus (CS).
The true CS along the lateral mitral ring is normal caliber. The presence of a very dilated
CS can distort normal landmarks during transseptal puncture. Lat = lateral; PA = posteroanterior.

diameter, and catheters will enter and advance very easily along its length, with unexpected deviation toward the left neck rather than following the lateral mitral ring.[7] Failure to recognize an LSVC-to-CS can complicate transseptal puncture since the true septum is foreshortened and the needle falls easily into the CS orifice where advancement can be hazardous. Accurate orientation for septal puncture in these cases can be obtained with the aid of angiography, intracardiac echocardiography (ICE), or transesophageal echocardiography.

Transseptal catheterization in patients with repaired atrial septal defects (ASD) can range from straightforward to very demanding depending on size of the original defect and the method of closure. Patients who had a small ASD repaired surgically with primary suture closure can be regarded as having nearly normal anatomy. Their septum may be slightly thicker than usual and more resistant to needle advancement, but it is unnecessary to modify technique to any significant degree. A larger ASD closed with a surgical patch is another matter. Various materials are used for this purpose, including glutaraldehyde-fixed pericardium, GORE-TEX, and on rare occasion, Dacron. All three materials become covered with endothelial tissue of unpredictable thickness after implant, and with time will become stiff or even calcified. More recently, a growing number of patients with a small- to moderate-sized ASD are being treated with transcatheter devices, including the Amplatzer wire mesh design (AGA Medical Corporation, Plymouth, MN) and the STARFlex or CardioSEAL double-umbrella designs (NMT Medical, Inc, Boston, MA).[8,9] As will be discussed in detail later in this chapter, atrial patches and occlusion devices do not preclude transseptal catheterization, although some modification in technique is usually required.

Gross distortion of atrial anatomy and septal configuration can occur after CHD operations that involve large intraatrial baffles to redirect systemic and pulmonary venous return. The Mustard and Senning procedures for transposition of the great arteries are illustrative examples of this challenge, and because these repairs result in a very high incidence of postoperative atrial tachyarrhythmias, transseptal ablation procedures are required commonly.[10] As part of both operations, blood return from the superior vena cava (SVC) and inferior vena cava (IVC) is channeled to the mitral valve, leaving the pulmonary veins and tricuspid valve on the left side of the circulation (Figure 9.3). Importantly, the cavotricuspid isthmus (the most common target for atrial flutter ablation in these cases) is longitudinally transected by the baffle suture line;

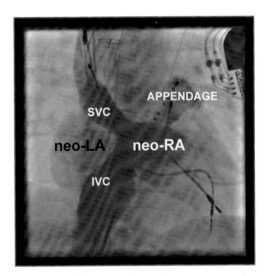

FIGURE 9.3   Atrial angiogram in a patient who underwent the Mustard operation for transposition of the great arteries. A pericardial patch has baffled blood flow from the superior and inferior vena cava (SVC and IVC) into a modified right atrial chamber (neo-RA) that empties across the mitral valve. Pulmonary venous blood returns to a right-sided modified left atrium (neo-LA) that empties across the tricuspid valve.

as a result, complete isthmus interruption will typically require ablation within the left heart (Figure 9.4). The tricuspid valve isthmus region can sometimes be reached with a retrograde arterial approach,[11-13] but baffle puncture[14] has recently become the preferred option in our institution.

The Fontan operation for CHD patients with single ventricle is another situation where extensive atrial baffling is performed, in this case to redirect SVC and IVC return into the pulmonary arteries. Similar to the Mustard and Senning populations, a high postoperative atrial tachycardia burden results in the frequent need for ablation therapy in these patients.[15] There have been several variations on the Fontan procedure over the years (Figure 9.5). Older surgical techniques retained the RA chamber in its entirety on the right side of the circulation, and although this resulted in a massively thickened and dilated RA, most arrhythmias could be mapped and ablated within this chamber without

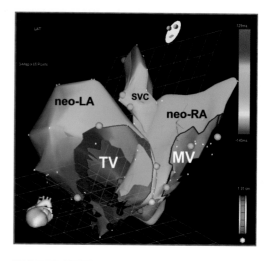

FIGURE 9.4   Electroanatomic map of atrial flutter in a patient who underwent the Mustard operation. The circuit propagates in a counterclockwise fashion around the tricuspid valve (TV). In order to reach the peritricuspid isthmus for ablation, the catheter can either be directed retrograde into the modified left atrium (neo-LA), or by transbaffle puncture from the neo-RA directly into the neo-LA. MV = mitral valve; SVC = superior vena cava.

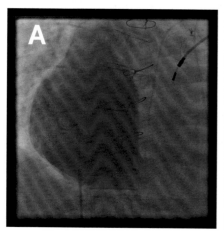
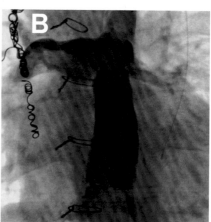

FIGURE 9.5   Variations on the Fontan operation for patients with single ventricle. **A.** Older style Fontan connection between the right atrium and pulmonary artery, showing the markedly dilated atrial chamber. **B.** Newer variation of Fontan connection with a GORE-TEX cavopulmonary baffle that bypasses the right atrium. Although the atrium is spared hemodynamic stress, a transbaffle puncture is needed to reach any atrial tissue for ablation.

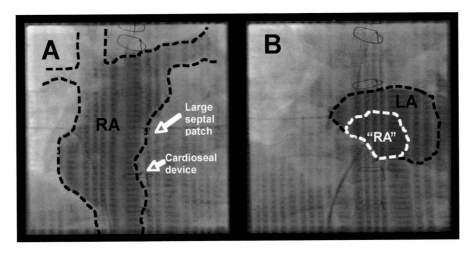

FIGURE 9.6   Example of the complex atrial anatomy that results from new varieties of the Fontan operation. **A.** Angiogram in the right atrium (RA) shows a moderately dilated chamber with its medial wall constructed of a large patch. A CardioSEAL occlusion device was also implanted to seal off a small patch leak. **B.** The patch and device sequester a small portion of the right atrium ("RA") on the left side of the circulation along with the normal left atrium (LA).

resorting to transseptal access. However, in efforts to reduce hemodynamic stress on RA tissue, surgery has now evolved toward a system of baffles or tubes that channel SVC and IVC flow more directly to the lungs, and, in so doing, sequesters large portions of the RA on the left side of the circulation (Figure 9.6). These newer surgical designs have significantly reduced arrhythmia incidence in Fontan patients,[16] but have not eliminated the problem entirely. Thus, on those occasions when ablation does become necessary, a transseptal approach is almost invariably required. These are without a doubt the most difficult transseptal procedures in the CHD population. Even when the baffle or tube is crossed successfully, the atrial architecture on the left side involves a complex maze of RA and LA tissue, along with remnants of the atrial septum, all of which can seriously confound catheter movement and mapping (Figure 9.7). In its most extreme

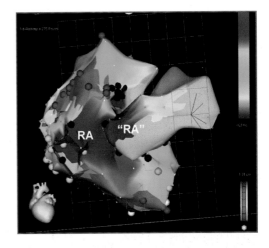

FIGURE 9.7   Same patient shown in Figure 9.5 during ablation for atrial flutter. Mapping revealed a complex circuit that involved both the right- and left-sided portions of the right atrium (RA and "RA"). Ablation on the right side of the patch slowed tachycardia but never terminated the circuit. It was only after entering the sequestered "RA" by trans-patch puncture that successful ablation could be accomplished.

form, the Fontan operation can bypass the RA completely using an extracardiac conduit running from the IVC to SVC that is then attached into the pulmonary arteries. This conduit may be sufficiently close and adherent to the lateral wall of the RA to permit a cautious attempt at needle puncture between the tube and the atrial wall, and some centers have even gone so far as to recommend needle puncture through the anterior chest wall directly into the LA when the caval return is connected in this fashion,[17] but experience with these rather daunting techniques remains extremely limited.

Basic Techniques for Transseptal Access in Pediatric Patients

This section will describe in detail the methodology currently in use at Children's Hospital Boston[18] for transseptal access during EP procedures. These recommendations stem from an institutional experience with more than 1000 transseptal ablation procedures involving children and CHD patients since 1990.

Most procedures in our laboratory are performed under general anesthesia, which may improve safety in anxious youngsters by eliminating unpredictable body motion at times when a transseptal needle is extended out of the sheath.[19] However, we do not hesitate to perform transseptal punctures in children under carefully titrated conscious sedation should the need arise.[3,20]

We do not feel obligated to stop anticoagulant medications, such as Coumadin, in preparation for EP procedures that involve transseptal puncture if there are legitimate concerns regarding prosthetic valves or atrial thrombus that support its use. We may elect to hold some doses just before the planned procedure, but are comfortable proceeding with any INR value of 2.9 or less. Likewise, during all our routine ablation cases, we elect to administer standard doses of heparin as soon as baseline EP catheters have been inserted, even when it is apparent transseptal puncture will be required later in the case. We aim to maintain activated clotting times around 300 seconds while any catheters are in the heart, and have never hesitated to perform transseptal puncture with values of this sort. Our overriding concern has always been minimizing thromboembolic risks, and even with this policy in place, we have never encountered a significant bleeding complication directly related to transseptal puncture.

All procedures are performed in a dedicated EP laboratory equipped with biplane fluoroscopy. On occasion we have enlisted the aid of transesophageal echocardiography to help direct the needle during difficult punctures, and have recently begun using ICE for a similar purpose, but the vast majority of our cases continue to be performed using X-ray alone. While acknowledging the utility of these alternate imaging modalities,[21,22] as described elsewhere in this textbook, we have acquired a high degree of confidence in fluoroscopic guidance, particularly for very young children in whom insertion of ICE catheters as currently sized would be undesirable because of small venous caliber. The posterior-anterior and lateral projections are our generally preferred starting points because of their familiarity; the oblique projections are reserved for select CHD cases where unusual anatomic features might be better displayed. Should septal orientation and LA position ever remain questionable by fluoroscopy, we advance an angiographic catheter out the pulmonary artery and perform a power injection with 0.5 cc of contrast per kilogram of body weight to visualize the outline of the LA and associated structures during the levophase (Figure 9.8).

The proper sheath/dilator and Brockenbrough needle are chosen according to patient size, as discussed earlier in this chapter. Both the sheath and dilator should be flushed thoroughly with heparinized solution before use. Because most transseptal sheaths are thin-walled and register poorly on fluoroscopy, some brands are equipped with a radiopaque tip marker to improve localization. Other brands (including the popular Mullins sheath) lack this marker, but instead have a centimeter ruler printed on the dilator shaft that allows one to gauge how far the sheath has slid over the dilator. Before insertion of a Mullins sheath, it is important to measure the distance that guarantees the sheath has extended beyond the dilator tip (usually about 2.5 cm to 3.0 cm). The obturator wire that comes packaged with the Brockenbrough needle is hardly ever needed in our experience, and can be removed to allow a 3-cc syringe of contrast to be affixed to the needle's stopcock. A small amount of contrast is injected through the needle to displace the air within. It is much preferred that the transseptal procedure be performed from the right femoral vein, though not infrequently we encounter CHD patients in whom this vessel is occluded after multiple prior catheterizations, and we are forced to work via the left femoral vein. This route is acceptable under most circumstances, but may require that the Brockenbrough needle be reshaped slightly by hand to increase the degree of curvature.

Once the guidewire is advanced from the femoral vein to a position in the SVC, the sheath/dilator is introduced and maneuvered so that the tip settles freely into the innominate vein. After the guidewire is withdrawn, it is always wise to aspirate the dilator to remove any air. Between 0.5 cc and 1.0 cc of air are routinely removed with this step, an amount

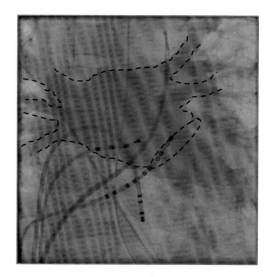

FIGURE 9.8   Levophase of a pulmonary artery angiogram in a 7-year-old girl. The dotted line outlines the contour of the left atrium prior to transseptal puncture.

that would be of trivial consequence in an adult with an intact atrial and ventricular septum, but could be hazardous if it embolized in a small child or any CHD patient with right-to-left shunting.

The needle is then advanced into the dilator/sheath. With certain equipment (particularly in pediatric sizes), it may be necessary to separate the stiff hubs of the sheath and dilator by several centimeters to accommodate the curve of the needle. This should be done by sliding the sheath forward along the dilator and not by pulling the dilator back in the sheath, since in a small heart the latter move invites dislodgment out of the innominate vein and SVC. The hubs are reapproximated after the curve has passed. The needle should advance very smoothly as it enters the body and passes along the pelvis, where the venous angles are most acute in pediatric patients. Any snag or resistance should prompt an immediate look by fluoroscopy to be sure the tip remains within the lumen of the dilator. If the needle does not advance smoothly, it sometimes helps to carefully advance the sheath/dilator along with the needle as a single unit for a centimeter or so to slide beyond an acute pelvic angle. If the needle still meets resistance despite this maneuver, it must never be forced. It should instead be removed, and a second attempt should be made with the obturator wire or another thin guidewire out the needle tip.

Beyond the level of the pelvis, the needle will travel easily through the sheath/dilator in children. The curve should be allowed to rotate freely as it moves past the abdomen and heart into the innominate vein. The needle tip at this stage is kept positioned just 1 mm to 3 mm back inside the dilator tip. While holding the needle and the sheath/dilator hubs in a fixed relationship to prevent needle slippage, the whole system is then turned and oriented so that the directional arrow on the needle hub is pointed between the patient's legs at about a 45° angle. A slow steady withdraw is then commenced under fluoroscopic guidance, alternating periodically between the posterior-anterior and lateral views to maintain spatial orientation.

We recognize two levels of "jump" as the system is withdrawn. The first occurs at the transition from the SVC to the RA, and is nearly always heralded by one or more atrial premature beats from mechanical stimulation. Slow withdrawal down the septum then continues while maintaining the 45° angle on the needle indicator arrow. The second level of jump occurs just as the system falls beneath the ridge corresponding to the limbus fossa ovalis and into the fossa proper. In about three-quarters of pediatric cases, this jump under the limbus is sufficiently distinctive to reassure the operator that the desired level on the septum has been reached, but in the remaining cases, can be so subtle as to be missed, causing the system to be withdrawn too low where it risks falling into the CS.

Whenever the jump into the fossa seems too vague for comfort, perhaps the best indicator for the true level of the limbus is to examine the position of the His-bundle catheter. As it turns out, for a normal pediatric heart viewed in the posterior-anterior projection, the limbus and the His bundle occupy the same horizontal plane (Figure 9.9). Thus, if the limbus is not easily located during the initial withdrawal exercise, it can be helpful to probe with the dilator tip along the atrial septum on the same plane as the His catheter, advancing the system slowly up and down the septum while feeling for a point where the dilator tip catches and engages under the ridge of the limbus. With enough experience, this maneuver is remarkably effective in locating the fossa when the jump technique fails. If uncertainty remains, imaging with echocardiography or angiography will be required.

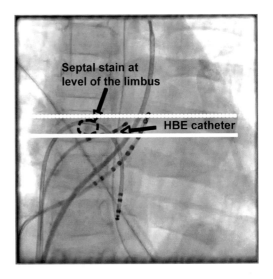

FIGURE 9.9   Relationship between the limbus of the fossa ovalis and the level of the His bundle electrogram (HBE) catheter. In this case, a small stain of contrast has been used to "tag" the septum at the site where transseptal puncture will be performed. Note that the contrast tag and the His catheter occupy the same horizontal plane.

Once the system has been positioned at the fossa, gentle forward pressure with the dilator tip (still keeping the needle a few millimeters inside) can be used to test for the possibility of a small PFO that may have been missed on earlier exploration. The distal taper on the dilator may indeed cross a PFO that seemed closed to the blunt tip of a deflectable electrode catheter. If no PFO is found, gentle forward pressure is maintained on the whole apparatus, and the needle tip is then advanced out the end of the dilator. Some operators prefer to deploy the needle with a quick stab, others with a more gentle motion, but either is acceptable as long as careful control is preserved. A small amount of contrast (about 0.2-0.5 cc) is then injected out the needle tip while observing carefully with fluoroscopy. We strongly prefer contrast injections to atrial pressure monitoring when attempting to predict needle location. There

are several possible observations during this injection. If the contrast exits the needle without resistance and simply swirls into the RA, it indicates that contact with the septum was poor, and the system needs to be repositioned. If the contrast exits without resistance and swirls into the LA, the hard work is done; the septum has been crossed successfully by the needle tip, but a second contrast injection using a larger volume (about 1.0 cc) is usually recommended to confirm this. When there is resistance to injection, it indicates that the needle tip is likely embedded in septal tissue. A bit of contrast is then forced out the needle to tag the area with a small stain that marks the site where more aggressive puncture efforts will subsequently be focused (Figure 9.10).

The stain location should be scrutinized carefully for its relationship to the back wall of the atrium and to the aortic root, since

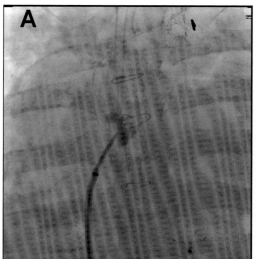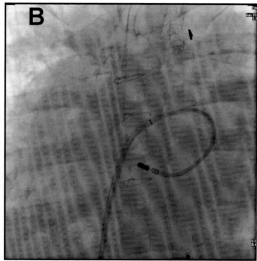

FIGURE 9.10   Staining the septum with a contrast injection through the needle tip. **A.** This patient had a Fontan operation for single ventricle, with a large patch closing the atrial septum. The contrast tag clearly marks the patch and gives some appreciation for the degree of thickness. Trans-patch puncture was facilitated by observing when the needle tip, and subsequently the dilator and sheath, passed through this tag area. **B.** Ablation catheter safely in the left atrium. The contrast tag is now barely visible, since it tends to dissipate within a few minutes of the injection.

excessive needle force directed toward either of these two regions could be hazardous. In our 18-year experience with transseptal puncture for EP procedures, we can recollect a total of 3 cases involving small patients where the needle tip entered the pericardial space, and 1 case where it entered the aorta. In all instances, the misdirection was recognized promptly with a contrast injection through the needle before the dilator was advanced, and the needle was withdrawn without serious harm to the patients. A small rim of pericardial effusion containing dilute contrast was apparent in 2 of these cases, but it did not expand or require drainage, and all 4 ablations were completed successfully. Though it can and should be avoided, we are presently unaware of any major consequence for inadvertent puncture by the needle alone in either our hemodynamic or EP laboratories over the last 2 decades, but reports certainly do exist of catastrophic bleeding when a dilator or sheath was mistakenly advanced through an incorrect channel. If there are ever concerns about the exact stain location, angiographic or echocardiographic guidance should be obtained before proceeding further.

If a properly positioned needle did not puncture into the LA up to this point, either because the septum is thick or very elastic, greater force will need to be applied. This should be done while keeping both hands on the apparatus; one on the shaft near the groin puncture site to prevent excessive forward excursion, with the second holding the needle hub to maintain the proper angle. Short jabs are then delivered by thrusting the whole system forward in a controlled fashion until the needle tip is seen to poke through the contrast stain tagging the septum. Additional contrast should be injected out the needle to confirm safe LA entry. Holding the needle stationary, the dilator is then advanced until it likewise passes beyond the contrast stain

into the LA; it should go into the chamber far enough to completely cover the needle point. The sheath is then advanced over the dilator. This last step can sometimes be the most difficult part of the process because the sheath may hang up on the rim of the puncture site, particularly when equipped with a radiopaque tip marker that actually adds a small ridge to its profile. Pushing too hard with the sheath against very resistant septal tissue may displace the septum far to the left beyond the dilator tip in a small heart, resulting in total loss of LA access. Therefore, it is critical to watch the septal contrast tag to be sure the sheath passes through it successfully instead of just forcing it to bow into the LA. Steady forward pressure on the sheath and a slight rotary motion should result in eventual success. The final sheath position can be confirmed by a fluoroscopic check of its tip marker, or if the sheath is not so equipped, by consulting the ruler on the dilator shaft to ensure it has advanced well into the LA.

With the end of the sheath safely in the LA, the dilator and needle are removed together in a slow, steady motion. Care must be taken to ensure the lumen end hole of the sheath is not obstructed by contact against the LA wall, since this will result in a vacuum as the dilator and needle are removed, and the sheath can fill with air. Some (but not all) sheaths are designed with a side hole near the tip to minimize this risk, but the best practice is simply to make certain the sheath tip is free-floating in the LA. The sheath is then carefully aspirated and flushed with heparinized solution. Some sheath designs include an integrated hemostatic backstop with an infusion side arm, but others require that a separate adapter be added to the hub for this purpose. The desired electrode catheter is then advanced through the sheath. As a precaution against clot formation, it has long been our policy to infuse heparinized flush solution at a slow rate through the sheath side arm whenever there is a mismatch between sheath and catheter size that creates the potential for stagnant blood within the sheath lumen (eg, a 6 F catheter through a 7 F sheath). If the French size of the catheter and sheath are identical, we elect not to run this infusion because we have encountered difficulty aspirating fluid back through the sheath to satisfactorily clear all small air bubbles from the system.

Advanced Transseptal Techniques for Patients with Congenital Heart Disease

Transseptal catheterization poses unique challenges in patients with CHD whenever prosthetic materials (patches, baffles, and occlusion devices) have been incorporated into atrial septal structure. Although it may be feasible in some cases to perform retrograde placement of catheters into the LA, this can be technically demanding and imposes substantial restrictions on catheter manipulation. In response to frustration with retrograde access in CHD patients, methods are evolving to cross these unusual septal barriers directly.

Published information regarding puncture through prosthetic material is still somewhat limited. Several small series have documented the feasibility and apparent safety of this approach. El-Said et al[23] reviewed their institutional experience over nearly 20 years with transseptal puncture through baffles and patches for hemodynamic (non-EP) indications; they reported that in 39 such patients, access without significant complications was achieved in all but 1 patient. Perry et al[14] later reported 2 patients

in which this approach was used successfully after the Mustard operation to achieve pulmonary venous access for ablation of atrial flutter. More recently, Lakkireddy et al[22] have added a series of 45 patients with ASD closure (22 surgical closures, 23 device closures); in 98% of the patients, successful transseptal access was achieved under ICE guidance for AF ablation. Our own institutional experience with transseptal technique for EP mapping and ablation through prosthetic barriers now exceeds 40 cases, including patients with Mustard and Senning baffles, various forms of the Fontan operation, and ASD repairs. We have observed procedural outcomes similar to those reported by El-Said and Lakkireddy, with successful LA entry in more than 95% of patients and no major complications attributable to the transseptal procedure.

Although we are presently pursuing the use of ICE and RF-assisted patch puncture[24] for our CHD cases, the vast majority of our procedures over the years have been performed using standard transseptal equipment and X-ray guidance. Careful understanding of patient-specific anatomy, as outlined earlier in this chapter, is the proper first step in planning an appropriate catheter trajectory. Both the underlying defect and details of the repair must be reviewed using surgical notes and any available noninvasive imaging studies. At a minimum, a careful pre-procedure echocardiogram should be performed. We do not insist upon cardiac MRI or CT scans in anticipation of patch puncture, but as these studies are being acquired with increasing frequency for merge applications with 3-D mapping systems, we have begun to appreciate their contribution to our visualization of the spatial anatomy.

As soon as it becomes apparent that a prosthetic barrier may need to be crossed in a CHD case, we perform biplane angiography of the RA, using a power injection with an adequate contrast volume to allow dense opacification for levophase study of the LA. This image is first reviewed for the possibility of a small baffle or patch leak that may be a suitable alternative to needle puncture. The position of a previously implanted occlusion device (eg, Amplatzer and CardioSEAL) is noted with a view to avoid, if at all possible. It is also important to note areas of patch calcification that may be evident on fluoroscopy, as these are typically impenetrable.

Assuming no fortuitous patch leaks are discovered, the operator must then elect a potential needle course offering the safest and most direct route to the tissue of interest. The needle must obviously point toward an open area of the pulmonary venous atrium that possesses adequate "depth" to allow for deformation of the baffle until the needle tip has crossed it completely. Some manual adjustment of the needle curve may be necessary before it is placed in the body. During normal transseptal puncture, force is applied

coaxially along the sheath and needle, and because of the mild curvature of the apparatus, some of that force is lost to puncture and is instead applied as a bending force to the needle. The straighter the course of the transseptal needle, the more force can be successfully transmitted without bending it. When attempting to penetrate woven or thickened baffle or patch material, this may be an important technical factor. In Mustard and Senning patients where the IVC portion of the baffle runs inferior to the LA, the geometry of the baffle allows the transseptal needle to be straightened to a considerable degree, facilitating the procedure by providing a favorable vector of force to the needle (Figure 9.11). In contrast, for patients with a massively enlarged RA after a Fontan operation or a large ASD closure, additional curvature of the needle may be necessary simply to engage the septal surface, and pushing on the system to achieve puncture may result in additional bending of the shaft. Excessive

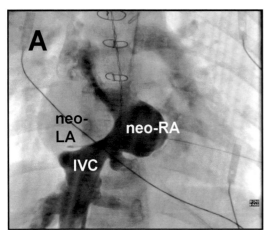 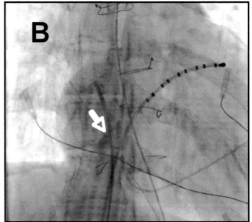

FIGURE 9.11   Transbaffle puncture in a patient after the Mustard operation to reach the tricuspid isthmus area for ablation of atrial flutter. **A.** Angiogram in the inferior vena caval (IVC) portion of the reconstructed right atrium (neo-RA). As was shown in Figures 9.2 and 9.3, the reconstructed left atrium (neo-LA) is located to the right side of the heart, with the IVC baffle running beneath it. **B.** Transbaffle puncture was accomplished successfully from the IVC limb in the neo-LA. The contrast stain used to tag the puncture site can be seen (white arrow).

curve must be avoided if the needle has to penetrate thick material.

Advancement of the needle across a patch or baffle will typically require greater-than-normal force. However, we have found that "sampling" of the engagement site with very small motions of the needle tip will frequently reveal a spot where the material is relatively thin and can be traversed without undue pressure (Figure 9.12). In cases where a comfortable puncture site cannot be located, the recently described technique for RF-assisted septal perforation could be considered.[25,26] This may be done using a standard Brockenbrough needle through which RF energy is delivered by activating a electrocautery pen for a short burst while in contact with the metal shaft. Alternately, new commercial transseptal needles are now available with an integrated system for RF delivery, using an insulated wire built into the needle hub and a dedicated RF generator specifically designed for this purpose. We have recently used RF energy for puncture through a particularly difficult GORE-TEX patch in a Fontan patient, and were impressed by the ease at which the needle could be advanced (Figure 9.13). Puncture with RF might offer a real advantage over a standard needle in CHD cases, and we have now begun an organized appraisal of the technique.

Transseptal puncture through a septal occlusion device is a new challenge with very restricted clinical experience.[22] We routinely try to avoid the device itself and find an alternate site for puncture, but in some recent cases where this was not feasible, we were able to cross successfully through the fabric material of double-umbrella CardioSEAL devices without great difficulty (Figure 9.14). Colleagues at our center performing hemodynamic interventions also report successful puncture through the wire mesh of Amplatzer devices, but we have no personal

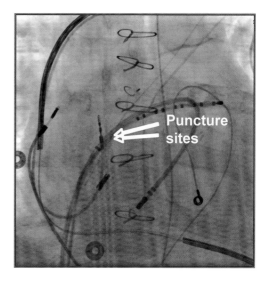

FIGURE 9.12   Patient with complex congenital heart disease (combined tetralogy of Fallot and atrioventricular canal defect) undergoing ablation for refractory atrial flutter of left atrial origin. A double-transseptal puncture for both a reference catheter and a mapping catheter was accomplished successfully through patch material without complication. Although the atrial patch was initially very resistant, a small region was eventually located by probing with the needle tip where the punctures could be done area safely. Transvenous ICD leads, as well as multiple abandoned epicardial leads are present.

experience with an EP procedure through such material. Perhaps one caution worthy of mention is that all these devices can take several months to fully scar and endothelialize within the heart, and dislodging could occur if a transseptal EP intervention was attempted too early after implant.

Getting the needle across the barrier is only part of the battle. The dilator, and especially the sheath, may not follow through tough septal materials. Whenever the biggest stumbling block is the sheath, it is important to consider whether the sheath chosen for the case has a radiopaque tip marker that distorts its contour. Simply switching to a sheath

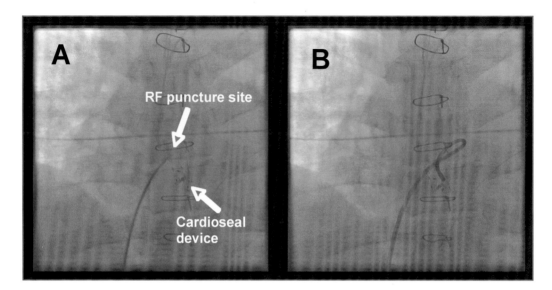

FIGURE 9.13   Transseptal puncture in an adult patient after the Fontan operation for single ventricle undergoing ablation for atrial flutter. **A.** The thick GORE-TEX patch proved resistant to conventional needle puncture, but could ultimately be crossed with the assistance of radiofrequency (RF) energy delivered through the needle tip. Note that the puncture site was chosen to avoid a CardioSEAL septal occlusion device. **B.** Ablation catheter on the left side of the septum at the site of successful ablation.

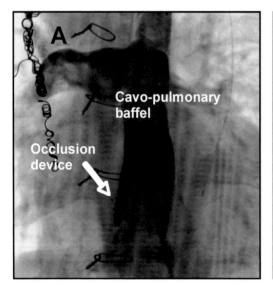
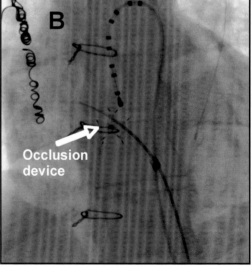

FIGURE 9.14   Patient with a complex Fontan operation involving a cavopulmonary baffle. **A.** There was no direct contact with atrial tissue from the baffle in this patient who required ablation for atrial flutter. An occlusion device was present in baffle at the site of an old surgical fenestration. **B.** The safest trajectory for transbaffle puncture appeared to be directly through the occlusion device. The needle tip is shown here after successful puncture through the baffle between the spokes of the device.

without a tip marker can make all the difference in some cases. In patients where we have been unsuccessful advancing the dilator and/or sheath despite prolonged efforts, we have occasionally resorted to placing a thin exchange wire through the needle lumen, removing the transseptal system, and then progressively enlarging the hole with a series of dilators, angioplasty balloons, and cutting balloons (Figure 9.15), resulting in easy passage for the dilator/sheath.

Most clinical experience suggests the risk of creating a persistent atrial-level shunt by transseptal puncture is negligible, whether

have we been forced to intervene to close the small defect.

Conclusions

Young children and patients with CHD present many unique challenges during transseptal EP interventions. Expanded experience, improved imaging modalities, and new technologies for puncture through prosthetic material should all contribute to improved safety and efficacy for these procedures.

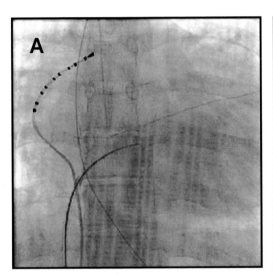 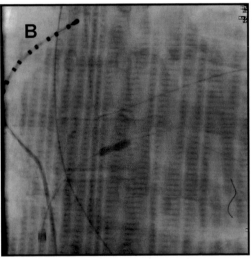

FIGURE 9.15   Transseptal puncture technique in a patient with Fontan operation and a very thick septal
patch. **A.** Although the needle tip entered left atrium successfully, neither the dilator or
sheath could be advanced despite long efforts. **B.** Dilation of puncture site using a high pressure angioplasty
balloon which then permitted easy advancement of the dilator and sheath.

it involves natural septal tissue, or prosthetic material.[22,27] Anecdotally, we have noted persistence of small baffle leaks on follow-up echocardiography and/or angiography after transseptal puncture in 2 CHD patients who had dramatic atrial pressure differentials after the Fontan operation, but never in a patient with normal atrial pressures, and in no case

References

1. Duff DF, Mullins CE. Transseptal left heart catheterization in infants and children. *Cathet Cardiovasc Diagn* 1978;4:213-223.
2. Mullins CE. Transseptal left heart catheterization: experience with a new technique in 520 pediatric and adult patients. *Pediatr Cardiol* 1983;4:239-245.

3. Walsh EP, Saul JP, Hulse JE, Rhodes LA, Hordof AJ, Mayer JE, Lock JE. Transcatheter ablation of ectopic atrial tachycardia in young patients using radiofrequency current. *Circulation* 1992;86:1138-1146.

4. Lesh MD, Van Hare GF, Scheinman MM, Ports TA, Epstein LA. Comparison of the retrograde and transseptal methods for ablation of left free wall accessory pathways. *J Am Coll Cardiol* 1993;22:542-549.

5. Saul JP, Hulse JE, De W, Weber AT, Rhodes LA, Lock JE, Walsh EP. Catheter ablation of accessory atrioventricular pathways in young patients: use of long vascular sheaths, the transseptal approach and a retrograde left posterior parallel approach. *J Am Coll Cardiol* 1993;21:571-583.

6. Hagen PT, Scholz DG, Edwards WD. Incidence and size of patent foramen ovale during the first 10 decades of life: an autopsy study of 965 normal hearts. *Mayo Clin Proc* 1984;59:17-20.

7. Gonzalez-Juanatey C, Testa A, Vidan J, Izquierdo R, Garcia-Castelo A, Daniel C, Armesto V. Persistent left superior vena cava draining into the coronary sinus: report of 10 cases and literature review. *Clin Cardiol* 2004;27:515-518.

8. Han YM, Gu X, Titus JL, Rickers C, Bass JL, Urness M, Amplatz K. New self-expanding patent foramen ovale occlusion device. *Catheter Cardiovasc Interv* 1999;47:370-376.

9. Nugent AW, Britt A, Gauvreau K, Piercey GE, Lock JE, Jenkins KJ. Device closure rates of simple atrial septal defects optimized by the STARFlex device. *J Am Coll Cardiol* 2006;48:538-544.

10. Walsh EP, Cecchin F. Arrhythmias in adult patients with congenital heart disease. *Circulation* 2007;115:534-545.

11. Van Hare GF, Lesh MD, Ross BA, Perry JC, Dorostkar PC. Mapping and radiofrequency ablation of intraatrial reentrant tachycardia after the Senning or Mustard procedure for transposition of the great arteries. *Am J Cardiol* 1996;77:985-991.

12. Triedman JK, Bergau DM, Saul JP, Epstein MR, Walsh EP. Efficacy of radiofrequency ablation for control of intraatrial reentrant tachycardia in patients with congenital heart disease. *J Am Coll Cardiol* 1997;30:1032-1038.

13. Kanter RJ, Papagiannis J, Carboni MP, Ungerleider RM, Sanders WE, Wharton JM. Radiofrequency catheter ablation of supraventricular tachycardia substrates after Mustard and Senning operations for d-transposition of the great arteries. *J Am Coll Cardiol* 2000;35:428-441.

14. Perry JC, Boramanand NK, Ing FF. "Transseptal" technique through atrial baffles for 3-dimensional mapping and ablation of atrial tachycardia in patients with d-transposition of the great arteries. *J Interv Card Electrophysiol* 2003;9:365-369.

15. Walsh EP. Interventional electrophysiology in patients with congenital heart disease. *Circulation* 2007;115:3224-3234.

16. Stamm C, Friehs I, Mayer JE, Zurakowski D, Triedman JK, Moran AM, Walsh EP, Lock JE, Jonas RA, DelNido PJ. Long-term results of the lateral tunnel Fontan operation. *J Thorac Cardiovasc Surg* 2001;121:28-41.

17. Nehgme RA, Carboni MP, Care J, Murphy JD. Transthoracic percutaneous access for electroanatomic mapping and catheter ablation of atrial tachycardia in patients with a lateral tunnel Fontan. *Heart Rhythm* 2006;3:37-43.

18. Lang P. Other catheterization laboratory techniques and interventions, including transseptal puncture. In: Lock JE, Keane JF, Perry SB, eds. *Diagnostic and Interventional Catheterization in Congenital Heart Disease.* 2nd ed. Boston: Kluwer; 2000:245-269.

19. Lavoie J, Walsh EP, Burrows FA, Laussen P, Lulu JA, Hansen DD. Effects of propofol or isoflurane anesthesia on cardiac conduction in children undergoing radiofrequency cath-

eter ablation for tachydysrhythmias. *Anesthesiology* 1995;82:884-887.

20. Walsh EP. Catheter ablation in young patients: special considerations. In: Wilber DJ, Packer DL, Stevenson WG, eds. *Catheter Ablation of Cardiac Arrhythmias: Basic Concepts and Clinical Applications.* 3rd ed. Malden, Mass.: Blackwell Futura; 2008:91-104.

21. Shalganov TN, Paprika D, Borbás S, Temesvári A, Szili-Török T. Preventing complicated transseptal puncture with intracardiac echocardiography: case report. *Cardiovasc Ultrasound* 2005;3:5.

22. Lakkireddy D, Rangisetty U, Prasad S, Verma A, Biria M, Berenbom L, Pimentel R, Emert M, Rosamond T, Fahmy T, Patel D, Biase LD, Schweikert R, Burkhardt D, Natale A. Intracardiac echo-guided radiofrequency catheter ablation of atrial fibrillation in patients with atrial septal defect or patent foramen ovale repair: a feasibility, safety, and efficacy study. *J Cardiovasc Electrophysiol* 2008;19:1137-1142.

23. El-Said HG, Ing FF, Grifka RG, Nihill MR, Morris C, Getty-Houswright D, Mullins CE. An 18-year experience with transseptal procedures through baffles, conduits, and other intra-atrial patches. *Catheter Cardiovasc Interv* 2000;50:434-439.

24. Sakata Y, Feldman T. Transcatheter creation of atrial septal perforation using a radiofrequency transseptal system: novel approach as an alternative to transseptal needle puncture. *Catheter Cardiovasc Interv.* 2005;64:327-332.

25. Bidart C, Vaseghi M, Cesario DA, Mahajan A, Fujimura O, Boyle NG, Shivkumar K. Radiofrequency current delivery via transseptal needle to facilitate septal puncture. *Heart Rhythm* 2007;4:1573-1576.

26. Casella M, Dello Russo A, Pelargonio G, Martino A, De Paulis S, Zecchi P, Bellocci F, Tondo C. Fossa ovalis radiofrequency perforation in a difficult case of conventional transseptal puncture for atrial fibrillation ablation. *J Interv Card Electrophysiol* 2008;21:249-253.

27. Fitchet A, Turkie W, et al. Transeptal approach to ablation of left-sided arrhythmias does not lead to persisting interatrial shunt: a transesophageal echocardiographic study. *Pacing Clin Electrophysiol* 1998, 21:2070-2072.

10

CHALLENGING TRANSSEPTAL CATHETERIZATIONS

Yu-Feng Hu, Ming-Hsiung Hsieh, Shih-Ann Chen

Although the transseptal puncture (TSP) technique has been shown to be safe in the vast majority of cases, this procedure can result in life-threatening complications, such as a cardiac tamponade, systemic emboli, or aortic perforation. The reported complication rate has ranged from 0.74% to 1.3%.[1] Complications during TSP are more likely when the cardiac anatomy is unusual or distorted, as in cases of congenital heart disease with or without surgical correction. However, TSP has become important for delivering modern therapeutic options to patients with cardiovascular diseases. To further improve the success rate and to avoid any complications, several imaging techniques have been developed to clarify the anatomy and to guide the TSP, including atriography, transesophageal echocardiography (TEE), and intracardiac echo-cardiography (ICE). Several new methods have recently been proposed to overcome any difficulty during the transseptal puncture; these methods include the use of a radiofrequency-assisted transseptal puncture or access through a patent foramen ovale (PFO).[2]

In this chapter we will describe some caveats regarding transseptal catheterization in patients with normal anatomy, discuss tips on TSP in patients with challenging anatomy, and, finally, provide guidelines for the use of ancillary imaging modalities to prevent complications in challenging cases.

Caveats for Transseptal Catheterization in the Normal Heart

Different modalities and instruments are used to perform TSP. Knowing the different instruments and methods for TSP helps the operator

Transseptal Catheterization and Interventions.
© 2010 Ranjan Thakur MD and Andrea Natale MD, eds.
Cardiotext Publishing, ISBN 978-0-9790164-1-7.

to overcome difficulties by choosing the most effective approach. In Figure 10.1, various steps and tools for TSP are listed. The general principles for TSP are described as follows.

Before TSP, the anatomical landmarks need to be clarified. The inferior margin of the interatrial septum is delineated by the coronary sinus catheter. The anterior roof of the interatrial septum is the aortic root, which can be marked either by a catheter at the His bundle, advanced through the venous systems, or by a pigtail catheter in the aorta, inserted retrogradely. Some centers use the right atriography routinely to delineate the interatrial septum, right atrium, and associated anatomical details. The left atrial border, pulmonary vein, and sometimes the aortic root can be clarified in the venophase of the right atriography. The use of ICE and TEE can be very helpful in defining the anatomy of both the atria and the interatrial septum.

To guide TSP, most centers use fluoroscopy, which may be biplane or single-plane with different projections. A variety of preshaped sheaths, such as the SL1 and SR0, are commonly used for catheter ablation of atrial fibrillation. Each curvature of the sheath can facilitate manipulation in different regions of the left upper chamber. Brockenbrough (BRK) transseptal needles have different lengths (71 cm for the adults and 56 cm for the pediatrics). Two different transseptal needles are commonly used: A BRK (small-curved, the angle between the distal curved portion and the shaft is ~19°) and a BRK-1 (large-curved, the angle between the distal curved portion and the shaft is ~53°). The small-curved needle is the best first choice in most patients. However, for older patients or patients with large right and/or left atria, the large-curved needle may be the best first choice. If required, the curve of the transseptal needle can be modified manually.

Confirmation of the location of the fossa ovalis is a critical step for TSP. The sudden medial drop of the needle tip moving from the superior vena cava (SVC) to the fossa ovalis and contrast staining of the septum are 2 common methods. ICE and TEE are very helpful in showing the contact between the transseptal needle and the interatrial septum as well as tenting of the septum.

Once transseptal catheterization is performed and the sheath is placed in the left atrium, a thrombus may form within a very short time (see Chapter 12). To prevent this, patients are often heparinized prior to transseptal catheterization. This may seem counterintuitive given the risk of aortic puncture and cardiac perforation. Different intensities of heparinization are used. In our center, an activated clotting time (ACT) from 200 seconds to 300 seconds is considered appropriate. However, in some centers, an ACT higher than 300 seconds is used, while others give a bolus of 5000 units of heparin without measuring the ACT at this stage of the procedure.

The penetration of the needle through the interatrial septum is achieved by manual force. Electrocautery or radiofrequency energy may be used to facilitate this part of the procedure. It is very important to confirm that the needle is within the left atrium before advancing the dilator or the sheath. Recoding the left atrial pressure waveform or contrast injection are 2 common methods. Oxygen saturation analysis to show high oxygen content may be useful. For the passage of the dilator and the sheath, some operators simply advance the sheath and dilator after the penetration of the transseptal needle, while others prefer to pass a guidewire through the transseptal needle to guide the direction before the advancement of the sheath and dilator.[3] For mitral valvuloplasty and balloon-based ablation devices, a large-size vascular dilator (up to 14 F) may be required for passage of the catheter.

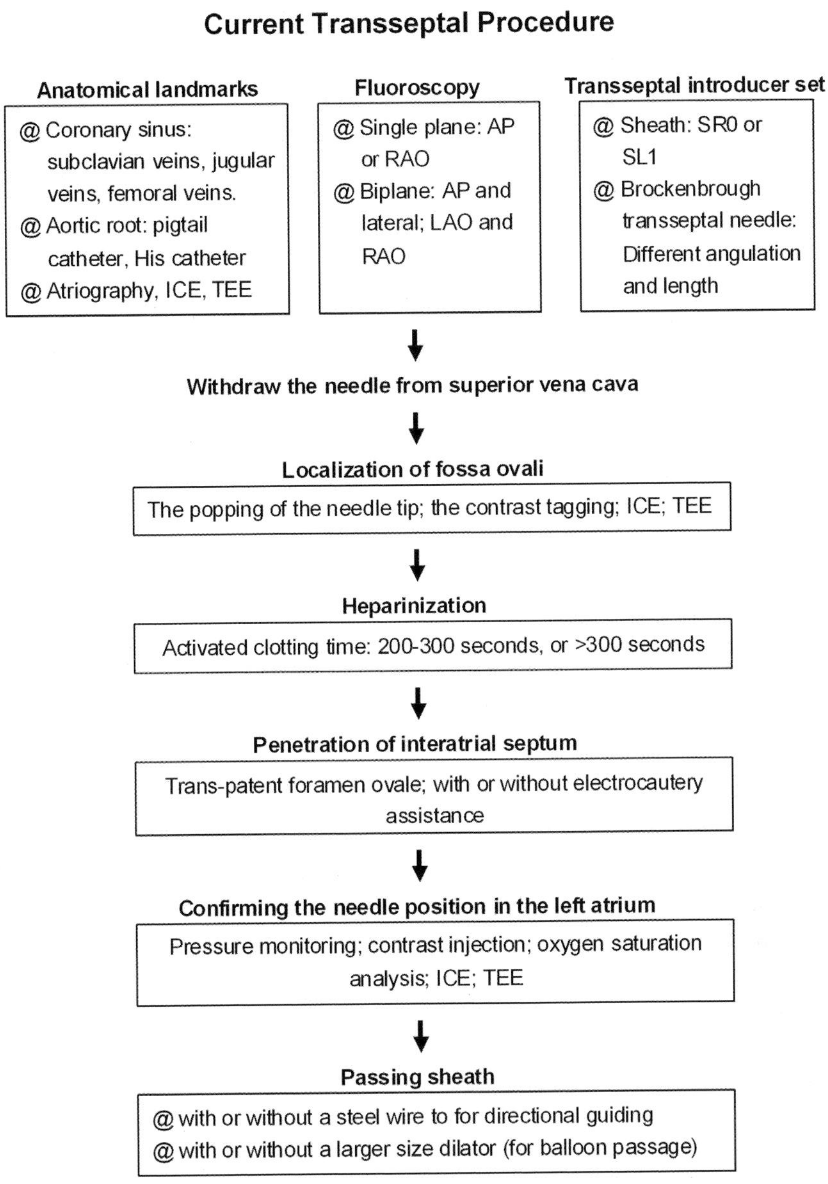

Current Transseptal Procedure

Anatomical landmarks	Fluoroscopy	Transseptal introducer set
@ Coronary sinus: subclavian veins, jugular veins, femoral veins. @ Aortic root: pigtail catheter, His catheter @ Atriography, ICE, TEE	@ Single plane: AP or RAO @ Biplane: AP and lateral; LAO and RAO	@ Sheath: SR0 or SL1 @ Brockenbrough transseptal needle: Different angulation and length

Withdraw the needle from superior vena cava

Localization of fossa ovali

The popping of the needle tip; the contrast tagging; ICE; TEE

Heparinization

Activated clotting time: 200-300 seconds, or >300 seconds

Penetration of interatrial septum

Trans-patent foramen ovale; with or without electrocautery assistance

Confirming the needle position in the left atrium

Pressure monitoring; contrast injection; oxygen saturation analysis; ICE; TEE

Passing sheath

@ with or without a steel wire to for directional guiding @ with or without a larger size dilator (for balloon passage)

FIGURE 10.1   *Current Transseptal Procedure*

AP = anteroposterior; ICE = intracardiac echocardiography; LAO = left anterior oblique; RAO = right anterior oblique; TEE = transesophageal echocardiography.

Complex Congenital Heart Diseases

Although it is thought to be highly risky to perform TSP in patients with complex congenital heart diseases, Mullins and his colleagues reported a series of studies that demonstrated TSP is safe in these patients.[4-6] From February 1975 to October 1976, TSP was reported in 80 patients using the original Brockenbrough technique. Moreover, using the modified technique with a long sheath developed by Mullins, TSP was reported in 520 patients from July 1978 to June 1982, and in 217 patients from October 1983 to September 1998. The majority of patients in these 3 studies were infants and children, many with congenital heart disease. Cardiac defects in these patients included 158 with ventricular septal defects; 141 with aortic valve disease; 91 with tetralogy of Fallot, truncus arteriosus, pseudotruncus arteriosus, or postoperative tetralogy; 88 with coarctation of the aorta; 61 with a patent ductus arteriosus; 48 with multiple left heart obstructive lesions; 45 with transpositions including ventricular inversions; 48 with mitral valve disease; 23 with double outlet right ventricles; 28 with cardiomyopathies; 8 with hypertrophic subaortic stenosis; 6 with pulmonary stenosis; and 42 with miscellaneous abnormalities. In summary, a total of 787 procedures were associated with a complication rate of 4.3%: 33 pericardial punctures (2 with cardiac tamponade) and 1 ascending aorta puncture. There were 6 failed procedures. The cardiac defects of 4 of the patients in whom a failed TSP was reported included pseudotruncus arteriosus, aortic stenosis with aortic insufficiency, coarctation of the aorta and aortic stenosis, and gigantic right atrium. Two TSPs were abandoned due to pericardial puncture. The complication rate of the TSP in patients with complex congenital heart disease seems to be acceptable and only a little higher than that in the general population. On the other hand, operator experience is a major determinant of procedural success and safety, and the vast experience reported by Mullins et al is unlikely to be accrued in most laboratories today. Before the procedure, several issues that contribute to safe and successful TSP need to be addressed.

Steps for Avoiding Major Complications with an Unusual Anatomy

1. Operator skill and experience are of considerable importance for transseptal puncture in patients with an unusual anatomy.
2. Delineate bi-atrial anatomy with auxiliary images, such as atriography, intracardiac echocardiography, or transesophageal echocardiography.
3. Continuously monitor the intracardiac pressures throughout the procedure, or use a contrast tag to confirm the needle position if needed.
4. Never advance the needle until the catheter has been perfectly positioned on the fossa ovalis.
5. Never advance the catheter until the needle has clearly entered the left atrium, as confirmed by a distinct left atrial pressure recording, contrast injection, and a free position of the needle on fluoroscopy.

First, because the cardiac anatomy, especially of the interatrial septum, changes after cardiac operations, auxiliary images to clarify the atrial anatomy are necessary, such as right atriography, ICE, or TEE. Second, confirming the puncture site with contrast tagging ("staining" the septum), continuous pressure monitor, or auxiliary images (ICE,

TEE) are important before penetrating the septum. At times, the direction of the needle may need to be modified, based on the altered anatomy of the interatrial septum. Third, sometimes, it is very difficult to penetrate prosthetic material. This may require electrocautery or other instruments. Finally, the needle position needs to be confirmed before advancing the sheath.

The Position of the Transseptal Needle in Complex Congenital Heart Disease

The position of the needle will differ because the cardiac anatomy changes after a cardiac operation. Figure 10.2 illustrates a patient after a Mustard procedure in our center who presented with typical atrial flutter. The TSP was performed successfully, as well as the catheter ablation of the atrial flutter. Right atriography was performed, using 30° right anterior oblique (RAO) and 60° left anterior oblique (LAO) views, which delineated the position of the interatrial septum. The transseptal set was withdrawn until the transseptal tip dropped off the native septum, onto the patch. The tip of the transseptal needle was directed anterior in the LAO view and aimed at the right shoulder in the RAO view. The transseptal needle successfully passed the inferior limb of the patch in the RAO view, requiring some force. In patients with a total anomalous pulmonary vein return or an atrial septal patch, using the anteroposterior and lateral projections, the needle is directed posteriorly and leftward toward the expected position of the left atrium. With Fontan baffles, the transseptal needle is oriented, as in patients with a normal heart, medially to the left and slightly posterior (Figure 10.3). Knowing the direction of the transseptal needle will help the operator perform the TSP more

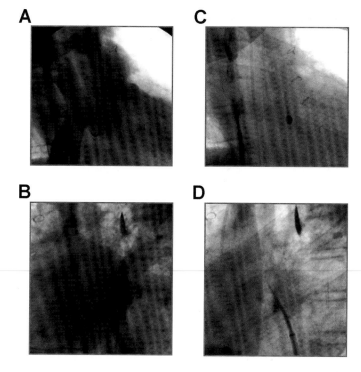

A

B

C

D

FIGURE 10.2 *Transseptal Puncture in a Patient with a Mustard Repair* **A.** 30° RAO projection. Contrast-opacified superior and inferior limbs of the baffle. **B.** 60° LAO projection. Opacification of the left atrium during levophase. **C.** 30° RAO projection. The transseptal needle is directed almost vertically, pointing toward the pulmonary venous atrium, and passes through the septum via the inferior limb of the baffle. **D.** 60° LAO projection. The transseptal needle is directed anteriorly. LAO = left anterior oblique; RAO = right anterior oblique.

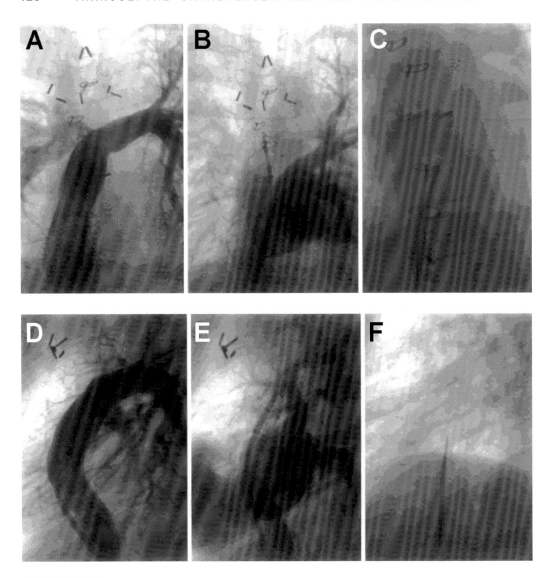

FIGURE 10.3   *Posteroanterior Projection of an Angiogram of a Lateral Tunnel Fontan (A-C) and Lateral Projection of an Angiogram of a Lateral Tunnel Fontan (D-F).*
A. The contrast filled the lateral tunnel. **B.** The left atrium opacified during the levophase. **C.** The transseptal needle was directed medially toward the left shoulder. **D.** The contrast opacified the lateral tunnel. **E.** Opacification of the left atrium during the levophase. **F.** The transseptal needle was directed medially and slightly posterior. From El-Said HG, Ing FF, Grifka RG, et al. 18-year experience with transseptal procedures through baffles, conduits, and other intra-atrial patches. *Catheter Cardiovasc Interv* 2000;50:434-439. Reprinted with permission from John Wiley and Sons.

efficiently. Table 10.1 lists the changes in the needle position relative to anatomical variations, which helps to localize the needle when a TSP is performed under fluoroscopy.

Transseptal Puncture Through Prosthetic Material

TSP in postoperative patients with complex congenital heart disease has been considered

TABLE 10.1

The Change in the Needle Position Due to Anatomical Variations

Anatomical Variation	The Change of Needle Position, Compared to Normal Position
Transposition of the great arteries after a Mustard or Senning procedure	Posterior in the AP view, anterior in the lateral view; low-lateral and anterior portion of the baffle over the combined systemic venous site
Total anomolous pulmonary vein return or atrial septal defect patches	Leftward in the AP view; posterior in the lateral view
Fontan baffles	Leftward in AP view; slightly posterior in the lateral view
A bulging LA	Anterior to the aorto-septal groove or far posterior in the right atrium-septal groove adjacent to the pericardium
Dilated aorta	Higher and posterior in the AP view
Atrial septal occluder	Below the rim of the device
Cardiac malposition or thoracic spine anomalies	Depends on the anatomical variation. Need auxiliary images to guide the needle position.
Large atrial septal aneurysm	Leftward in the AP view, close to the posterior free wall. Sometimes, not possible to achieve a stable position of the transseptal needle in the fossa itself. The needle slides and points to the aorta.
Thick and fibrotic septum	Higher in the AP view

more challenging. However, according to previous reports, it can be performed safely without any sequelae. Guided by fluoroscopy, El-Said et al[7] reported 39 patients (1-31 years old) with intraatrial patches, including 16 with a D-transposition of the great arteries after a Mustard or Senning procedure, 4 with single ventricle variants post-Fontan operation, 4 with total anomalous pulmonary venous return repairs, 9 with atrioventricular canal repairs, and 6 with atrial septal defects with patch repairs. The material for the repairs included pericardium, native atrial tissue repair, Dacron, GORE-TEX, and Teflon. Only 1 transseptal puncture in a 17-month-old child with a status post-Senning repair failed because the intraatrial patch could not be traversed. Echocardiographic follow-up was available in 30 patients, and no residual shunts were noted in 28 patients. In 2 patients, the shunts were created intentionally (a fenestration). No complications were reported. Similarly, Perry et al reported 2 successful TSP procedures in 2 patients with a D-transposition of the great arteries, using a fluoroscopy-guided transseptal approach.[8] One underwent a Mustard procedure, and the other underwent a Senning operation. More recently, Lakkireddy et al reported TSP procedures in 45 post-atrial septal defect (ASD)/patent foramen ovale (PFO) repair patients using intracardiac echocardiography.[9] In the patients who had undergone an ASD (24 secundum defect and 4 primum defect) repair, 22 had a surgical repair (7 with pericardial patch, 4 with septal stitch, 10 with Dacron, 1 with GORE-TEX), and 6 had a CardioSEAL closure. Direct sutures without any patches are often used when the septal defects are not large enough to use a patch. There were 17 PFO patients, in whom either a CardioSEAL device (12 patients) or an Amplatzer closure device (5 patients) were used. The TSPs were successfully performed in 98% (44/45) of the patients. One patient had a wide GORE-TEX patch covering a significant area of the interatrial septum, leaving insufficient interatrial septal tissue to negotiate the transseptal needle through the septum. A prolonged attempt at safely crossing the interatrial septum through the GORE-TEX patch was not successful. No complications related to the transseptal puncture were reported. Echocardiography

at 3 months revealed an interatrial communication in 2 (4.5%) patients, which resolved by the 12 months of follow-up. Thus, it seems safe to puncture through either the patches or the surrounding native interatrial septum (Figure 10.4).

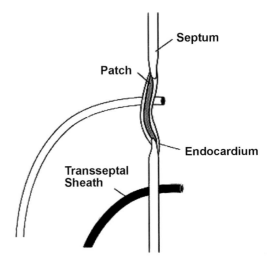

FIGURE 10.4   *Illustration of How a Transseptal Puncture Can Be Made through the Surgical Closure Patch or Native Interatrial Septum*

From Lakkireddy D, Rangisetty U, Prasad S, et al. Intracardiac echo guided radiofrequency catheter ablation of atrial fibrillation in patients with atrial septal defect or patent foramen ovale repair: a feasibility, safety, and efficacy study. *J Cardiovasc Electrophysiol* 2008;19:1137-1142. Reprinted with permission from John Wiley and Sons.

Similarly, Yamada et al reported 2 patients after direct suture closure of a congenital atrial septal defect who received transseptal procedures for catheter ablation of atrial fibrillation.[10] The procedures were guided by intracardiac echocardiography in 1 patient who underwent repeated procedures and by fluoroscopy in the other. In those 2 patients, the atrial transseptal procedure was feasible, and no residual iatrogenic shunts were observed, even after multiple procedures. This is consistent with Lakkireddy et al,[9] which included 4 patients with direct closure without any significant residual shunts. The problem with TSP in patients post direct suture closures of an ASD is that the membranous portion of the septum is often nonexistent, and a jump of the needle position will not be clear when one pulls down from the superior vena cava into the atrium. Ancillary imaging using ICE or TEE can be immensely helpful in such cases.

Although the aforementioned studies included only limited numbers of patients, the results consistently showed that the prosthetic materials do not pose a higher risk for complications or post-procedural new shunts.

Difficult Penetration of the Needle Due to IntraAtrial Patches

Schneider et al reported 2 children with progressively thickened autologous pericardial patches.[11] A specially sharpened transseptal needle was used to cut into the surface of the patch and reduce the force required during the perforation. Some force was required to perforate the patch by the needle, but it was not possible to advance the dilator of the long sheath over the needle into the left atrium due to the thickening of the interatrial septum. A cutting balloon was used to dilate the orifice and help the long sheath pass (Figure 10.5). Lakkireddy et al[9] reported that prosthetic materials like Dacron can easily be punctured in order to achieve transseptal access. GORE-TEX is a harder material to penetrate. Calcification of the surgical patch can make transseptal puncture arduous, and it carries the risk of embolization of calcified material. In such cases, application of the

electrocautery to the transseptal needle can be used to facilitate penetration into the left atrium.

Anatomical Variations Leading to Challenging TSP

Some unusual anatomical variations are more commonly seen in practice than complex congenital heart disease. These variations include thickened or fibrotic septum, atrial septal aneurysm (ASA), enlarged left or right atrium, and dilated aorta. The methods used for TSP for each of these anatomical variations are discussed next.

Atrial Septal Occluder

Using only fluoroscopic guidance, 3 cases of TSP through an ASD occluder were reported.[12,13] A 52-year-old female received a transseptal left ventricular assist device because of cardiogenic shock 4 days after multivessel stenting and closure of a PFO with a 25-mm Amplatzer occluder.[12] The transseptal puncture was performed at the lower rim of the occluder easily and without any complications (Figure 10.6). Zaker-Shahrak et al reported 2 transseptal punctures for catheter ablation of atrial fibrillation 6 to 7 months after a percutaneous closure of a foramen ovale with the Amplatzer occluders.[13] One of the sizes was 25 mm, and the other, 35 mm. Rather than complicating or preventing a safe transseptal puncture to access the left atrium, the PFO occluder provided a handy marker. Usually, there was a safe area of thin septum primum used for the puncture right below the caudal rim of the device. Both reports suggested that the TSP was safe, at least with the Amplatzer occluder. Recently,

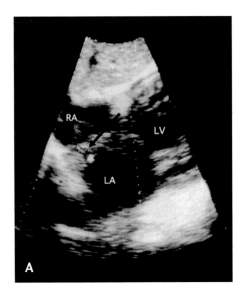
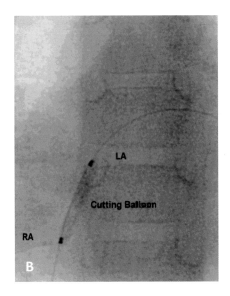

FIGURE 10.5   *Transseptal Approach in Children After Patch Occlusion of Atrial Septal Defect*
A child with a supracardiac total anomalous pulmonary venous drainage to the innominate vein received an atrial septal defect repair using an autologous pericardial patch. The transseptal puncture was performed to achieve left atrial access for a balloon dilation of an occluded left superior pulmonary vein. **A.** Progressive thickening of the patch was noted; the thickening made it difficult for the transseptal needle to penetrate the septum. A special sharpened needle was used to penetrate the septum with strong force. Due to the thickening, however, the sheath could not be passed. Dilation of the thickened interatrial patch was performed with a cutting balloon after the transseptal puncture. A residual shunt was noted after the procedure. **B.** Dilation of the thickened interatrial patch with the cutting balloon. RA = right atrium; LA = left atrium; LV = left ventricle. From Schneider MB, Zartner PA, Magee AG. Transseptal approach in children after patch occlusion of atrial septal defect: first experience with the cutting balloon. *Catheter Cardiovasc Interv* 1999;48:378-381. Reprinted with permission from John Wiley and Sons.

using ICE guidance, transseptal procedures in 23 patients (18 CardioSEAL and 5 Amplatzer closure devices) were reported.[9] Most of the ASD or PFO closure devices typically occluded the anterosuperior aspect of the interatrial septum, leaving behind a wide posteroinferior area for safe transseptal access. Similar to the previous report, among those with closure devices, the left atrium was accessed through a septal puncture in the periphery of the device inferoposteriorly (Figure 10.7). The 12-month follow-up revealed no occluder dysfunction or left-to-right shunts.

Atrial Septal Aneurysm

An atrial septal aneurysm (ASA) is an intrinsically thin-walled and saclike protrusion involving the fossa ovalis, which may be potentially problematic during the TSP. First, an ASA may either increase the difficulty in securing a transseptal access or prevent the selection of an optimal puncture site. Second, a localized thrombus within the ASA might increase the risk of an embolic event during the TSP. Third, as reported by Shalganov et al,[14] intracardiac echocardiography revealed a small fossa ovalis abutting against an enlarged aorta anteriorly. A very small

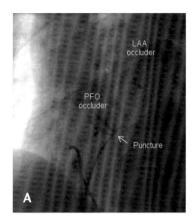
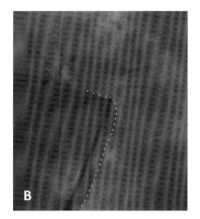

FIGURE 10.6   *Transseptal Puncture for Catheter Ablation of Atrial Fibrillation*
After Device Closure of Patent Foramen Ovale

A. Left anterior oblique projection depicting a PFO occluder in profile. The transseptal puncture (arrow) is performed just caudal to the occluder. **B.** Safe zone (dotted line) for the transseptal puncture caudal to a 25-mm Amplatzer occluder. Tenting of the thin septum primum was delineated by contrast medium injection into the right atrium in the left anterior oblique projection. LAA = left atrial appendage; PFO = patent foramen ovale. From Zaker-Shahrak R, Fuhrer J, Meier B. Transseptal puncture for catheter ablation of atrial fibrillation after device closure of patent foramen ovale. *Catheter Cardiovasc Interv* 2008;71:551-552. Reprinted with permission from John Wiley and Sons.

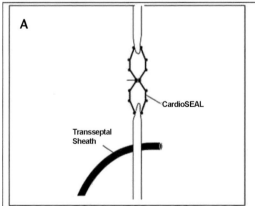
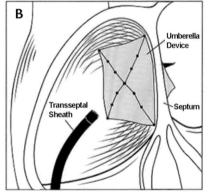

FIGURE 10.7   *A Cross Section of the Interatrial Septum Showing the Transseptal Sheath*
Inferior and Posterior to the Closure Device

A. The transspetal sheath is inferior to the closure device. **B.** The transseptal sheath is posterior to the closure device. From Lakkireddy D, Rangisetty U, Prasad S, et al. Intracardiac echo guided radiofrequency catheter ablation of atrial fibrillation in patients with atrial septal defect or patent foramen ovale repair: a feasibility, safety, and efficacy study. *J Cardiovasc Electrophysiol* 2008;19:1137-1142. Reprinted with permission from John Wiley and Sons.

distance from the interatrial septum to the left atrial free wall was seen. The latter 2 conditions predisposed to complications during the transseptal puncture. According to the fluoroscopy, the transseptal needle was correctly positioned, but the intracardiac echo image showed that it was actually pointing toward the aortic root, and, most importantly, it was virtually impossible to stabilize it in the fossa itself (Figure 10.8). The transseptal puncture was aborted.

By contrast, TSPs were performed successfully for mitral balloon valvotomy in 4 reported cases.[15-17] Fluoroscopy and right atrial angiography were used in 2 patients, and intraprocedural transesophageal echocardiography was used in the remaining 2 patients. The transseptal sites in 2 cases were within the ASA, and within the border of the ASA in another 2 cases (both transseptal sites were superior to the ASA). No cardiac ruptures, cardiac tamponades, aortic punctures, or strokes were reported. A left-to-right shunt was noted in only 1 patient, in whom the TSP was via the inner zone of the ASA, and the shunt was no longer evident after 10 weeks of follow-up.

Bidart et al reported on TSP using radiofrequency current delivery via a transseptal needle in order to facilitate the puncture using fluoroscopic guidance as well as ICE imaging[18]; 2 of 5 patients had an ASA. No short-term sequelae from the transseptal access using the radiofrequency (RF) current was noted. However, 3 patients had a left-to-right shunt after the procedure. The

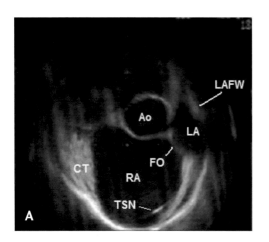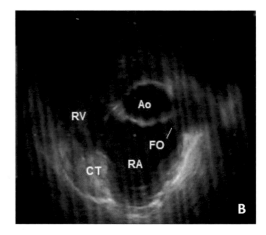

FIGURE 10.8   *Preventing Complicated Transseptal Puncture with Intracardiac Echocardiography*
A. An intracardiac echocardiography (ICE) image during atrial diastole before the jump of the transseptal needle into the oval fossa. In this patient the left atrial (LA) cavity had a crescent-like shape at that time point of the cardiac cycle. **B.** An ICE image during atrial systole before the jump of the transseptal needle into the oval fossa. The LA cavity is virtually missing at this time point of the cardiac cycle. Ao = noncoronary sinus of the aorta; CT = terminal crest; FO = fossa ovalis; ICE = intracardiac echocardiography; LA = left atrium; LAFW = left atrial free wall; RA = right atrium; RV = right ventricle; TSN = transseptal needle.
From Shalganov TN, Paprika D, Borbás S, et al. Preventing complicated transseptal puncture with intracardiac echocardiography: case report. *Cardiovasc Ultrasound* 2005;3:5. This work is licensed under the Creative Commons Attribution 2.0 Generic License. To view a copy of this license, visit http://creativecommons.org/licenses/by/2.0/ or send a letter to Creative Commons, 171 Second Street, Suite 300, San Francisco, California, 94105, USA.

TSP in patients with an ASA needs to be individualized, and the variable size of the aneurysm may have a differing influence on the risk. The prevalence of a patent foramen ovale is higher in the presence of an ASA, and ranges from 33% to 70%, which makes the trans-PFO method clinically relevant. Using the foramen ovale as the access to the left atrium might provide an alternative that can avoid complications in patients with ASA.

Thick or Fibrotic Septum

In spite of increasing operator experience and better visualization when performing transseptal catheterizations, there are several clinical settings in which crossing the septum remains very difficult. These include patients undergoing repeat transseptal accesses and patients with cardiac surgical repairs involving the interatrial septum. Repeat left atrial procedures are required in 26% of cases after catheter ablation of paroxysmal atrial fibrillation and in 30% to 50% after catheter ablation of persistent atrial fibrillation.[19] Marcus et al reported 16 patients undergoing repeat transseptal procedures.[20] Of the 4 patients in whom the first procedure was performed with an ablation catheter across a PFO, 3 required a transseptal puncture for their repeat procedure because the PFO closed after the catheter ablation. The remaining 12 patients underwent a transseptal puncture without any difficulty during their first procedure, and, despite the same operators performing the procedure in each patient, the repeat transseptal procedure was noted to be difficult in 5 of the procedures. Potential mechanisms were proposed to explain the more difficult second transseptal procedures and the PFO closures. First, a series of ablation applications over the septum, especially in the area of the PFO resulted in sufficient scarring to close the PFO. Second, simple catheter manipulation across the transseptal puncture site over an extended period of time might have produced enough irritation to cause inflammation and chronic scarring (Figure 10.9). Similarly, our previous report also supported the observation that repeat transseptal catheterizations after AF ablation are more difficult than the first transseptal procedure (Figure 10.10).[21] Part of these issues might be overcome by changing the needle curve from a small-curve to a large-curve design, resulting in increasing structural support and allowing more pressure to be delivered to the needle tip. RF current delivery to the septum using the needle as the ablation device facilitated the transseptal access (Figure 10.11).[18,22]

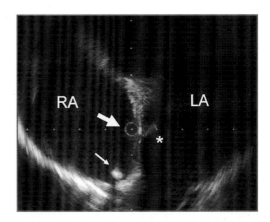

FIGURE 10.9   *Intracardiac Echocardiogram of Thinnest Aspect of the Interatrial Septum in a Patient 517 Days After a Transseptal Puncture*

The intracardiac echocardiography (ICE) catheter (large arrow) and an electrode catheter recording the His-bundle electrogram (small arrow) are positioned in the right atrium. Due to significant scarring at the previous transseptal site (*), a second attempt at a transseptal puncture was unsuccessful. From Marcus GM, Ren X, Tseng ZH, et al. Repeat transseptal catheterization after ablation for atrial fibrillation. *J Cardiovasc Electrophysiol* 2007;18:55-59. Reprinted with permission from John Wiley and Sons.

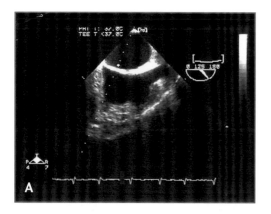

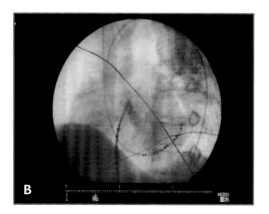

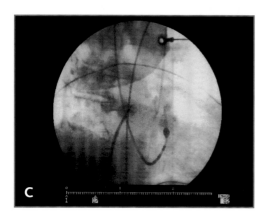

FIGURE 10.10   *A Resistant Transseptal Puncture Due to a Thick Interatrial Septum*

A. Transesophageal echocardiography revealed a thick interatrial septum. **B.** Staining of the interatrial septum and bowing of the transseptal apparatus in left anterior oblique view. **C.** Right anterior oblique view.

This was used when the needle force alone could not achieve the puncture because of fibrosis or increased compliance of the septum. The transmission of the radiofrequency energy from the ablation catheter up to the tip of the transseptal needle provides an easy and safe method for piercing the fossa ovalis when the conventional approach fails due to a resistant septum. However, RF puncture of the aorta, for instance, is a devastating complication that could occur if direct visualization is not used. The potential long-term impact of this procedure on the interatrial septum is unknown at this point. There are concerns regarding the long-term impact, including the possibility of persistent iatrogenic atrial septal defects or, conversely, greater fibrosis and scarring as a result of the application of RF current, making further access to the LA even more difficult in the future.

Abnormal Atrium or Aorta

A number of conditions, such as a very small or large left atrium, a large dilated aortic root, a large coronary sinus with a left-sided superior vena cava, cardiac malposition, and thoracic spine deformities, need extra attention during the TSP in order to avoid any complications. In patients with a dilated aorta and in those with a bulging LA, the fossa ovalis can be located more superiorly or inferiorly, respectively. The large, dilated, and usually tense left atrium produces a marked convex bulging of the interatrial septum into the right atrium (Figure 10.12).[23] It is very difficult to position the needle at the center of the interatrial septum. The tendency is for the needle tip to slide either anteriorly into a newly created aorto-atrial septal groove or far posteriorly into a posterior right atrium-septal groove. Similarly, a very large dilated aortic root (for example, in Marfan's syndrome) may exaggerate the aorto-septal groove and

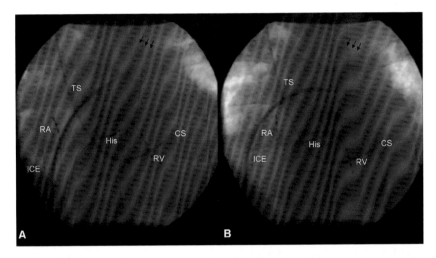

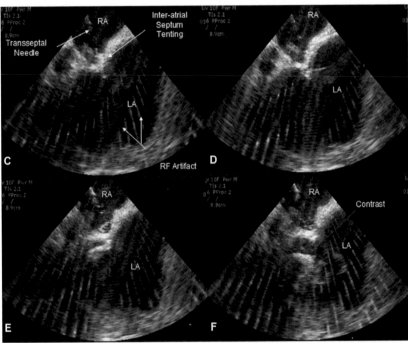

FIGURE 10.11   *Transseptal Catheterization Using Radiofrequency*

A. The left anterior oblique view of the catheter and transseptal apparatus seen fluoroscopically before the transseptal puncture. **B.** The panels show the "bowing" of the transseptal apparatus due to resistance at the level of the fossa, which made the needle unable to puncture the septum at that location. The transseptal needle was located in the fossa (confirmed by intracardiac echocardiography [ICE]). The arrows point to the location of the left main stem bronchus. **C-F.** ICE images of the transseptal catheterization using electrocautery. Images show progression from the initiation of the radiofrequency energy until the puncture through the interatrial septum. CS = coronary sinus catheter; His = His-monitoring catheter; LA = left atrium; RA = right atrial catheter (A and B); RA = right atrium (C-F); RV = right ventricular catheter; TS = transseptal sheath and needle. From Bidart C, Vaseghi M, Cesario DA, et al. Radiofrequency current delivery via transseptal needle to facilitate septal puncture. *Heart Rhythm* 2007;4:1573-1576. Reprinted with permission from Elsevier.

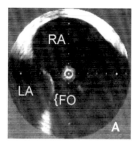 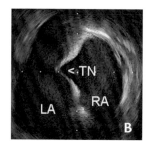

FIGURE 10.12 *Transseptal Puncture during Percutaneous Transvenous Mitral Commissurotomy in Patients with Distorted Anatomy of the Fossa Ovalis*

A 75-year-old woman with a long history of rheumatic and ischemic heart disease underwent a transseptal puncture for a percutaneous transvenous mitral commissurotomy. **A.** The positioning of the transseptal needle becomes difficult due to the fossa ovalis protruding into the right atrium secondary to left atrial dilation and elevated left atrial pressure. **B.** Under intracardiac echocardiographic (ICE) guidance, the transseptal needle was directed into the fossa ovalis with tenting. Thereafter, the transseptal needle was advanced smoothly. FO = fossa ovalis; LA = left atrium; RA = right atrium; TN = transseptal needle. From Cafri C, de la Guardia B, Barasch E, et al. Transseptal puncture guided by intracardiac echocardiography during percutaneous transvenous mitral commissurotomy in patients with distorted anatomy of the fossa ovalis. *Catheter Cardiovasc Interv* 2000;50:463-467. Reprinted with permission from John Wiley and Sons.

lead to an unstable needle and a higher risk of aortic puncture. The use of a large-curve needle might help to stabilize the needle. However, auxiliary images should be used to avoid puncturing the aorta or the free wall of the left atrium. In case of a small left atrium, the operator should pay special attention to use less force while advancing the needle, in order to decrease the possibility of puncturing

through the posterior wall. The use of radio-frequency energy may help to penetrate the septum with less force.

The problem with a giant right atrium is that the needle cannot be positioned on the septum due to the long distance between the inferior vena cava and interatrial septum. A large-curve needle, in which the curve may sometimes need to be modified by the opera-

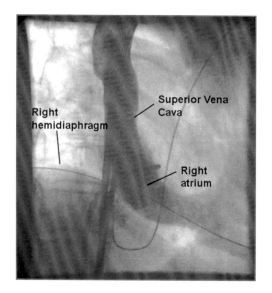

FIGURE 10.13   *Right Atrial Angiography Facilitates Transseptal Puncture for Complex Ablation in Patients with Unusual Anatomy*

In a patient in whom the target fossa ovalis area was not apparent during manipulation of the transseptal sheath, right atrial (RA) angiography revealed markedly reduced RA dimensions and enabled the safe identification of the puncture site. With kind permission from Springer Science+Business Media: *Journal of Interventional Cardiac Electrophysiology,* Right atrial angiography facilitates transseptal puncture for complex ablation in patients with unusual anatomy, 17, 2006, 29-34, Rogers DP, Lambiase PD, Dhinoja M, et al.

tor in order to match the atrial size, may help overcome the problem. In such conditions, auxiliary imaging with ICE may be necessary to define the foramen ovale (Figure 10.13).[24]

Thoracic Deformity

With thoracic spine deformities, the anatomy may change accordingly, which could result in a higher risk of complications. For example, a complicated transseptal puncture was reported in a patient with straight back syndrome.[25] The left atrium has a "pancake-shaped" deformity, and the plane of the atrial septum becomes narrow and is curved due to the cardiac distortion (Figure 10.14). Therefore, the puncture needle cannot be accurately positioned and fixed on the fossa

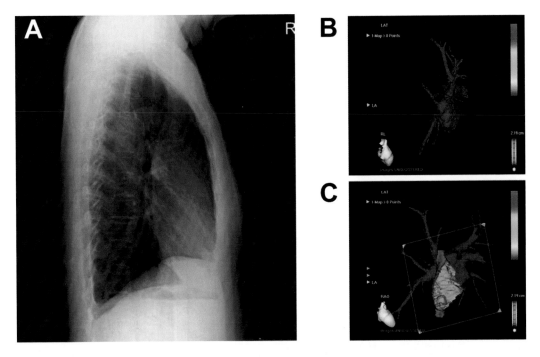

FIGURE 10.14   *Complicated Transseptal Puncture during Intervention Catheter Ablation on Atrial Fibrillation Concomitant with Straight Back Syndrome*

A patient with straight back syndrome who underwent a complicated transseptal puncture. The needle penetrated through the left atrial free wall due to cardiac distortion. Straight back syndrome is a thoracic deformity with the absence of upper thoracic spine kyphosis, heart compression, and a reduced anteroposterior diameter of the chest. **A.** Right lateral chest X-ray showing the straight thoracic spine and narrow antero-posterior diameter. **B.** A 64-slice contrast-enhanced computed tomography and 3-D reconstruction image showing a "pancake" deformity of the left atrium from the right lateral view. **C.** A clipping plane image and a right anterior oblique view, showing that the plane of the atrial septum for the puncture was narrow and curved. Note the clipped and exposed right atrium by the fictitious plane and the full manifestation of the position and configuration of the atrial septum. LA = left atrium; LAT = local activation time; RAO = right anterior oblique; RL = right lateral. With kind permission from Springer Science+Business Media: *Journal of Interventional Cardiac Electrophysiology*, Complicated transseptal puncture during intervention catheter ablation on atrial fibrillation concomitant with straight back syndrome, 19, 2007, 41-43, Tao H, Dong J, Yu R, Ma C.

ovalis. Furthermore, during TSP the atrial septum in straight back syndrome lies close to the posterior wall of the left atrium, and the orientation of the puncture needle becomes confusing. The aforementioned anomalies may contribute to a high likelihood of cardiac perforation and pericardial tamponade.

Alternative Venous Access— Left Femoral or Right Jugular Vein

When the left femoral vein is used, there will be a different bend in the transseptal needle, which will change the angle of the needle and could make it difficult to engage the transseptal needle on the interatrial septum. The difficulty can be overcome by bending, not twisting or rotating, the patient's thorax to his

or her right to 30° from the long axis, leaving the remainder of the trunk as straight as possible. This makes the interatrial septum more perpendicular to the tip of the needle and will facilitate engaging the needle and catheter on the interatrial septum. Another method is to modify the curve of the transseptal needle. A larger curve at a more proximal section of the needle may direct the needle more medially, allowing it to engage the septum. An unusual report described a TSP performed through the superior vena cava (superior approach). El-Said et al reported the superior approach of TSP in a Mustard repair patient due to a femoral vein occlusion.[7] The TSP needle was directed almost straight downwards, pointing toward the pulmonary venous atrium (Figure 10.15). No reports have been noted for a superior approach in a normal atrial septum. Although it does seem applicable, it is still an

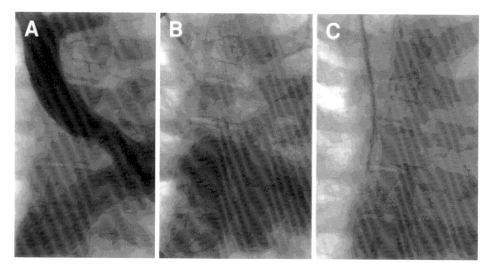

FIGURE 10.15   *Superior Approach in a Mustard Repair, Posteroanterior Projection*
A. Contrast-opacified superior and inferior limb of the baffle. **B.** Opacification of the left atrium during the levophase. **C.** The transseptal puncture needle is directed almost straight downwards, pointing toward the pulmonary venous atrium. From El-Said HG, Ing FF, Grifka RG, et al. 18-year experience with transseptal procedures through baffles, conduits, and other intra-atrial patches. *Catheter Cardiovasc Interv* 2000;50:434-439. Reprinted with permission from John Wiley and Sons.

undeveloped area. Possible contraindications and trouble-shooting for TSP are summarized in the following list and in Table 10.2.

Contraindications
of Transseptal Punctures

1. Left atrial tumor
2. Left atrial thrombus
3. Diffuse calcification of the interatrial septum or surgical patch
4. Uncooperative patient
5. Contraindication to anticoagulation, for example, bleeding tendency or intracranial bleed
6. Patients with active infections

Transseptal Puncture for Catheter Ablation of Atrial Fibrillation

AF ablation is increasingly performed in patients with complex anatomy and older age. We have found that the transseptal puncture site moves higher with the second procedure. In addition, because of a decreasing base-to-apex dimension, rightward shift, and dilation of the aortic root with age, the transseptal puncture site in the right anterior oblique view moves higher and more posteriorly, and the transseptal puncture angle in the left anterior oblique view decreases (Figure 10.16).[26] Crossing in the left atrium using a PFO will render catheter manipulation more difficult and should be discouraged.

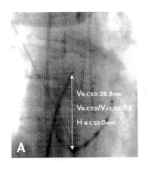
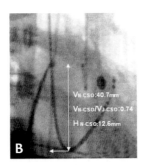
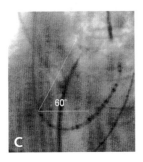
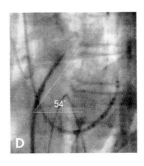

FIGURE 10.16 *Comparison of Transseptal Puncture Site by Age*

The older group exhibited a higher and more posterior successful transseptal puncture site (**B**) than did the younger group in the atrial end-diastolic phase (**A**). The angle of the puncture needle was smaller in the younger group (**D**) than in the older group (**C**). All parameters were measured during the atrial end-diastolic phase. In the 30° right anterior oblique (RAO) view, the definition of each parameter was (1) $V_{N\text{-}cso}$: the vertical distance between the transseptal puncture site and coronary artery ostium (CSO); (2) $H_{N\text{-}cso}$: the horizontal distance between the transseptal puncture site and CSO; (3) $V_{J\text{-}cso}$: the vertical distance between the superior vena cava-right atrial junction and CSO; (4) In the 60° left anterior oblique (LAO) view, the angle of the direction of the transseptal needle (N-angle) was measured as the angle between the direction of the needle at the puncture site and a horizontal line. From Hu YF, Tai CT, Lin YJ, et al. The change in the fluoroscopy-guided transseptal puncture site and difficult punctures in catheter ablation of recurrent atrial fibrillation. *Europace* 2008;10:276-279. Reprinted with permission from John Wiley and Sons.

TABLE 10.2

Trouble-Shooting

Problems	Causes
Difficult penetration of the septum	Thick, fibrotic, or calcified septum, artificial materials after a surgical repair
Difficult to pass the sheath	Thick or fibrotic septum, artificial materials after a surgical repair
Narrow space between the needle and left atrial free wall	Large atrial septal aneurysm, or small or flat left atrium
Difficult to localize the needle on the fossa ovalis	Giant right or left atrium, after a surgical repair, dilated aorta, or malformation of the fossa ovalis
Narrow window between the fossa ovalis and aorta	Dilated, and transverse aorta
Hard to engage the needle on the septum while accessing through the left femoral vein	Different bends in the transseptal needle between that through the right and left femoral veins will change the angle of the needle
Uncertain or unusual transseptal site	No jump due to an altered anatomy of the fossa ovalis and septum, for example after a surgical repair, heart rotation, or deformity of the chest
Damping left atrial pressure curve as both needle and catheter are advanced	The engagement of the needle tip on the posterior wall of the left atrium
Flat non-oscillating pressure curves from within what was apparently the left atrium	Thrombotic mass in the left atrium[25]
Wire can not be passed through IVC or right femoral vein	Femoral vein or inferior vena cava thrombosis or occlusion

Solution

Radiofrequency-assisted; excimer laser catheter; sharp and large curve needle

Pre-dilation with a dilator, standard angioplasty balloon, or cutting balloon; use of a support wire into LA; smaller sheath

Be cautious and apply less force while passing the needle; auxiliary images to define the space; access through a patent foramen ovale; radiofrequency-assisted puncture; steel wire for directional guiding

Large curve needle, ICE-assisted procedure

Auxiliary images to define the course of the aorta; large curve needle

Bending the patient's thorax to his or her right to 30°; change the curve of the transseptal needle manually

Confirm the atrial anatomy: venophase in the right atriography, ICE, or TEE
Confirm the puncture site: contrast tagging, continuous pressure monitor, ICE, or TEE

Withdraw the needle and catheter

Withdraw the needle and catheter; anticoagulation

Superior vena cava or left femoral vein access

Conclusion

Transseptal catheterization has become important because of the advances in interventional electrophysiology and interventional cardiology, where the technique is increasingly being applied in patients with altered anatomy. Transseptal catheterization can be safely performed even in the most complex anatomy by the use of a tailored puncture technique according to the anatomical variation. The use of additional imaging information to ascertain the needle position before performing the transseptal catheterization will ultimately make this a safer procedure.

References

1. De Ponti R, Cappato R, Curnis A, Della Bella P, Padeletti L, Raviele A, Santini M, Salerno-Uriarte JA. Trans-septal catheterization in the electrophysiology laboratory: data from a multicenter survey spanning 12 years. *J Am Coll Cardiol* 2006;47:1037-1042.

2. Knecht S, Wright M, Lellouche N, Nault I, Matsuo S, O'Neill MD, Lomas O, Delplagne A, Bordachar P, Sacher F, Derval N, Hocini M, Jaïs P, Clementy J, Roudaut R, Haïssaguerre M. Impact of a patent foramen ovale on paroxysmal atrial fibrillation ablation. *J Cardiovasc Electrophysiol* 2008;19:1236-1241.

3. Cheng A, Calkins H. A conservative approach to performing transseptal punctures without the use of intracardiac echocardiography: stepwise approach with real-time video clips. *J Cardiovasc Electrophysiol* 2007;18:686-689.

4. Ali Khan MA, Mullins CE, Bash SE, al Yousef S, Nihill MR, Sawyer W. Transseptal left heart catheterisation in infants, children, and young adults. *Cathet Cardiovasc Diagn* 1989;17:198-201.

5. Mullins CE. Transseptal left heart catheterization: experience with a new technique in 520 pediatric and adult patients. *Pediatr Cardiol* 1983;4:239-245.

6. Duff DF, Mullins CE. Transseptal left heart catheterization in infants and children. *Cathet Cardiovasc Diagn* 1978;4:213-223.

7. El-Said HG, Ing FF, Grifka RG, Nihill MR, Morris C, Getty-Houswright D, Mullins CE. 18-year experience with transseptal procedures through baffles, conduits, and other intra-atrial patches. *Catheter Cardiovasc Interv* 2000;50:434-439.

8. Perry JC, Boramanand NK, Ing FF. "Transseptal" technique through atrial baffles for 3-dimensional mapping and ablation of atrial tachycardia in patients with d-transposition of the great arteries. *J Interv Card Electrophysiol* 2003;9:365-369.

9. Lakkireddy D, Rangisetty U, Prasad S, Verma A, Biria M, Berenbom L, Pimentel R, Emert M, Rosamond T, Fahmy T, Patel D, Biase LD, Schweikert R, Burkhardt D, Natale A. Intracardiac echo guided radiofrequency catheter ablation of atrial fibrillation in patients with atrial septal defect or patent foramen ovale repair: a feasibility, safety, and efficacy study. *J Cardiovasc Electrophysiol* 2008;19:1137-1142.

10. Yamada T, McElderry HT, Muto M, Murakami Y, Kay GN. Pulmonary vein isolation in patients with paroxysmal atrial fibrillation after direct suture closure of congenital atrial septal defect. *Circ J* 2007;71:1989-1992.

11. Schneider MB, Zartner PA, Magee AG. Transseptal approach in children after patch occlusion of atrial septal defect: first experience with the cutting balloon. *Catheter Cardiovasc Interv* 1999;48:378-381.

12. Cook S, Meier B, Windecker S. Transseptal TandemHeart implantation through an Amplatzer atrial septal occluder. *J Invasive Cardiol* 2007;19:198-199.

13. Zaker-Shahrak R, Fuhrer J, Meier B. Transseptal puncture for catheter ablation of atrial fibrillation after device closure of patent foramen ovale. *Catheter Cardiovasc Interv* 2008;71:551-552.

14. Shalganov TN, Paprika D, Borbás S, Temesvári A, Szili-Török T. Preventing complicated transseptal puncture with intracardiac echocardiography: case report. *Cardiovasc Ultrasound* 2005;3:5.

15. Rittoo D, Sutherland GR, Shaw TR. Transseptal mitral balloon valvotomy in patients with atrial septal aneurysms. *Cardiology* 1997;88:300-304.

16. Lau KW, Ding ZP, Johan A. Percutaneous transseptal mitral valvuloplasty in the presence of atrial septal aneurysm. *Cathet Cardiovasc Diagn* 1994;31:337-340.

17. Yeh KH, Fu M, Wu CJ, Chua SO, Chen YC, Hung JS. Transseptal balloon mitral valvuloplasty in mitral stenosis with atrial septal aneurysm. *Am Heart J* 1993;126:474-475

18. Bidart C, Vaseghi M, Cesario DA, Mahajan A, Fujimura O, Boyle NG, Shivkumar K. Radiofrequency current delivery via transseptal needle to facilitate septal puncture. *Heart Rhythm* 2007;4:1573-1576.

19. Natale A, Raviele A, Arentz T, Calkins H, Chen SA, Haïssaguerre M, Hindricks G, Ho Y, Kuck KH, Marchlinski F, Napolitano C, Packer D, Pappone C, Prystowsky EN, Schilling R, Shah D, Themistoclakis S, Verma A. Venice Chart international consensus document on atrial fibrillation ablation. *J Cardiovasc Electrophysiol* 2007;18:560-580.

20. Marcus GM, Ren X, Tseng ZH, Badhwar N, Lee BK, Lee RJ, Foster E, Olgin JE. Repeat transseptal catheterization after ablation for atrial fibrillation. *J Cardiovasc Electrophysiol* 2007;18:55-59.

21. Hu YF, Tai CT, Lin YJ, Chang SL, Lo LW, Wongcharoen W, Udyavar AR, Tuan TC, Chen SA. The change in the fluoroscopy-guided transseptal puncture site and difficult punctures in catheter ablation of recurrent atrial fibrillation. *Europace* 2008;10:276-279.

22. Knecht S, Jaïs P, Nault I, Wright MJ, Matsuo S, Madaffari A, Lellouche N, Derval N, O'Neill MD, Deplagne A, Bordachar P, Sacher F, Hocini M, Clémenty J, Haïssaguerre M. Radiofrequency puncture of the fossa ovalis for resistant transseptal access. *Circ Arrhythm Electrophysiol* 2008; 1:169-174.

23. Cafri C, de la Guardia B, Barasch E, Brink J, Smalling RW. Transseptal puncture guided by intracardiac echocardiography during percutaneous transvenous mitral commissurotomy in patients with distorted anatomy of the fossa ovalis. *Catheter Cardiovasc Interv* 2000;50:463-467.

24. Rogers DP, Lambiase PD, Dhinoja M, Lowe MD, Chow AW. Right atrial angiography facilitates transseptal puncture for complex ablation in patients with unusual anatomy. *J Interv Card Electrophysiol* 2006;17:29-34.

25. Tao H, Dong J, Yu R, Ma C. Complicated transseptal puncture during intervention catheter ablation on atrial fibrillation concomitant with straight back syndrome. *J Interv Card Electrophysiol* 2007;19:41-43.

26. Hu YF, Tai CT, Lin YJ, Chang SL, Lo LW, Wongcharoen W, Udyavar AR, Tuan TC, Chen SA. Does the age affect the fluoroscopy-guided transseptal puncture in catheter ablation of atrial fibrillation? *Pacing Clin Electrophysiol* 2007; 30:1506-1510.

11

Transcatheter Atrial Septal Defect Device Closure

Sawsan M. Awad, Qi-Ling Cao, Ziyad M. Hijazi

Transcatheter closure of secundum atrial septal defects (ASD) has become an accepted alternative to surgical repair. With more advances in device manufacturing and the availability of a broad array of devices, decreasing complications and higher closure rates have been reported. In this chapter, we will discuss the technique of percutaneous ASD device closure and the commonly encountered complications and problems during the procedure.

Equipment

Performing interventional cardiac catheterization for congenital heart diseases (CHD), both in adults and children, requires well-trained cardiologists and a well-equipped

cardiac catheterization laboratory. Biplane fluoroscopy imaging is preferred, but not essential, for ASD device closure, as it allows the interventional cardiologist to have better assessment of the anatomy and location of the defect, and it minimizes the amount of contrast agent given during the procedure. All types of wires, catheters, balloons, retrieval catheters/snares, and devices (in an array of sizes) should be readily available in the catheterization laboratory that does this type of procedure. The use of the wrong-size device or a failed procedure or complication due to a lack of the proper equipment is unacceptable.

Atrial Septal Defect

Closure atrial septal defects (ASDs) represents a communication between the right and the left atria. Surgical repair of simple ASDs was among the first congenital cardiac abnormalities to be corrected. This became

Transseptal Catheterization and Interventions.
© 2010 Ranjan Thakur MD and Andrea Natale MD, eds.
Cardiotext Publishing, ISBN 978-0-9790164-1-7.

more common after the advent of cardio-pulmonary bypass. However, surgical correction entailed a small risk of morbidity and mortality. With the advent of closure devices that could be delivered via a catheter in the 1990s, non-surgical closure of these defects became possible.

Anatomical Defects

ASD accounts for approximately 19% of all CHD.[1] The ostium secundum defect is the most common type, and accounts for 60% to 70% of all ASDs and for 30% to 40% of all CHD in patients older than 40 years. This is the type of ASD that is amenable for percutaneous device closure. Another type, the ostium primum defect, accounts for 15% to 20% of ASDs, and a third type, the sinus venosus defect, is seen in 5% to 15% of ASD patients. The latter 2 types are not amenable for percutaneous closure using the currently available devices/techniques.

Procedure Indications

Indications for closure of secundum ASD are related to patient symptoms and the risks of having atrial level shunting. Patients with ASDs are usually asymptomatic in the first 2 decades of life. We believe the most important criterion of shunt significance is the presence of right ventricle volume overload as shown by transthoracic echocardiography. If the Qp:Qs ratio (pulmonary to systemic flow ratio) is more than 1.5:1, such patients may experience symptoms of shortness of breath and fatigue.[2] However, calculation of the Qp:Qs ratio is not required to judge the significance of the shunt and may have some flaws. The presence of left-to-right shunting across the defect will lead to the development of right ventricular volume overload and, later, right ventricular dysfunction, progres-

sive pulmonary vascular disease, and atrial dysrhythmias. In addition, patients with an atrial communication may be at risk of development of paradoxical embolus, leading to stroke, transient ischemic attack, or peripheral emboli.[2-4]

Contraindications for Transcatheter Device Closure

Only secundum type defects with appropriate rims are eligible for device closure. The presence of at least a 5-mm rim of tissue around the defect is needed to be able to anchor the device. The superior, inferior, and posterior rims are essential; however, absence of the anterior rim is not required when using the Amplatzer device. Size of the defect by itself does not constitute an indication or contraindication for device closure. However, one needs to be careful placing large devices that occupy the entire septum. We have placed devices in children that occupied the entire septum; as these patients grow in size, the device becomes smaller for that septum (personal observation).

Other types of ASDs are not appropriate for the currently available devices. These include sinus venosus defects (of the superior and inferior type) and ostium primum defects. Other contraindications for closure include the presence of active infection (within 1 month of closure) and the inability to take antiplatelet therapy.

Available Devices

The first successful transcatheter closure of a secundum ASD was performed by King and Mills in the early 1970s.[5] The devices currently approved by the U.S. Food and Drug Administration (FDA) for clinical use are the Amplatzer Septal Occluder (AGA Medical Corporation, Plymouth, MN), and the GORE HELEX Septal Occluder (W. L. Gore and Associates, Inc, Flagstaff, AZ).

Amplatzer Septal Occluder (ASO) devices provide good closure rates (97%) with comparable complication rates to open-heart surgery.[6,7] The GORE HELEX Septal Occluder consists of an expanded polytetra-fluoroethylene patch material with hydro-philic coating, supported by a nickel-titanium (nitinol) super-elastic wire frame in the shape of a coil. This device is not suitable for defects larger than 18 mm as sized by a balloon cath-eter.[8] Various modifications of the ASO have been reported, including the fenestrated ASO and the cribriform ASO devices for multi-fenestrated ASDs or ASDs with septal aneurysms.[9,10] There are other devices avail-able outside the United States for device clo-sure of secundum ASDs. These include the Occlutech Figulla device and its new gen-eration the Figulla Flex (Occlutech, Jena, Germany), the Cardia ATRIASEPT device (Cardia, Inc, Eagan, MN), and the Solysafe Septal Occluder (Swissimplant, Solothum, Switzerland). Figure 11.1 depicts some of the devices that are available both in and outside the United States.

Imaging During ASD Device Closure

In addition to fluoroscopic imaging, intracar-diac echocardiography (ICE) is the tool pre-ferred for guiding ASD closure in both adults and children[11]; however, due to the cost of the ICE catheters, many centers still use trans-esophageal echocardiography (TEE) to guide the closure procedure.

Operator Training

When embarking on a transcatheter closure of an ASD, it is imperative that the operator has very good experience and is versed in all aspects of interventional cardiology and that the laboratory is equipped with all types of catheters, snares, and delivery sheaths and has a surgical team in-house for bailout situa-tions. When the devices were approved in the early 2000s, the manufacturer, along with the FDA, required operators to be trained (proc-tored) on the use of these devices. Training is supervised by the manufacturer and involves didactic lectures, simulation, and live cases. For more information on training require-ments, the reader can visit the Web site of any of the manufacturers.

Closure Protocol

The procedure is performed under con-scious sedation with the use of continuous ICE imaging for guidance. Vascular access is usually through the right femoral vein. For patients >35 kg in weight, the right femoral vein is accessed via 2 separate punctures, a few millimeters apart, 1 for the delivery sys-tem and 1 for the 8 F ICE catheter. Rou-tine right and left heart catheterization is performed, followed by assessment of the degree of left-to-right shunt. Full assessment of the defect, surrounding rims, and remain-ing cardiac structures should be performed prior to device insertion (Figures 11.2 and 11.5). Heparin is administered routinely in all patients to achieve activated clotting time (ACT) >200 seconds at the time of device deployment. Angiography is performed in the right upper pulmonary vein in the hepa-toclavicular projection to assess the size and location of the defect. This step is an optional one. We usually do this in our laboratory, and use this angiogram as a road map when we deploy the device. Selection of the device size is performed according to the "stop flow" diameter of the defect (Figures 11.3a, 11.6a). This is performed under echocardiography with color Doppler. The balloon is inflated across the defect until there is cessation of

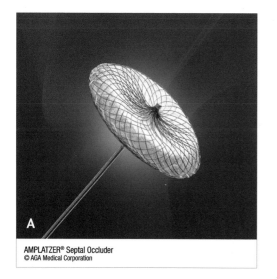

AMPLATZER® Septal Occluder
© AGA Medical Corporation

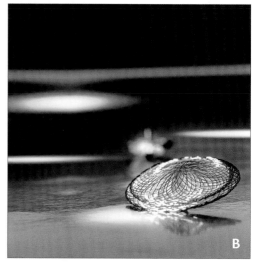

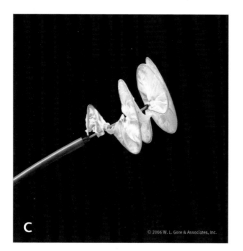

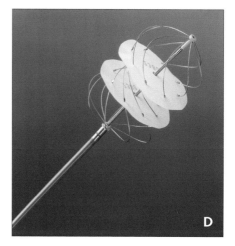

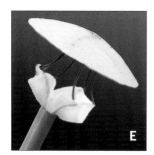

FIGURE 11.1   *Most Frequently Used Transcatheter Closure*
Devices for Secundum Atrial Septal Defects,
in the United States (US) and Outside the United States (OUS)
A. Amplatzer Septal Occluder (available in US and OUS). Courtesy of AGA
Medical Corporation. **B.** Occlutech Figulla Flex ASD Occluder (available
only OUS). Courtesy of Occlutech. **C.** GORE HELEX Septal Occluder
(available both US and OUS). Courtesy of W. L Gore & Associates.
D. Solysafe Septal Occluder (available OUS). Courtesy of Swissimplant.
E. Cardia ATRIASEPT device (available OUS). Courtesy of Cardia, Inc.

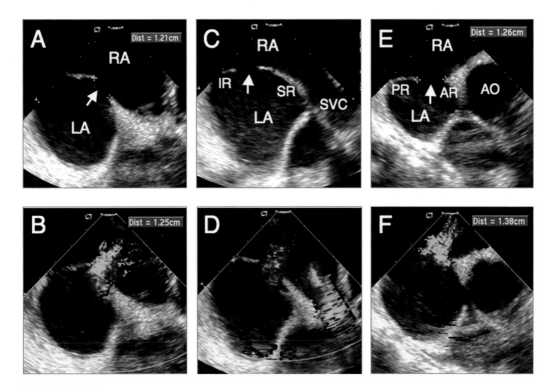

FIGURE 11.2   *Intracardiac Echocardiographic Images of Patient with Secundum Atrial Septal Defect*

These intracardiac echocardiographic (ICE) images were obtained during assessment for device suitability. **A, B.** Septal view without and with color Doppler showing moderate size atrial septal defect measuring 12.5 mm (arrow) with left-to-right shunt. **C, D.** Caval view without and with color Doppler showing the defect (arrow), superior rim (SR) and inferior rim (IR). **E, F.** Short-axis view without and with color Doppler showing the defect (arrow), anterior rim (AR), and posterior rim (PR). AO = aorta; LA = left atrium; RA = right atrium; SVC = superior vena cava.

shunt. Once there is cessation of shunt, a freeze-frame by echocardiography (Figures 11.3a, 11.6a) and cine-fluoroscopy (Figures 11.4b, 11.7b) is performed to measure the size of the balloon. For the ASO, a device no more than 2 mm larger than this diameter is chosen for closure, and for the GORE HELEX, a ratio of 1.7-2X this size is chosen. Balloon sizing in our center is optional. We usually use a device 25% to 30% larger than the 2-D diameter by ICE for the ASO device.

A long, proper size delivery sheath (AGA Medical Corporation, Plymouth, MN) is then introduced over an exchange guidewire into the left upper pulmonary vein. The delivery cable is passed through the loader, and the proper size device is screwed clockwise into the tip of the delivery cable. The device and the loader are immersed in saline as the ASO device is pulled into the loader. The loader is introduced into the delivery sheath, and without rotation, the device is advanced into the left atrium (LA). The sheath is retracted until the left atrial disc is opened in the middle of the LA. The sheath with the delivery cable in it is pulled back as a single unit close to the left atrial side of the septum. The sheath is retracted further until the waist and part of the right atrial disc are deployed very close to the left atrial side of the septum. With further

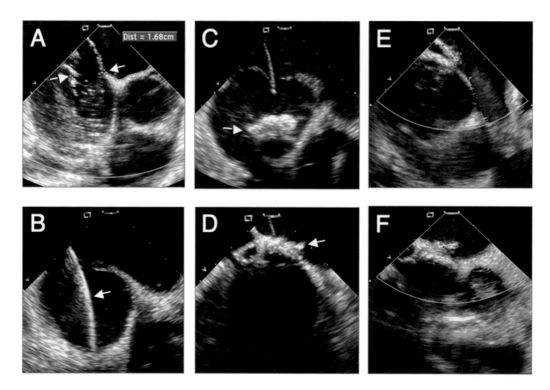

FIGURE 11.3   *Intracardiac Echocardiographic Images During Deployment*
of a 25-mm GORE HELEX Device for the Patient in Figure 11.2

A. Intracardiac echocardiographic (ICE) image during balloon sizing demonstrating the "stop flow" diameter (arrows), measuring 16.8 mm. **B.** ICE image showing the delivery sheath (arrow) through the defect into the left upper pulmonary vein. **C.** ICE image after the left atrial desk (arrow) was deployed in the mid-left atrium. **D.** ICE image during deployment of the right atrial desk (arrow) in right atrial side of the septum. **E.** ICE image in caval view after the device was released showing good device position. **F.** ICE image in short-axis view after the device was released showing good device position.

retraction of the sheath while maintaining constant tension on the delivery sheath and cable, the right atrial disc is deployed in the right atrium. To confirm correct placement, the delivery cable still attached to the device is pushed forward and pulled backward ("Minnesota Wiggle"),[12] ie, correct placement will be manifested by stable device position. ICE also is used to visualize both discs on their respective sides. If there is device misplacement, the device can be retracted back inside the delivery sheath, and the steps are repeated. The device and adjacent structures are then examined by ICE to ensure

that there has been no encroachment of the device on the atrioventricular valves or on the right pulmonary veins. Once proper device position is confirmed, the device is released by turning the cable counterclockwise using the pin vise. Assessment of device position and residual shunt is performed using ICE. Figures 11.6 and 11.7 demonstrate various steps of device deployment in a patient with secundum ASD by ICE and cine-fluoroscopy using the ASO device for closure. Figures 11.3 and 11.4 demonstrate various steps of device deployment in a patient with secundum ASD by ICE and cine-fluoroscopy using

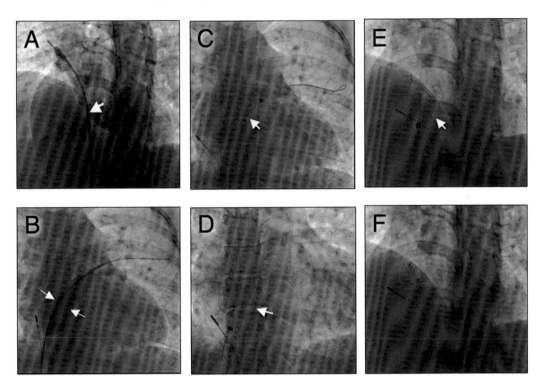

FIGURE 11.4   *Cine-fluoroscopic Images During Device Deployment*
A. Angiogram in the hepatoclavicular view showing left-to-right shunt via the defect (arrow). **B.** Image in frontal projection showing the sizing balloon and the "stop flow" diameter (arrows). **C.** Image of the delivery sheath (arrow) over a guidewire positioned in the left upper pulmonary vein. **D.** Image in frontal projection of the left atrial desk (arrow) during deployment in the mid-left atrium. **E.** Hepatoclavicular projection showing the right atrial disk (arrow) prior to device release. **F.** Hepato-clavicular view after release. Device is parallel to the septum. (Compare with image **A.**)

the GORE HELEX device. Hemostasis is assured, and the patient recovers overnight at the hospital. Ancef (1 gram) is given intravenously during the procedure, and 2 doses, 8 hours apart, are given in the hospital. The following day, an electrocardiogram and a transthoracic color Doppler echocardiogram (TTE) are performed prior to discharge.

Technical Tips/Tricks
During ASD Device Closure

1. Extreme care must be exercised not to allow passage of air inside the delivery sheath. An alternative technique to minimize air embolism is passage of the sheath with the dilator over the wire until the tip of the sheath is in the inferior vena cava. Then the dilator is removed, and the sheath is advanced over the wire into the left atrium while continuously flushing the side arm of the sheath.

2. Be alert for "cobra-head" formation, when the left disk maintains a high profile when deployed, mimicking a cobra head. This can occur if the left disk is opened in the pulmonary vein or left atrial appendage, or if the LA is too small

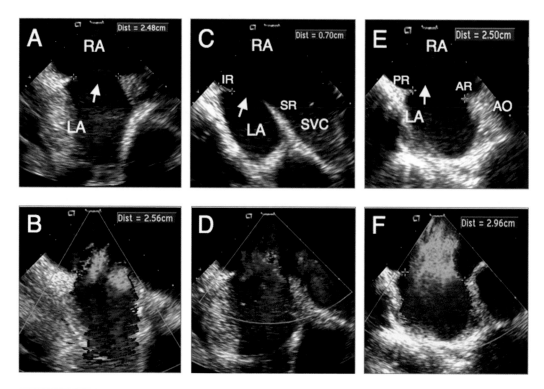

FIGURE 11.5   *Intracardiac Echocardiographic Images of a Patient*
with Secundum Atrial Septal Defect Measuring about 24mm to 26mm

These images were obtained during assessment for device suitability. **A, B.** Septal view without and with color Doppler showing large-size ASD measuring 24mm to 26mm (arrow) with left-to-right shunt. **C, D.** Caval view without and with color Doppler showing the defect (arrow), superior rim (SR), and inferior rim (IR). **E, F.** Short-axis view without and with color Doppler showing the defect (arrow), anterior rim (AR), and posterior rim (PR). In this view the defect by color measures 29.6 mm. AO = aorta; LA = left atrium; RA = right atrium; SVC = superior vena cava.

to accommodate the device size. It can also occur if the device is defective or if the device has been loaded with unusual strain on it. Should the formation occur, check the site of deployment, and, if appropriate, recapture the device, remove it, and inspect it. If the cobra head forms outside the body, use a different device. If the disk forms normally, try deploying the device again. Do not release a device that has a cobra head appearance to the left disk. Figure 11.8 is a photograph of a cobra head formation of the Amplatzer device.

3. If using a device with a prominent eustachian valve, avoid the possibility of cable entrapment during release by advancing the sheath to the hub of the right disk, so that when the cable is released it will be inside the sheath. Hence, there will be no chance of entrapment in the eustachian valve.

4. A large ASD defect (>25 mm by 2-D ICE in the adult patient), especially when associated with deficient rims, is still challenging. When deploying the left atrial disk in such circumstances, the disk often becomes perpendicular to the atrial sep-

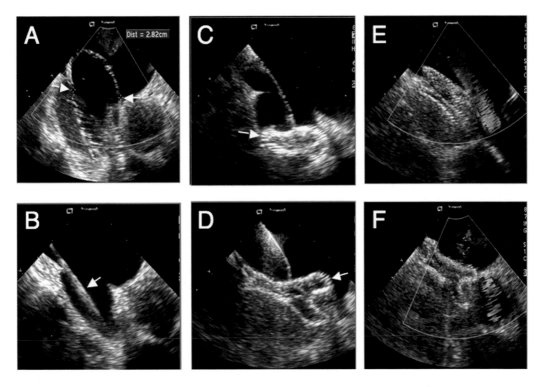

FIGURE 11.6   *Intracardiac Echocardiographic Images During Deployment of a 30-mm Amplatzer Septal Occluder (ASO) for the Patient in Figure 11.4*

A. ICE image during balloon sizing demonstrating the "stop flow" diameter (arrows), measuring 28.2 mm. **B.** ICE image showing the delivery sheath (arrow) through the defect into the left upper pulmonary vein. **C.** ICE image after the left atrial desk (arrow) was deployed in the mid-left atrium. **D.** ICE image during deployment of the right atrial desk (arrow) in right atrial side of the septum. **E.** ICE image in caval view after the device was released showing good device position and no obstruction to superior vena cava flow. **F.** ICE image in short-axis view after the device was released showing good device position.

tum, resulting in prolapse into the right atrium. There are several techniques that can be used to overcome such difficulties in aligning the left atrial disk to be parallel to the atrial septum that will result in a successful procedure.[13]

    i. *The Hausdorf sheath* (Cook, Inc, Bloomington, IN) *technique.* This technique involves a specially designed long sheath with two curves at its end. The two posterior curves help align the left disk parallel to the septum. This sheath is available in sizes 10 F to 12 F. Under fluoroscopic

and echocardiographic guidance, if the initial deployment of the left disk is not ideal, counterclockwise rotation of the sheath will orient the tip posterior, and further deployment of the left disk will be parallel to the septum.

    ii. *Right upper pulmonary vein technique.* This technique is only recommended in large patients. The delivery sheath is carefully positioned in the right upper pulmonary vein, the device is advanced to the tip of the sheath, and then the left disk is partially deployed in the right upper

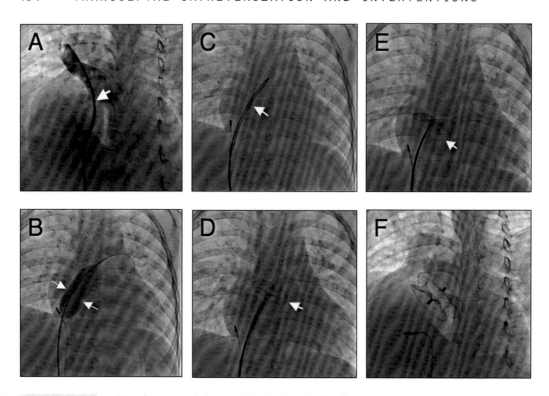

FIGURE 11.7   *Cine-fluoroscopic Images During Device Deployment*
A. Angiogram in the hepatoclavicular view showing left-to-right shunt via the defect (arrow). **B.** Image in frontal projection showing the sizing balloon and the "stop flow" diameter (arrows). **C.** Image of the delivery sheath (arrow) in the mid-left atrium. **D.** Image in frontal projection of the left atrial desk (arrow) during deployment in the mid-left atrium. **E.** Frontal projection showing the right atrial desk (arrow) prior to device release. **F.** Hepatoclavicular projection showing the 2 disks are parallel to the septum. (Compare with image **A.**)

pulmonary vein. The sheath is quickly retracted to deploy the remainder of the left disk; this will result in the disk jumping from that location to be parallel to the atrial septum. Quick and successive deployment of both the connecting waist and the right disk is carried out before the sheath may change its position or prior to the left disk prolapsing through the defect to the right atrium.

    iii. *Left upper pulmonary vein technique.* This technique can be used in children as well as in adults. The delivery sheath is carefully posi-

tioned in the left upper pulmonary vein. The device is advanced to the tip of the sheath, and the left disk is then deployed inside the vein. Deployment of the waist and right disk is continued to create an "American football" appearance within the vein. As the sheath reaches the right atrium, the left disk disengages from the pulmonary vein, and the disk jumps to be parallel to the atrial septum. Continuous retraction of the sheath over the cable with pulling of the entire assembly toward the right atrium will result in parallel alignment of the left disk to the septum.

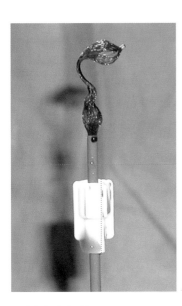

FIGURE 11.8   *Amplatzer Device Removed from a Patient After It Formed a "Cobra Head"*

The device was recaptured and tested outside the body, and it still formed the cobra head. The patient received another device.

iv. *Dilator assisted technique.*[14] After deployment of the left disk, a long dilator (usually of the delivery sheath being used) is advanced into the left atrium by an assistant to hold the superior-anterior part of the left disk, preventing it from prolapsing into the right atrium. At the same time, the operator continues to deploy the waist and right disk in their respective locations. Once the right disk is deployed in the right atrium, the assistant withdraws the dilator back to the right atrium.

v. *Balloon assisted technique.* Dalvi et al[15] reported a balloon-assisted technique to facilitate device closure of large ASDs and to prevent prolapse of the left disk into the right atrium. In essence, it is similar in concept to the dilator technique. During device deployment, they used a balloon catheter to support the left disk of the ASO device, preventing its prolapse into the right atrium.

vi. *Right coronary Judkins guide catheter technique.* This technique is used only if the device size is < 16 mm. An 8 F delivery sheath is positioned in the left atrium. The device is then pre-loaded inside the 8 F Judkins coronary guide catheter (inner lumen 0.098 inch). The entire assembly (device/cable/guide catheter) is then advanced inside the delivery sheath until the catheter reaches the tip of the sheath. The sheath is brought back to the inferior vena cava, keeping the coronary catheter in the left atrium. Due to the curve of the catheter, once the left disk is deployed in the left atrium, counterclockwise rotation of the guide catheter will result in alignment of the left disk to be parallel to the septum. Deployment of the waist and right disk in their respective locations is continued. We found this technique to be of help in small children.

5. The need to perform transseptal left heart catheterization may arise in those patients who had ASD repaired surgically or using one of the available devices (Amplatzer, GORE HELEX, etc). Patients who had surgical repair using pericardial or Gore-Tex patch may undergo successful transseptal puncture using the Brockenbrough needle. However, patients who had a device in the septum may encounter difficulties, especially if the device is occupying the entire septum. If the device is small, it is feasible to puncture the septum outside the area of the device by employing the conventional technique or the radiofrequency perforation technique[16] using the Baylis Medical system

(Baylis Medical Company, Inc, Montreal, Canada). If the septum is occupied by an Amplatzer device, it may be very difficult to perform the puncture using the conventional or radiofrequency technique due to the amount of metal inside the device (personal experience). It is perhaps feasible to perform the puncture with a device that does not have much metal in the middle of it (GORE HELEX device).

Another new technology that also may improve the safety of transseptal puncture is the excimer laser catheter (0.9-mm CLiRpath X-80, Spectranetics Corporation, Colorado Springs, CO).[17-19] This catheter can puncture the septum after a brief 2- to 5-second application of laser energy.

Complications Encountered During/After ASD Device Closure

1. Device migration/embolization. This rare complication (1%) is usually encountered in percutaneous device closure of large ASDs and deficient rims. Assessment of the stability of the device by the "Minnesota Wiggle" technique is of great importance prior to device release. Migrated devices are usually snared and retrieved percutaneously. If percutaneous retrieval fails, surgical retrieval should take place without delay.

2. Cardiac erosion/perforation. In contrast to device migration, this complication tends to occur if one uses an oversized device compared to the defect size. It has been also reported in cases with multiple ASDs requiring multiple devices for closure. Awad et al[20] reported 1 case of device protrusion into the aortic root with resultant chest pain and pericardial effusion. The device tends to erode into the left atrial wall and the adjacent aorta.

Appropriate sizing of the defect using all available tools (fluoroscopy, ICE, and/or transesophageal echocardiography) is crucial to avoid device oversizing. Amin et al[21] reported on potential factors that may increase the risk of erosion. Defects with deficient anterior-superior rim that may receive a device >150% of the defect native diameter is a setup for this complication. Using the stop-flow technique may decrease this serious complication. Close follow-up of high-risk patients with transthoracic echocardiography is important for early diagnosis of such a complication.

3. Arrhythmias. Atrioventricular block is a rare complication (<1%), and is usually encountered in cases of large ASDs requiring large devices for closure. The inferior part of the device tends to cause continuous mechanical pressure on the atrioventricular node (AVN), which results in variable degrees of atrioventricular block.

Hill et al[22] reported the incidence of abnormal atrioventricular (AV) conduction to be 7%. Complete AV block is a potential risk, but rare (<1%). Suda et al[23] reported that 10 of 162 (6.2%) patients presented with new-onset (N = 9) or aggravation of pre-existing (N = 1) AV block. Three of the AV blocks occurred during the procedure, and 7 were first noted in patients 1 to 7 days later. All AV blocks (first-degree in 4, second-degree in 4, and third-degree in 2) resolved or improved spontaneously, with no recurrence at mid-term follow-up.

In our center, a 12-lead electrocardiogram is obtained in every patient after ASD device closure and prior to discharge. First-degree atrioventricular block (AVB) may be secondary to temporary edema/inflammation post-device placement and usually resolves spontaneously. These patients need more frequent follow-up until normalization of their atrioventricular conduction is evident.

In more severe cases with a resultant second- and third-degree AVB, there may be a transient mechanical compression on the AVN or temporary edema/inflammation. In such patients, a trial of steroids and nonsteroidal anti-inflammatory drugs should take place for a few days in an inpatient hospital setting with close cardiorespiratory monitoring. If no improvement of the conduction is noticed, surgical removal of the device and surgical repair of the defect is mandated. Patients usually resume their normal sinus rhythm with 1:1 atrioventricular conduction after removal of the device.

Permanent pacemaker placement for patients with complete AVB after ASD device closure has not been reported in the literature. This complication is usually temporary and resolves by medical treatment or after elimination of the mechanical compression on the AV node (removal of the device). We do not believe it is appropriate to implant a permanent pacemaker in such patients. This would limit their lifestyle and subject them to lifelong follow-up and pacemaker complications (acute and chronic). In the same study by Hill et al,[22] supraventricular ectopy was noted in 26 (63%) of 41 patients immediately after device closure, including 9 patients (23%) with non-sustained supraventricular tachycardia.

4. Stroke/transient ischemic attack. This is a rare complication. To avoid this complication, we start antiplatelet therapy at least 48 hours prior to the procedure and give a heparin dose to achieve ACT >200 seconds at the time of device deployment. Post closure, all patients should receive aspirin (81-325 mg/day) and clopidogrel (75 mg/day). The aspirin is for 6 to 12 months, and the clopidogrel is for 2 to 3 months. Clot formation on the devices is rare using the ASO or the GORE HELEX device.[24]

5. Headaches/migraines. Up to 5% to 10% of patients may encounter unusual headaches/migraines after device closure. The exact mechanism is not fully understood. Since we have been using clopidogrel, the incidence of this complication has decreased significantly.

Conclusion

Availability of several closure devices has made percutaneous transcatheter closure of a secundum ASD an alternative to surgical repair. Patients should be evaluated carefully as to the indication for ASD closure. The catheterization laboratory should be staffed and fully equipped with a broad range and many sizes of closure devices and delivery tools. The use of the wrong size device or a failed procedure or complication due to a lack of the proper equipment is unacceptable. The operator should be well trained in the deployment of the particular device being used (its limitations and its merits) as well as in transseptal catheterization and the use of intracardiac or transesophageal echocardiography image interpretation particular to this procedure. While the procedure has a low complication and failure rate in experienced hands, a high index of suspicion for complications and vigilance are key to a safe procedure.

Acknowledgments
Ziyad M. Hijazi would like to thank the cath lab and echo lab staff at the Rush Center for Congenital & Structural Heart Disease for their hard work and dedication.

References

1. Miyague NI, Cardoso SM, Meyer F, et al. Epidemiological study of congenital heart defects in children and adolescents. *Arq Bras Cardiol* 2003;80:269-278.

2. Inglessis I, Landzberg MJ. Interventional catheterization in adult congenital heart disease. *Circulation* 2007;115:1622-1633.

3. Andrews RE, Tulloh RM. Interventional cardiac catheterization in congenital heart disease. *Arch Dis Child* 2004;89:1168-1173.

4. Mullen MJ, Hildick-Smith D, De Giovanni JV, et al. BioSTAR Evaluation STudy (BEST): a prospective, multicenter, phase I clinical trial to evaluate the feasibility, efficacy, and safety of the BioSTAR bioabsorbable septal repair implant for the closure of atrial-level shunts. *Circulation* 2006;114:1962-1967.

5. King TD, Mills NL. Nonoperative closure of atrial septal defects. *Surgery* 1974;75:383-388.

6. Du ZD, Hijazi ZM, Kleinman CS, et al. Comparison between transcatheter and surgical closure of secundum atrial septal defect in children and adults: results of a multicenter non-randomized trial. *J Am Coll Cardiol* 2002;39:1836-1844.

7. Diab KA, Cao QL, Bacha EA, et al. Device closure of atrial septal defects with the Amplatzer septal occluder: safety and outcome in infants. *J Thorac Cardiovasc Surg* 2007;134:960-966.

8. Jones TK, Latson LA, Zahn E, et al; Multicenter Pivotal Study of the HELEX Septal Occluder Investigators. Results of the U.S. multicenter pivotal study of the HELEX septal occluder for percutaneous closure of secundum atrial septal defects. *J Am Coll Cardiol* 2007;49:2215-2221.

9. Amin Z, Danford DA, Pedra CA. A new Amplatzer device to maintain patency of Fontan fenestrations and atrial septal defects. *Catheter Cardiovasc Interv* 2002; 57:246-251.

10. Cheatham JP, Hill SL, Chisolm JL. Initial results using the new cribriform Amplatzer septal occluder for transcatheter closure of multifenestrated atrial septal defects with septal aneurysm. *Catheter Cardiovasc Interv* [abstract] PICS-VII suppl. 2003;60:126.

11. Patel A, Cao QL, Koenig PR, et al. Intracardiac echocardiography to guide closure of atrial septal defects in children less than 15 kilograms. *Catheter Cardiovasc Interv* 2006;68:287-291.

12. Fischer G, Stieh J, Uebing A, et al. Experience with transcatheter closure of secundum atrial septal defects using the Amplatzer septal occluder: a single centre study in 236 consecutive patients. *Heart* 2003;89:199-204.

13. Fu YC, Cao QL, Hijazi ZM. Device closure of large atrial septal defects: technical considerations. *J Cardiovasc Med (Hagerstown)* 2007;8:30-33.

14. Wahab HA, Bairam AR, Cao QL, Hijazi ZM. Novel technique to prevent prolapse of the Amplatzer septal occluder through large atrial septal defect. *Catheter Cardiovasc Interv* 2003;60:543-545.

15. Dalvi BV, Pinto RJ, Gupta A. New technique for device closure of large atrial septal defects. *Catheter Cardiovasc Interv* 2005;64:102-107.

16. Sherman W, Lee P, Hartley A, Love B. Transatrial septal catheterization using a new radiofrequency probe. *Catheter Cardiovasc Interv* 2005;66:14-17.

17. Bommer WJ, Lee G, Riemenschneider TA, et al. Laser atrial septostomy. *Am Heart J* 1983;106:1152-1156.

18. Galal O, Weber HP, Enders S, et al. Transcatheter laser atrial septostomy in rabbits. *Int J Cardiol* 1993;42:31-35.

19. Elagha AA, Kim AH, Kocaturk O, Lederman RJ. Blunt atrial transseptal puncture using excimer laser in swine. *Catheter Cardiovasc Interv* 2007;70:585-590.

20. Awad SM, Garay FF, Cao QL, et al. Multiple Amplatzer septal occluder devices for multiple atrial communications: immediate

and long-term follow-up results. *Catheter Cardiovasc Interv* 2007;70:265-273.

21. Amin Z, Hijazi ZM, Bass JL, Cheatham JP, Hellenbrand WE, Kleinman CS. Erosion of Amplatzer septal occluder device after closure of secundum atrial septal defects: review of registry of complications and recommendations to minimize future work. *Catheter Cardiovasc Interv* 2004;63:496-502.

22. Hill SL, Berul CI, Patel HT, et al. Early ECG abnormalities associated with transcatheter closure of atrial septal defects using the Amplatzer septal occluder. *J Interv Card Electrophysiol* 2000;4:469-474.

23. Suda K, Raboisson MJ, Piette E, et al. Reversible atrioventricular block associated with closure of atrial septal defects using the Amplatzer device. *J Am Coll Cardiol* 2004;43:1677-1682.

24. Krumsdorf U, Ostermayer S, Billinger K, Trepels T, Zadan E, Horvath K, Sievert H. Incidence and clinical course of thrombus formation on atrial septal defect and patent foramen ovale closure devices in 1,000 consecutive patients. *J Am Coll Cardiol* 2004;43:302-309.

12

Transseptal Left Heart Interventions

Mehul B. Patel, Tahmeed Contractor, Samin K. Sharma

Transseptal catheterization (TSC) was first introduced in 1959 by Ross and Cope, and later modified by Brockenbrough and Mullins.[1,2] There was a significant decline in the utilization of this technique after the introduction of the balloon flotation pulmonary artery catheter in 1970 by Swan and Ganz.[3] With the advent of mitral and aortic valvuloplasty along with catheter ablation for left atrial tachycardia and left-sided accessory pathways, there was a renewed interest in transseptal catheterization worldwide. Transseptal catheterization has seen a further resurgence because of catheter ablation for atrial fibrillation and cardiac interventions on the left side of the heart.

Due to the limited working space of the fossa ovalis and the potential for life-threatening complications, the operator must have a thorough knowledge of the anatomy of the interatrial septum (IAS) along with the contraindications of the procedure.[4-6] The fundamental principles of transseptal catheterization along with the indications, contraindications, and complications are described in accompanying chapters in this book. An elaborative description of individual procedures is beyond the scope of this chapter. This chapter has detailed the salient technical steps of left heart interventions that require transseptal access and focuses on the variations in transseptal puncture (TSP) sites. Left atrial appendage (LAA) closure with the WATCHMAN device (Atritech, Inc, Plymouth, MN) is discussed in Chapter 13. Most of these procedures are fairly complex and require real-time transesophageal echocardiography (TEE) or intracardiac echocardiography (ICE) guidance for transseptal puncture, catheter manipulation, and precise placement of devices.

Transseptal Catheterization and Interventions.
© 2010 Ranjan Thakur MD and Andrea Natale MD, eds.
Cardiotext Publishing, ISBN 978-0-9790164-1-7.

Left Heart Interventions via Transseptal Puncture

1. Percutaneous mitral valve interventions
   a. Percutaneous transluminal mitral commissurotomy
   b. Direct mitral valve repair
   c. Mitral paravalvular leak repair
2. Pulmonary vein stenosis: venoplasty and stenting
3. Percutaneous aortic valve implantation and aortic valvuloplasty
4. Percutaneous left ventricular assist: TandemHeart device (CardiacAssist, Inc, Pittsburgh, PA)
5. Left atrial appendage closure: LAA WATCHMAN device

Percutaneous Mitral Valve Interventions

Transseptal catheterization plays a pivotal role for mitral valve interventions. The individual procedures are described in Charts 12.1 and 12.2, which are supported by two schematic representations, Figures 12.1 and 12.2.

Percutaneous Transluminal Mitral Commissurotomy (PTMC) or Mitral Valvuloplasty

Indications
Moderate to severe symptomatic mitral stenosis with a favorable mitral anatomy in the absence of a left atrial (LA) clot.

Pre-catheterization Planning
All patients should undergo a regular transthoracic echocardiogram (TTE) along with a transesophageal echocardiogram (TEE) using standard views to rule out left atrial or left atrial appendage thrombus prior to the procedure. The mitral valve should be evaluated and scored using the standard Wilkins scoring system for risk stratification.

Hardware
Standard transseptal catheterization hardware as described in Chapter 5 is used. An Inoue balloon should also be available, along with such auxiliary instruments as a 14 F dilator, a spring wire, a preshaped left ventricular (LV) stylet with a pre-marked syringe for balloon inflation, and Vernier calipers to measure the balloon waist diameter.

Procedure
The salient steps of percutaneous transluminal mitral commissurotomy are shown in Chart 12.1.[7-14]

Problems and Precautions
The precautions and special circumstances are described in Chapter 15 ("Complications of Transseptal Catheterization").

Current Status
PTMC is a well-established procedure with efficacy equivalent to closed mitral commissurotomy. It remains the treatment of choice for stenotic mitral valves without commissural calcification or extensive subvalvular fusion.

Percutaneous Direct Edge-to-Edge Mitral Valve Repair ("The Percutaneous Alfieri Stitch")

Indications
Symptomatic severe mitral regurgitation with a favorable mitral valve anatomy in a patient deemed at an unacceptably high risk for sur-

gical correction. A logistic EuroSCORE predicted surgical mortality of greater than 20% is considered as a reasonable indication for percutaneous intervention.

Pre-catheterization Planning

All patients should undergo a TTE along with a TEE to assess the mitral valve morphology. The working views include a regular short-axis TEE at the base, a long-axis four-chamber view, and a mid-esophageal five-chamber view. The fluoroscopic views include the standard fluoroscopic views for TSP. The device deployment and withdrawal are done strictly using real-time TEE imaging.[15]

Hardware

The hardware consists of the regular TSP hardware, along with the clip and the clip-delivery system (CDS). The Evalve repair device (Abbott Laboratories, Abbott Park, IL) contains a single-plane steerable guide catheter and a CDS, which includes a dual-plane steerable sleeve, a clip delivery catheter, and a clip (MitraClip, Abbott Laboratories, Abbott Park, IL).

Procedure

The salient steps for direct mitral valve repair are shown in Chart 12.2 and illustrated in Figure 12.1. In 40% of patients an additional clip may be required to achieve success.

Current Status

The clips for mitral valve repair are still in clinical trials. Following enrollment completion of the EVEREST trials, patients who receive the MitraClip are being treated in a continued access registry called REALISM.

Mitral Paravalvular Leak Repair

Indications

Symptomatic paravalvular leak after prosthetic mitral valve replacement.

Paravalvular leak can present early or late. Clinical presentation can be with heart failure or incessant hemolysis. The defect can be small or large, and it can be circular, crescent, or tunnel-like in shape.

Pre-catheterization Planning

All patients should have a regular TTE along with TEE to assess the mitral valve morphology. The fluoroscopic views include the standard fluoroscopic views for TSP, along with 30° left anterior oblique (LAO-30) and 30° right anterior oblique (RAO-30) projections.

Hardware

The hardware for a mitral paravalvular leak repair consists of a Judkins right 4.0 catheter, a 0.035 stiff, straight Terumo Glidewire (Terumo Medical Corporation, Somersset NJ), a patent ductus arteriosus (PDA) occluder, an Amplatzer PDA device (AGA Medical Corporation, Plymouth, MN), rigid coils, and small-sized atrial septal defect (ASD) closure devices.

Procedure

Vascular Approach. For leaks close to the IAS, an internal jugular approach is best suited for crossing the defect. For leaks further away from the IAS, a femoral approach is preferred.

Crossing the Defect with Leak. Due to high-pressure turbulent flow across the paravalvular leak, it may be difficult to cross the defect from the LA to the LV (Figure 12.2). The defect can be crossed from the left ventricle using a 0.35 straight, stiff Glidewire over

CHART 12.1

PTMC: Important Steps and Precautions

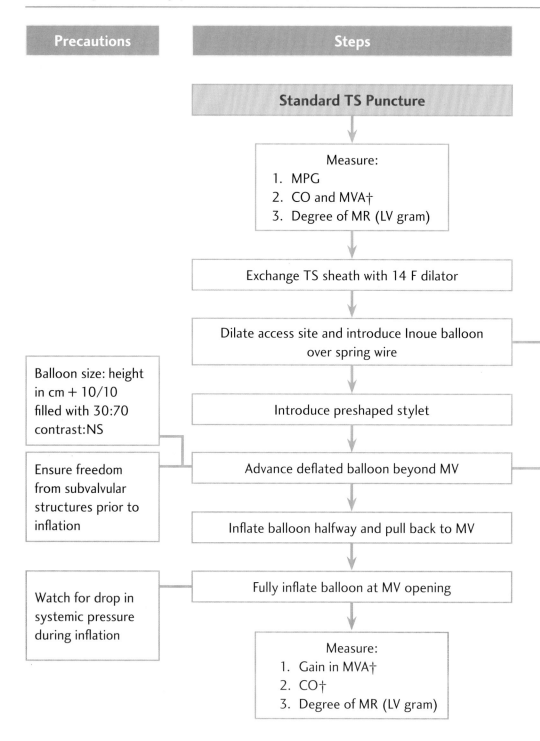

Precautions	Steps

Standard TS Puncture

Measure:
1. MPG
2. CO and MVA†
3. Degree of MR (LV gram)

Exchange TS sheath with 14 F dilator

Dilate access site and introduce Inoue balloon over spring wire

Balloon size: height in cm + 10/10 filled with 30:70 contrast:NS

Introduce preshaped stylet

Ensure freedom from subvalvular structures prior to inflation

Advance deflated balloon beyond MV

Inflate balloon halfway and pull back to MV

Fully inflate balloon at MV opening

Watch for drop in systemic pressure during inflation

Measure:
1. Gain in MVA†
2. CO†
3. Degree of MR (LV gram)

PTMC (continued)

Precautions

Introduce with big arc of circle to avoid LAA and PV

Look for the woodpecking sign: bobbing of balloon near MV

Remove hysteresis after crossing MV

CO = cardiac output; LAA = left atrial appendage;

LV = left ventricle; MPG = mean pulmonary gradient;

MR = mitral regurgitation; MV = mitral valve;

MVA = mitral valve area; NS = normal saline;

PV = pulmonary vein; TS = transseptal;

TTE = transthoracic echocardiogram;

† = Using Gorlin's formula

CHART 12.2

Percutaneous Direct Mitral Valve Repair: Important Steps and Precautions

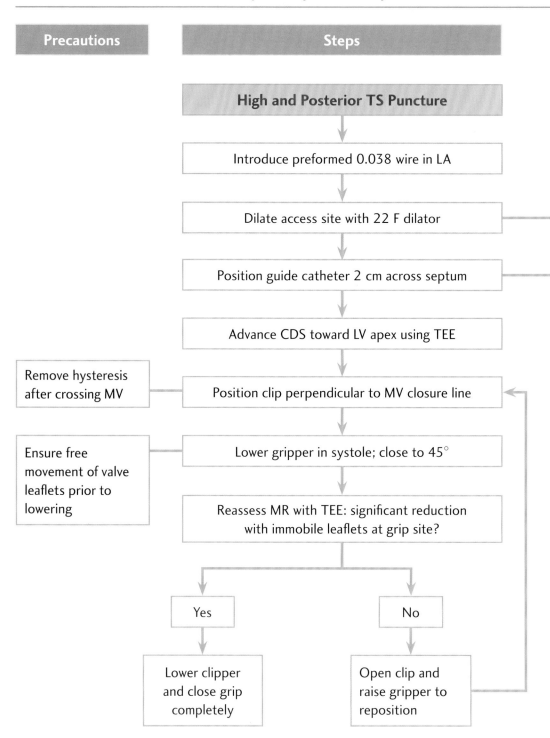

Percutaneous Direct Mitral Valve Repair (continued)

Precautions

Stretch for 30 seconds

De-air system before proceeding

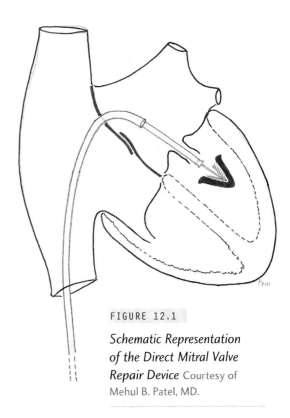

FIGURE 12.1

Schematic Representation of the Direct Mitral Valve Repair Device Courtesy of Mehul B. Patel, MD.

CDS = clip delivery system;
LA = left atrium; LV = left ventricle;
MR = mitral regurgitation; MV = mitral valve;
TEE = transesophageal echocardiogram;
TS = transseptal

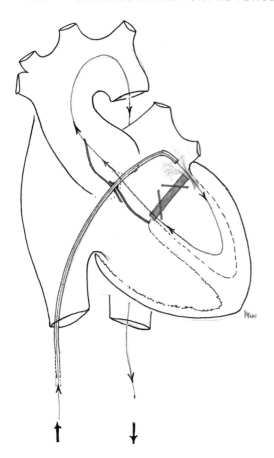

FIGURE 12.2 *Schematic Representation of Crossing the Paravalvular Defect from the Left Atrium (LA) to the Left Ventricle (LV)* Courtesy of Mehul B. Patel, MD.

a Judkins right 4.0 (JR 4) catheter (Figure 12.3). The wire is then snared from the LA into the inferior vena cava (IVC) and brought out through the femoral vein. A 0.035 compatible Swan-Ganz balloon catheter is then introduced over the wire and parked across the defect. The balloon is then inflated to define the waist, and the size of the defect measured under TEE guidance. The defect is then closed using coils, plugs, or small ASD closure devices depending on the size and shape of the defect.[16-19]

Pulmonary Vein (PV) Stenosis

Indications

Intervention should only be performed if a significant portion of the lung drainage is at jeopardy or if there are recurrent symptoms due to localized infections.

Causes

1. After atrial fibrillation (AF) ablation
2. After surgical correction of total anomalous pulmonary venous drainage (TAPVC) or partial anomalous pulmonary venous drainage (PAPVC) with suture line discrete stenosis
3. Mediastinal fibrosis
4. Congenital pulmonary vein stenosis
5. Restenosis after intervention

Pre-catheter Planning

Involvement of right pulmonary veins: The right femoral vein approach is preferred, as the internal jugular vein (IJV) approach is technically challenging.

Involvement of left pulmonary veins: either right femoral or right IJV approach can be used.

Fluoroscopic views: A frontal view for right pulmonary vein intervention and a hepatoclavicular view for left pulmonary vein intervention are preferred.

Hardware

1. Regular TSC hardware along with guide catheters, such as a Judkins right 2.0 catheter, a hockey stick catheter, a cobra 4.0 catheter, or a steerable sheath for directional entry in the pulmonary vein
2. 0.035 Terumo Glidewire
3. 5 F glide catheter for a pullback gradient
4. Intracoronary stenting (ICS) inventory including 4 to 5 mm cutting balloons

Procedure

The stent size matching the closest normal vessel diameter should be used, because any extent of undersizing or oversizing would accelerate restenosis.[20-28]

Problems

Ostial lesions and lesions smaller than 5 mm in diameter have a higher rate of restenosis. The current stenting technique has a reasonable outcome for postablation pulmonary vein stenosis. Results for other indications are not very encouraging due to high rates of restenosis requiring strict surveillance and repeated interventions. For bifurcation lesions, a simultaneous kissing stent technique has been reported with good success rates.

Follow-up

A follow-up catheterization should be considered after 6 months to prevent permanent loss of involved lung segments. Computerized tomography angiography and magnetic resonance angiography are poor modalities after stenting due to the metal artifacts produced by the stent.

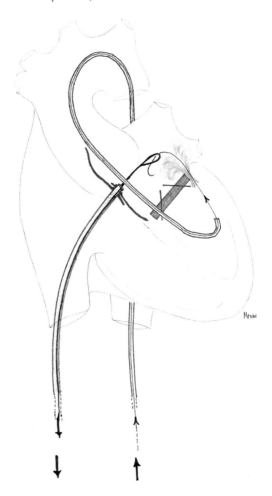

FIGURE 12.3   *Schematic Representation of Crossing the Paravalvular Defect from the Left Ventricle (LV) to the Left Atrium (LA)* Courtesy of Mehul B. Patel, MD.

Percutaneous Aortic Valve Implantation

Indications

Severe symptomatic aortic stenosis with extensive comorbidities considered very high risk for surgical replacement.

Hardware

The hardware for this procedure consists of a percutaneous heart valve (PHV), a 22-mm balloon catheter, a crimping device with metal housing, a measuring ring, and a rotary knob.

The PHV is an equine trileaflet bioprosthetic valve that is securely sutured to a stainless, balloon-expandable steel frame. The stent is 23 mm × 14 mm with a crimped diameter of <8 mm, and is stored in low concentrations of glutaraldehyde in the open position. The valve is available in two sizes. For an annulus of 18 mm to 22 mm, a 23-mm diameter prosthesis is preferred, and for an annulus of 21 mm to 25 mm, a 26-mm diameter prosthesis is considered suitable.

The manual crimping tool symmetrically compresses the PHV over the delivery balloon catheter in a metal housing with a hand-held rotary knob. The crimper is housed within a 24 F tube simulating the venous sheath through which the PHV is negotiated. A 22-mm measuring ring verifies the delivery balloon diameter at full inflation.

The delivery balloon catheter is a commercially available as 22 mm × 3 cm Z-MED II (NuMED, Inc, Hopkinton, NY) percutaneous transluminal balloon catheter. The catheter length is 120 cm, a size necessary for larger patients with significant vessel tortuosity. The balloon catheter is purged before mounting the stent. A 20-mL syringe filled with diluted contrast (1:9 contrast/saline) is attached to the distal hub for stent deployment.

Pre-catheter Planning

All patients should undergo TTE and TEE using standard views to assess the aortic valve morphology and aortic annulus. The fluoroscopic views include the standard fluoroscopic views for TSP along with LAO-30 and RAO-30. A coronary angiogram to define the coronary ostia is required to understand the possible displacement of any leaflet calcific nodule toward it. Assessment of the aorta along with the iliac and the femoral vessels helps to define the vascular course and suitability of 24 F sheath.

Procedure

The salient steps of PHV are shown in Chart 12.3 and illustrated in Figure 12.4.[29-32]

Percutaneous aortic valavulpolasty using the antegrade approach is usually limited in neonates to reduce the risk of femoral arterial injury. The foramen ovale is usually patent, making it easy to cross to the left atrium. The antegrade approach may also reduce the incidence of aortic insufficiency due to valve leaflet perforation.

Percutaneous Left Ventricular Assist (TandemHeart)

Indications

1. Acute myocardial infarction with mechanical complication
2. Cardiogenic shock
3. High-risk percutaneous coronary intervention (PCI)

Hardware

The hardware for this procedure consists of the standard TSC hardware, a TandemHeart transseptal cannula (THTC) with dilator and obturator, an LA cannula with 14 side holes and 1 large end hole, a femoral arterial cannula with a large single end hole, a centrifugal pump, Tygon tubings, and a controller (Figure 12.5).

Technique

The standard TSP hardware with 14 F IAS dilator is used. The interatrial septum is dilated with a 2-stage dilator and the Tandem-Heart transseptal LA cannula is advanced over the preshaped 0.035 guidewire.

The distal curve on the cannula ensures a safe location in the center of the LA, thereby avoiding the PV or the LAA. Centimeter markings at the proximal end of the cannula are used to reference the position of the cannula at the time of placement. Distal tip and side holes are configured to allow adequate blood flow and drainage of the LA, and care should be taken to ensure that all 14 holes are located in the LA. The tip of the transseptal cannula has a radiopaque marker for visualization under fluoroscopy.

The arterial cannula is placed percutaneously in the femoral artery (FA), and the size of this cannula determines the expected rise in cardiac output. The arterial access site may be pre-closed with the Perclose A-T device (Abbott Laboratories, Abbott Park, IL).

The TandemHeart controller consists of a pump drive motor circuit, flow estimator, air bubble detector, IV pump, and infusion system. The recently introduced TandemHeart Escort Controller with built-in batteries that last for 1 hour, weighs 21 pounds, allowing for easier transport within the hospital.[33,34] The LA and the FA cannula are inserted and clamped at the site specified to prevent any damage to the tubings. The pump is primed, and the arterial and venous cannulae are connected with a fluid-to-fluid interface at the time of attachment to prevent air embolism. Flushing normal saline with a 50-cc syringe at both the open ends of the tubing at the time of connection helps to prevent entrapment of air bubbles.

The pump, which uses a brushless DC motor back EMF detection algorithm, is initiated at slow speeds with gradual increments, to have a smooth increment in the cardiac output.

Conclusions

The contemporary interventional cardiologist can perform various procedures percutaneously that could be done only surgically just a few years ago. The procedures require access to the left heart via the IAS and presuppose an easy and expert facility with the transseptal technique. Such left heart interventions are likely to become more commonplace in the future. Transesophageal echocardiogram provides real-time images that are both unique and complementary to fluoroscopic images, and also provide guidance for deciding the candidacy of the specific defect for percutaneous device intervention. As these therapies expand to include more complex defects, collaboration of the interventional cardiologist and the cardiothoracic surgeon may see a remarkable evolution of hybrid strategies.

CHART 12.3

Percutaneous Heart Valve Replacement: Important Steps and Precautions

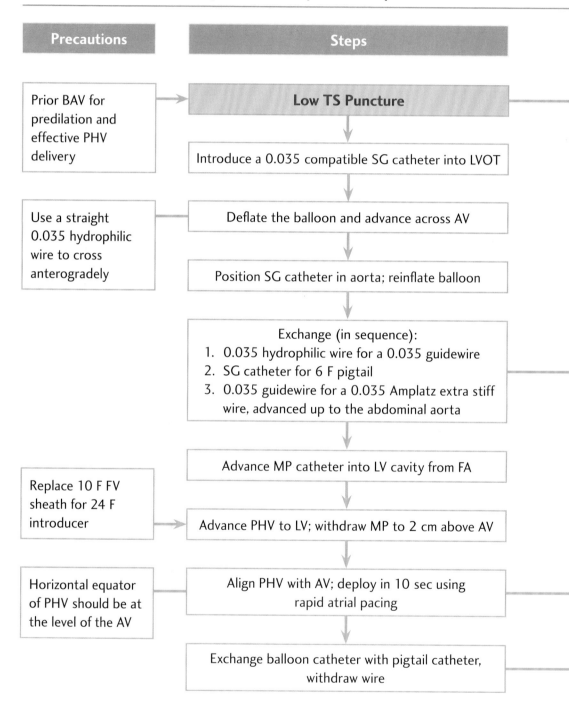

Precautions	Steps
Prior BAV for predilation and effective PHV delivery	**Low TS Puncture**
	Introduce a 0.035 compatible SG catheter into LVOT
Use a straight 0.035 hydrophilic wire to cross anterogradely	Deflate the balloon and advance across AV
	Position SG catheter in aorta; reinflate balloon
	Exchange (in sequence): 1. 0.035 hydrophilic wire for a 0.035 guidewire 2. SG catheter for 6 F pigtail 3. 0.035 guidewire for a 0.035 Amplatz extra stiff wire, advanced up to the abdominal aorta
	Advance MP catheter into LV cavity from FA
Replace 10 F FV sheath for 24 F introducer	Advance PHV to LV; withdraw MP to 2 cm above AV
Horizontal equator of PHV should be at the level of the AV	Align PHV with AV; deploy in 10 sec using rapid atrial pacing
	Exchange balloon catheter with pigtail catheter, withdraw wire

AV = aortic valve; BAV =balloon atrial valvuloplasty; FA = femoral artery;
FV = femoral vein; IAS = interatrial septum; LV = left ventricle;

Percutaneous Heart Valve Replacement (continued)

Precautions

Balloon dilation
of IAS: 10 mm
balloon for 10 secs

Careful push
and pull method,
*maintaining full alpha
loop in the LV*

Snare the free end
of the Amplatz wire
to the FA

Deploy with 20-ml
syringe filled with
30:70 diluted
contrast; stop
atrial pacing only
after balloon is
completely deflated

Check gradient
across AV

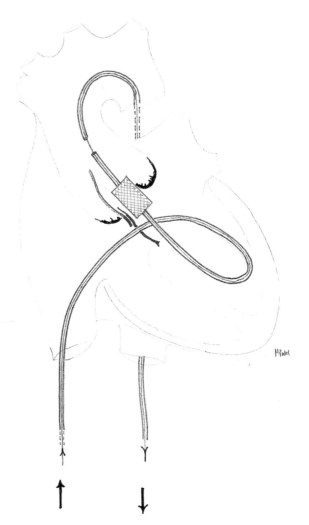

FIGURE 12.4   *Schematic Representation
of the Percutaneous Heart
Valve (PHV) Technique* Courtesy of Mehul B.
Patel, MD.

LVOT = left ventricular outflow tract; MP = multipurpose;
PHV = percutaneous heart valve; SG = Swan-Ganz; TS = transseptal

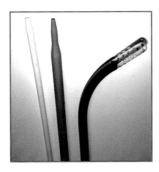
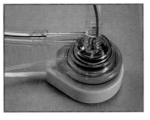
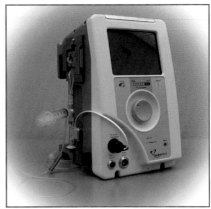

FIGURE 12.5   *The TandemHeart System*
The cannula set, the pump,
and the controller. Courtesy of CardiacAssist, Inc.

References

1. Ross J Jr, Braunwald E, Morrow AG. Transseptal left atrial puncture: a new technique for the measurement of left atrial pressure in man. *Am J Cardiol* 1959;3:653-655.

2. Cope C. Technique for transseptal catheterization of the left atrium: Preliminary report. *J Thorac Surg* 1959;37:482-486.

3. Swan HJC, Ganz W, Forrester J, et al. Catheterization of the heart in man with use of a flow-directed balloon-tipped catheter. *N Engl J Med* 1970;283:447-451.

4. Clugston R, Lau FYK, Ruiz C. Transseptal catheterization update 1992. *Cathet Cardiovasc Diagn* 1992;26:266-274.

5. Roelke M, Smith AJ, Palacios IF. The technique and safety of transseptal left heart catheterization: the Massachusetts General Hospital experience with 1,279 procedures. *Cathet Cardiovasc Diagn* 1994;32:332-339.

6. Babaliaros VC, Green JT, Lerakis S, Lloyd M, Block PC. Emerging applications for transseptal left heart catheterization old techniques for new procedures. *J Am Coll Cardiol* 2008;51:2116-2122.

7. Al Zaibag M, Al Kasab S, Ribeiro PA, Al Fagig MR. Percutaneous double-balloon mitral valvotomy for rheumatic mitral-valve stenosis. *Lancet* 1986;327:757-761.

8. Vahanian A, Michel PL, Cormier B, et al. Results of percutaneous mitral commissurotomy in 200 patients. *Am J Cardiol* 1989;63:847-852.

9. Palacios I, Block PC, Brandi S, et al. Percutaneous balloon valvotomy for patients with severe mitral stenosis. *Circulation* 1987;75:778-784.

10. Chen CR, Cheng TO, Chen IY, et al. Percutaneous mitral valvuloplasty with the Inoue balloon catheter. *Am J Cardiol* 1992;70:1455-1458.

11. Hung IS, Chern MS, Wu JJ, et al. Short- and long-term results of catheter balloon percutaneous transvenous mitral commissurotomy. *Am J Cardiol* 1991;67:854-862.

12. Cribier A, Eltchaninoff H, Koning R, et al. Percutaneous mechanical mitral commissurotomy with a newly designed metallic valvulotome. *Circulation* 1999;99:793-799.

13. Palacios IF, Sanchez PL, Harrell LC, et al. Which patients benefit from percutaneous mitral balloon valvuloplasty? Prevalvuloplasty and postvalvuloplasty variables that predict long-term outcome. *Circulation* 2002; 05(12):1465-1471.

14. Vahanian A, Palacios IF. Percutaneous approaches to valvular disease. *Circulation* 2004;109(13):1572-1579.

15. Piazza N, Asgar A, Ibrahim R, Bonan R. Transcatheter mitral and pulmonary valve therapy. *J Am Coll Cardiol* 2009;53(20): 1837-1851.

16. Sorajja P, Cabalka AK, Hagler DJ, et al. Successful percutaneous repair of perivalvular prosthetic regurgitation. *Catheter Cardiovasc Interv* 2007;70:815-23.

17. Hourihan M, Perry SB, Mandell VS, et al. Transcatheter umbrella closure of valvular and paravalvular leaks. *J Am Coll Cardiol* 1992;20(6):1371-1377.

18. Piechaud IF. Percutaneous closure of mitral paravalvular leak. *J Interv Cardiol* 2003;20(2):153-155.

19. Pate G, Webb J, Thompson C, et al. Percutaneous closure of a complex prosthetic mitral paravalvular leak using transesophageal echocardiographic guidance. *Can J Cardiol* 2004;20(4):452-455.

20. Caldarone CA, Najm HK, Kadletz M, et al. Relentless pulmonary vein stenosis after repair of total anomalous pulmonary venous drainage. *Ann Thorac Surg* 1998;66(5): 1514-1520.

21. Purerfellner H, Aichinger J, Martinek M, et al. Incidence, management, and outcome in significant pulmonary vein stenosis complicating ablation for atrial fibrillation. *Am J Cardiol* 2004;93(11):1428-1431, A10.

22. Packer DL, Keelan P, Munger TM, et al. Clinical presentation, investigation, and management of pulmonary vein stenosis complicating ablation for atrial fibrillation. *Circulation* 2005;111(5):546-554.

23. Latson LA, Prieto LR. Congenital and acquired pulmonary vein stenosis. *Circulation* 2007;115(1):103-138.

24. Barrett CD, Di Biase L, Natale A. How to identify and treat patient with pulmonary vein stenosis post atrial fibrillation ablation. *Curr Opin Cardiol* 2009;24:42-49.

25. McMahon CJ, Mullins CE, El Said HG. Intrastent sonotherapy in pulmonary vein restenosis: a new treatment for a recalcitrant problem. *Heart* 2003;89(2):E6.

26. Doyle TP, Loyd JE, Robbins IM. Percutaneous pulmonary artery and vein stenting: a novel treatment for mediastinal fibrosis. *Am J Resp Crit Care Med* 2001;164(4):657-660.

27. Dieter RS, Nelson B, Wolff MR, et al. Transseptal stent treatment of anastomotic stricture after repair of partial anomalous pulmonary venous return. *J Endovasc Ther* 2003;10(4):838-842.

28. Michel-Behnke I, Luedemann M, Hagel KJ, Schranz D. Serial stent implantation to relieve in-stern stenosis in obstructed total anomalous pulmonary venous return. *Pediatr Cardiol* 2002;23(2):221-223.

29. National Heart, Lung, and Blood Institute participants group. Percutaneous balloon aortic valvuloplasty: acute and 30-day follow up results in 674 patients from the NHLBI Balloon Valvuloplasty Registry. *Circulation* 1991;84(6):2383-2397.

30. Thielmann M, Wendt D, Eggebrecht H, et al. Transcatheter aortic valve implantation in patients with very high risk for conventional aortic valve replacement. *Ann Thorac Surg* 2009;88:1468-1474.

31. Patel JH, Mathew ST, Hennebry TA. Transcatheter aortic valve replacement: a potential option for the nonsurgical patient. *Clin Cardiol* 2009;32:296-301.

32. Cribier A, Eltchaninoff H, Tron C, et al. Early experience with percutaneous transcatheter implantation of heart valve prosthesis for the treatment of end-stage inoperable

patients with calcific aortic stenosis. *J Am Coll Cardiol* 2004;43(4):698-703.

33. Moliterno DJ. Left main and multivessel coronary artery stenting for patients deemed inoperable—a real need for a tandem approach. *Catheter Cardiovasc Interv* 2009;74(2):311-312.

34. Kar B, Adkins LE, Civitello AB, et al. Clinical experience with the TandemHeart percutaneous ventricular assist device. *Tex Heart Inst J* 2006;33(2):111-115.

Percutaneous Left Atrial Appendage Occlusion Devices

Rodney P. Horton, Javier E. Sánchez, Yan Wang, Andrea Natale

The left atrial appendage (LAA) is a curved, muscular structure connected to the left atrium (LA), located anterior to the left superior pulmonary vein. The majority of the structure extends anterior to the LA and superior to the left ventricle. It usually covers the left main coronary artery or the circumflex coronary artery. Its embryologic origin is derived from the primordial left atrium although its inner surface is derived from the primordial pulmonary vein. In contrast, the developed LA is almost entirely derived from the primordial pulmonary vein.[1] Structurally, the LAA differs from the LA considerably. While the entire endocardial surface of the LA is smooth, only the proximal tubular portion of the LAA is smooth.[2] Beyond this region, the LAA becomes highly pectinate and varies widely with regard to overall shape, length,

and degree of lobulation. At the cellular level, LAA cells appear similar to LA cells but distinct from pulmonary venous cells.[3] However, chronic atrial fibrillation (AF) appears to cause smoothing and thickening of the endocardium of the appendage, particularly in the portions overlying the left ventricle.[4]

The purpose of the LAA is not fully understood. The LAA is more distensible than the LA and possesses both sympathetic and parasympathetic afferent nervous tissue. Amputation of both right and left appendages results in decreases in parasympathetic afferent and sympathetic efferent reflexes.[5] Furthermore, the LAA tissue is a major source of atrial natriuretic peptide (ANP) and brain natriuretic peptide (BNP).[6] Distension of the LAA induces urine output, sodium excretion, and increased heart rate. This is thought to be mediated in part by release of ANP. During sinus rhythm the LAA accounts for a significant portion of active left ventricular diastolic filling.

Transsseptal Catheterization and Interventions.
© 2010 Ranjan Thakur MD and Andrea Natale MD, eds.
Cardiotext Publishing, ISBN 978-0-9790164-1-7.

The primary morbidity associated with AF is the development of a stroke. During AF, the LAA allows for intracavitary thrombus formation, which can subsequently embolize.[7-8] In the 1940s the LAA was thought to be responsible for 50% of strokes associated with AF.[9] More recent studies suggest a more prominent role of the LAA in the formation of thrombi; it may be responsible for more than 90% of strokes in nonvalvular AF cases.[10-13]

For decades, the gold standard for lowering stroke risk in AF patients has been oral anticoagulation (typically with warfarin). While this strategy is effective, it is still poorly tolerated by many patients. Bleeding risks, frequent dose titration and phlebotomy, and drug interactions with other medications and foods have led to the pursuit of alternatives to this treatment strategy.[14] In 1948, amputation of the LAA was first proposed as a means of lowering subsequent stroke risk during heart surgery. Over the subsequent 60 years, closure or removal of the LAA has become a focus of therapy for both surgeons and cardiologists alike to prevent embolic stroke in the setting of AF.[15-16]

LAA removal (obliteration) has been performed as a concomitant procedure to other open chest surgical procedures for 2 decades.[17-20] Although this appears effective in eliminating thrombus formation for a dysfunctional LAA, it is technically difficult and not possible in patients whose LAA ostium is broad. Also, fluid retention has been reported in the first few months following this procedure.[21] This is believed to be due to the loss of LAA-associated ANP production. Surgical ligation (closure at the base with suture or staples) has become more popular in recent years as it is less anatomically challenging and leaves a functioning organ for ANP release.[22-23] Though expedient, the incidence of incomplete closure is high (36-40%).[18,22] The risk of subsequent embolism from an incompletely closed LAA is concerning and appears to be higher than in intact LAAs.[19]

As an alternative to surgical treatment, closure of the LAA using a percutaneous, transseptal device had been performed for the last decade using the PLAATO device (ev3, Inc, Plymouth, MN).[24-25] While this device provided a less invasive procedure with a high degree of successful closure, complications, including tamponade and device migration, ultimately led to abandonment of the technology. The WATCHMAN LAA Closure Device (Atritech, Inc, Plymouth, MN) is a self-expanding device roughly the shape of an acorn, which is placed in the LAA in a similar fashion as the PLAATO device. It has shown promising safety and efficacy results in a randomized, controlled trial compared with warfarin therapy for prevention of strokes.[26-28] Because this device remains the only percutaneous device still undergoing clinical testing, the remainder of this chapter will focus on it.

Device Characteristics

The WATCHMAN LAA Closure Device consists of a self-expanding Nitinol metal frame with a porous 160 micron polyester membrane covering the proximal face. The membrane serves to filter blood, thereby preventing LAA thrombus embolization, and promotes endothelial growth over the device. Small barbs are positioned radially around the mid portion of the device to prevent migration following deployment. Prior to release, the device is mounted on a detachable deployment catheter, which is housed in a 12 F delivery catheter. The delivery catheter is required to prevent premature opening of the device. The WATCHMAN LAA Closure Device and delivery catheter are inserted into the heart within a 14 F access sheath. The access sheath is available in 2 shapes, a single and double curve (Figure 13.1). The single-curve access sheath has a single 30° distal bend. The double-curve access sheath has the same primary bend as the single curve but includes a secondary bend out of plane toward the right. The purpose of the secondary bend is to angle more toward the mitral valve and facilitate LAA engagement. The device is manufactured in sizes ranging from 21 mm to 33 mm (3 mm increments) in diameter and in long and short device lengths. Because the shorter device offers more versatility, the longer device type is no longer used. The size measurement represents the width of the device at the widest point (shoulder) upon deployment from the delivery catheter (Figure 13.2). While the device size relates to the uncompressed cross-sectional diameter at the widest point, each of the device sizes fit in a 12 F delivery catheter. The LAA dimensions seen during transesophageal echocardiography (TEE) are used to determine the appropriate device size.

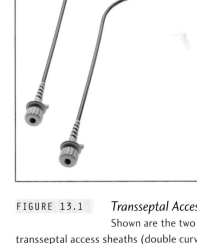

FIGURE 13.1 **Transseptal Access Sheaths** Shown are the two types of transseptal access sheaths (double curve on left, single curve on right) used for deployment of the WATCHMAN LAA Closure Device. The double curve sheath can be used for most conventionally shaped LAAs. The single curve sheath is less "self-guiding" but more versatile for device placement in LAAs with angled ostia or acute bends. Used with permission from Atritech, Inc.

Procedure

Patients usually arrive in the procedure room having withdrawn from warfarin therapy (INR <1.7) and in a fasting state. Aspirin or clopidogrel may be continued for this procedure. As with other medical device implants, strict sterile technique is followed, and prophylactic antibiotics are administered intravenously. Central venous access is obtained from the femoral vein; LA imaging is employed using transesophageal (TEE) or intracardiac echocardiography. With this imaging, all physical characteristics of the LAA are observed with particular focus on the ostial dimensions of the LAA in 2 obliquities, the length of the main structure from ostium to distal tip, the number and orientation of the appendage lobes, and orientation of the LAA to the left

pulmonary veins. Based on these observations, the device size and access sheath shape are determined. Selection of the device size is based on the largest ostial diameter of the LAA with a desired 10% to 20% approximate (company IFU guidelines) device compression. For example, a measured LAA ostial diameter of 20 mm would usually require a 24-mm WATCHMAN LAA Closure Device for adequate coverage with 20% device compression. While using echocardiographic guidance to visualize the fossa ovalis, transseptal catheterization is performed in the interatrial septum using a standard transseptal sheath and needle. While transseptal perforation anywhere along the fossa ovalis allows for LAA cannulation, a more superior puncture usually offers a more direct route to the appendage. Heparin anticoagulation is

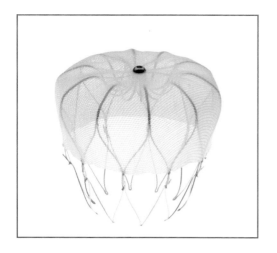

access sheath is advanced across the interatrial septum, and the wire and dilator are removed.

Accessing the LAA with the sheath can be operator dependent. The 2 recommended strategies involve a pigtail catheter approach or a direct sheath approach. For the pigtail catheter approach, a pigtail catheter is inserted into the access sheath, which is then advanced into the LAA. Once engaged, the sheath can be advanced over the pigtail catheter. The pigtail is then replaced by the WATCHMAN LAA Closure Device, which is housed in the delivery catheter. This approach has the benefit of using tools familiar to most operators. Disadvantages include the risk of air or thrombus introduction during the insertion and replacement of the pigtail with the WATCHMAN LAA Closure Device, and sheath migration as the device is advanced distally and a need for more contrast. (The access sheath takes 10 cc of contrast just to fill the lumen.) The migration issue is due to the greater stiffness of the sheath/device combination as compared to the sheath/pigtail combination. This stiffness differential can cause deformation of the LAA by the access sheath, which can result in sheath retraction as the WATCHMAN LAA Closure Device is advanced.

Our preferred approach is to directly advance the sheath into the LAA under fluoroscopic and echocardiographic guidance. Using this approach, the device is inserted into the access sheath and advanced under fluoroscopic guidance up to the level of the RA-IVC junction prior to LAA engagement. Because the stiffness of the device alters the

Device Size (uncompressed diameter)	Short Implant Overall Height (approximate)	Short Implant Crown to Barb (approximate)
21 mm	15.0 mm	9.0 mm
24 mm	17.0 mm	10.5 mm
27 mm	19.2 mm	12.5 mm
30 mm	21.0 mm	13.5 mm
33 mm	22.5 mm	14.2 mm

FIGURE 13.2   *Detailed Image of the WATCHMAN LAA Closure Device with Table of Deployed Device Sizes and Lengths*
Used with permission from Atritech, Inc.

administered either prior to or immediately following transseptal puncture with a target activated clotting time (ACT) range of 200 seconds to 300 seconds. Upon advancement of the sheath into the LA, a long exchange wire is advanced through the sheath and into the LA or left superior pulmonary vein. The sheath is then removed while maintaining the wire in the LA. Under fluoroscopy, the 14 F

curvature of the sheath, varying the position of the device in the sheath allows for dynamic control of sheath curve, as LAA anatomy can be variable. Contrast is then injected through the device, filling only the distal portion of the access sheath. Using fluoroscopic and echocardiographic guidance aided by contrast imaging, the sheath is advanced into the main lobe of the LAA.

Regardless of the LAA cannulation technique, the access sheath is positioned in the distal portion of the LAA. The access sheath position is maintained and the device/containment sheath combination is advanced to the end of the access sheath. Because the device shortens upon deployment, marker bands on the access sheath offer guidance as to the position on the proximal surface of the deployed device upon opening (Figure 13.3). After fluoroscopic confirmation of position, the access and containment sheaths are withdrawn en bloc while maintaining distal position of the WATCHMAN LAA Closure Device. This allows the device to spring into the open (deployed) position. Contrast fluoroscopy, echocardiographic, and mechanical (tug) tests are performed confirming proper position of the device, demonstrating adequate device compression, confirming acceptable LAA seal with color Doppler, and confirming stability of final position. Once these criteria are confirmed, the device is released from the delivery catheter by counterclockwise rotation of the deployment knob. Final echocardiographic measurements are recorded, and the access sheath and delivery catheter are withdrawn into the right atrium (Figure 13.4).

Following the procedure, the patient is placed on warfarin therapy with a target therapeutic INR range of 2.0-3.0. After 45 days, an outpatient TEE is performed to assess device closure. Once confirmed, warfarin may be discontinued and aspirin therapy initiated.

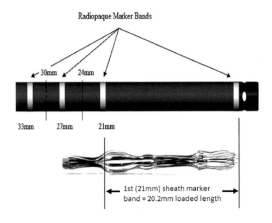

Device Size	Compressed Short Device
(uncompressed diameter)	Length
21 mm	20.2 mm
24 mm	22.9 mm
27 mm	26.5 mm
30 mm	29.4 mm
33 mm	31.5 mm

FIGURE 13.3   *Table of Predeployed Device Lengths and an Image of an Undeployed (Compressed) WATCHMAN LAA Closure Device*
The distal end of the access sheath includes radiopaque marker bands. By using these reference measurements, the deployed device position can be estimated. This offers a guide to sheath depth within the LAA prior to deployment. Used with permission from Atritech, Inc.

Complications

As can be seen with all invasive procedures, placement of the WATCHMAN LAA Closure Device is not without some inherent complication risks. Central venous access using a

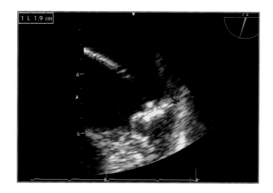

FIGURE 13.4   *TEE Image of an LAA with a Deployed Device*

Compression calculations are based on deployed device dimensions compared with known dimensions for the specific device size. The measurement of 19 mm (shown in the upper left) is obtained for a 24 mm device. This indicates a 21% compression ratio [1-(measured device width/fully expanded device size)].

14 F access sheath risks bleeding, hematoma, and pseudoaneurysm. Placement of an ipsilateral arterial access sheath during the procedure increases this risk slightly. Placement of catheters into the atria risks mechanical injury to the chambers. With the exception of the WATCHMAN LAA Closure Device and 14 F guiding sheath, standard catheters are employed for the procedure. The transseptal catheterization is performed in a standard fashion; however, upon LA access, the transseptal sheath is replaced with the 14 F access sheath. Because of the access sheath size, risk of perforation or residual atrial septal defect exists. Upon engagement of the LAA with the sheath and WATCHMAN LAA Closure Device, perforation risk is significant within the LAA if force is applied aggressively. Finally, device dislodgment and embolization are possible if device stability is not confirmed.

Anatomical Considerations

LAA anatomy varies widely in humans. Using computed tomography and TEE to analyze the different anatomical characteristics, the LAA may possess 1 lobe (71%), 2 lobes (4%), or multiple lobes (25%). Moreover, Figure 13.5 demonstrates the gross morphologic appearances, which can resemble a cauliflower (17%), a chicken wing (36%), a windsock (35%), or a cactus (13%). In addition to these variations in shape, the relationship of the LAA ostium to the left superior pulmonary vein (LSPV) varies as well. It connects to the LA above the LSPV (20%), at the level of the LSPV (71%), and below the LSPV (9%). Figure 13.6 illustrates LAA ostial position that originates superiorly and inferiorly.

The LAA anatomical characteristics should be considered when considering percutaneous closure. The different morphologies offer specific challenges. The "windsock" and "chicken wing" varieties are the easiest to close. Because both of these LAA types share a long primary lobe with branching occurring distally, they provide a long region for device placement with complete coverage. The "cauliflower" and "cactus" types offer much greater challenge, as these share proximal branching. As a result, a narrow window is provided that allows for complete coverage while ensuring adequate compression and stability. In rare cases, device deployment is not possible in some "cauliflower" LAA types that demonstrate a wide ostium and multiple short non-dominant lobes. In this situation, the LAA is simply too short to allow for an appropriately large device to be inserted that covers all lobes and that is stable enough for release.

The LAA ostial position should be considered when approaching the transseptal puncture. While the majority of LAA loca-

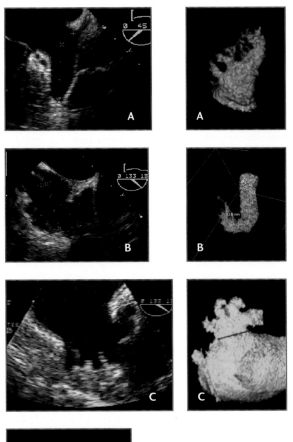

FIGURE 13.5   *The Four Most Common LAA Anatomic Variations*

A. The windsock-type left atrial appendage (LAA) is an anatomy in which 1 dominant lobe of sufficient length is the primary structure. Variations of this LAA type occur with the location and number of secondary lobes. **B.** The chicken wing–type LAA is an anatomy whose main characteristic is a sharp bend in the dominant lobe or the folding back of the LAA anatomy on itself at some distance from the perceived LAA ostium. Variations of this LAA type relate to the measured distance to this bend as well as to the orientation (anterior, superior, inferior, etc) of the bend relative to the main lobe. **C.** The cauliflower-type LAA is an anatomy whose main characteristic is an LAA that has limited overall length with more complex internal characteristics. Variations of this LAA type relate to the shape of the LAA ostium (oval versus round) and the number of significant lobes present. **D.** The cactus-type LAA is an anatomy whose main characteristic is a dominant central lobe with secondary lobes extending from the central lobe in both superior and inferior directions. Variations of this type relate to the number, location, and orientation of the secondary lobes.

tions are level with or superior to the LSPV, some are positioned lower in the LA. In this group, effort should be made to puncture the septum more inferiorly in the fossa ovalis. Engagement of an inferiorly positioned LAA is more difficult if the transseptal puncture occurs superiorly.

Access sheath selection also requires consideration of anatomy. The double-curved sheath tends to work best for engagement of most LAA anatomies. The main excep-

tion would be an LAA with a short tubular ostium with the dominant lobe located at a sharp angle in either direction. In this case, the double-curve sheath offers little control over which lobe ultimately becomes engaged. In this instance, the single-curve offers more versatility in sub-selecting the desired primary lobe.

Considering these anatomical variations, achieving consistent and complete closure of the appendage requires anatomic

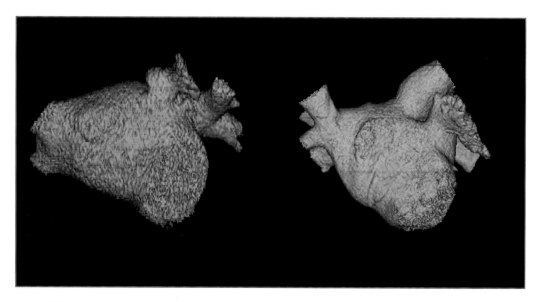

FIGURE 13.6   *3-D Computer Rendering of 2 LAs Illustrating Variations in LAA Position*
A superior and inferior left atrial appendage (LAA) orientation is demonstrated.
The latter requires a more inferior transseptal puncture to allow for easier LAA engagement.

consideration prior to device and access sheath selection. Because the WATCHMAN LAA Closure Device size range is 21 mm to 33 mm, very small and very large LAA may not be suitable for this procedure (Figure 13.2). The larger the deployed device, the longer the device length in the delivery catheter. Whether in the contained or open state, the device maintains a linear orientation. While the ideal device position would be coaxial, with the proximal face of the device at the level of the LAA ostium, this goal cannot always be achieved given orientation of the major lobe of the LAA, device size, angulation of the LAA, and ostial relationship of the LSPV.

Obviously, final device position is of greatest importance with this procedure. In many cases, final device placement may be angled with 1 shoulder just inside or outside the ostium. The primary criteria needed for safe and effective placement are device stability, coverage, and location. Device stabil-

ity at the final position is required to prevent subsequent device migration. This is assured when the final location demonstrates adequate device compression, remains stable during a mechanical tug test, and is located with all fixation barbs within the LAA structure. Conversely, coverage of all major lobes of the LAA is crucial for long-term efficacy. Any significant gap in coverage allowing for flow around the device risks inadequate closure of the LAA long term. Figure 13.7 shows an angled device with flow around the device and a well-positioned device with no leak. The final device location should not be too proximal, risking migration, or too distal, risking inadequate coverage (Figure 13.8).

Summary

In summary, the LAA is an anatomically and physiologically complex structure, which plays a key role in formation of LA thrombus

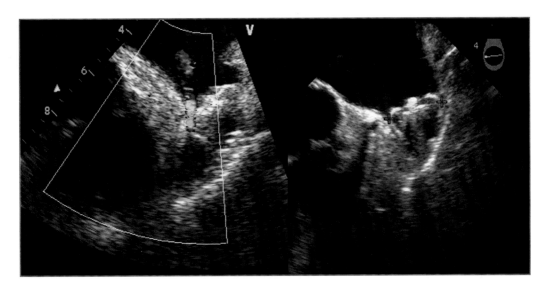

FIGURE 13.7   *Example of an Angled and Coaxial Device Position*
The angled device position (left) allows for flow around the device and incomplete closure, and it should ideally be repositioned more proximally. The coaxial device position (right) demonstrates proper position and occlusion.

in patients with AF. It is the site of thrombus formation in 90% of patients with AF. Numerous strategies have been pursued to prevent this complication, including surgical removal, surgical closure, and percutaneous closure. Surgical removal is invasive, technically challenging, and associated with changes in volume status due to loss of ANP. Surgical closure (over-sewing or stapling) is technically simpler, but invasive and often results in incomplete closure, which can paradoxically increase thrombus formation. Percutaneous transseptal closure appears to be an ideal approach, as it is less invasive, effective, and preserves the endocrine functions of the LAA while offering a high rate

of complete closure with a low complication rate. Results from a multicenter randomized trial demonstrated that the WATCHMAN LAA Closure Device was not inferior to warfarin therapy for stroke prophylaxis therapy.[29]

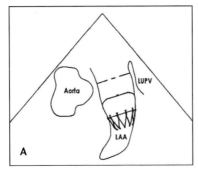

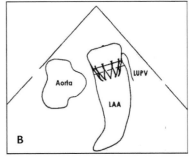

FIGURE 13.8   *Illustration of Incorrect WATCHMAN LAA Closure Device Positioning*
A. Distal device position risks incomplete coverage.
B. Proximal device position risks device migration.
Used with permission from Atritech, Inc.

Acknowledgments

Thanks are offered to George Latus of Atritech for providing images of the WATCHMAN system.

References

1. Moore KL. *The Developing Human: Clinically Oriented Embryology*. 6th ed. Philadelphia, PA: W B Saunders; 1998.

2. Ho SY, Anderson RH, Sánchez-Quintana D. Atrial structure and fibres: morphologic basis of atrial contraction. *Cardiovasc Res* 2002;54:325-336.

3. Perez-Lugones A, McMahon JT, Ratliff NB, et al. Evidence of specialized conduction cells in human pulmonary veins of patients with atrial fibrillation. *J Cardiovasc Electrophysiol* 2003;14(8):803-809.

4. Shirani J, Alaeddini J. Structural remodeling of the left atrial appendage in patients with chronic non-valvular atrial fibrillation: implications for thrombus formation, systemic embolism, and assessment by transesophageal echocardiography. *Cardiovasc Pathol* 2000;9(2):95-101.

5. Kappagoda CT, Linden RJ, Scott EM, et al. Atrial receptors and heart rate: the efferent pathway. *J Physiol* Aug 1975;249(3):581-590.

6. Inoue S, Murakami Y, Sano K, et al. Atrium as a source of brain natriuretic polypeptide in patients with atrial fibrillation. *J Card Fail* 2000;6(2):92-96.

7. Shively BK, Gelgand EA, Crawford MH. Regional left atrial stasis during atrial fibrillation and flutter: determinants and relation to stroke. *J Am Coll Cardiol* 1996;27(7): 1722-1729.

8. Fatkin D, Feneley MP. Patterns of Doppler-measured blood flow velocity in the normal and fibrillating human left atrial appendage. *Am Heart J* 1996;132(5):995-1003.

9. Madden J. Resection of the left auricular appendix; a prophylaxis for recurrent arterial emboli. *JAMA* 1949;140:769-772.

10. Verhorst PM, Kamp O, Visser CA, et al. Left atrial appendage flow velocity assessment using transesophageal echocardiography in nonrheumatic atrial fibrillation and systemic embolism. *Am J Cardiol* 1993;71(2):192-196.

11. Al-Saady NM, Obel OA, Camm AJ. Left atrial appendage: structure, function, and role in thromboembolism. *Heart* 1999;82(5):547-554.

12. Wolf PA, Dawber TR, Thomas HE Jr, et al. Epidemiologic assessment of chronic atrial fibrillation and risk of stroke: the Framingham study. *Neurology* 1978;28(10): 973-977.

13. Kannel WB, Wolf PA, Benjamin EJ, et al. Prevalence, incidence, prognosis, and predisposing conditions for atrial fibrillation: population-based estimates. *Am J Cardiol* 1998;82(8A):2N-9N.

14. Levine MN, Raskob G, Landefeld S, et al. Hemorrhagic complications of anticoagulant treatment. *Chest* 2001;119(1 suppl):108-121.

15. Schneider B, Stollberger C, Sievers HH. Surgical closure of the left atrial appendage—a beneficial procedure? *Cardiology* 2005;104(3):127-132.

16. Odell JA, Blackshear JL, Davies E, et al. Thoracoscopic obliteration of the left atrial appendage: potential for stroke reduction? *Ann Thorac Surg* 1996;61(2):565-569.

17. Lindsay BD. Obliteration of the left atrial appendage: a concept worth testing. *Ann Thorac Surg* 1996;61(2):515.

18. Katz ES, Tsiamtsiouris T, Applebaum RM, et al. Surgical left atrial appendage ligation is frequently incomplete: a transesophageal echocardiographic study. *J Am Coll Cardiol* 2000;36(2):468-471.

19. Kanderian AS, Gillinov AM, Pettersson GB, et al. Success of surgical left atrial appendage closure: assessment by transesophageal echocardiography. *J Am Coll Cardiol* 2008; 52(11):924-929.

20. Blackshear JL, Odell JA. Appendage obliteration to reduce stroke in cardiac surgical patients with atrial fibrillation. *Ann Thorac Surg* 1996;61(2):755-759.

21. Nishimura K. Does atrial appendectomy aggravate secretory function of atrial natriuretic polypeptide? *J Thorac Cardiovasc Surg* 1991;101(3):502-508.

22. Landymore R, Kinley CE. Staple closure of the left atrial appendage. *Can J Surg* 1984;27(2):144-145.

23. DiSesa VJ, Tam S, Cohn LH. Ligation of the left atrial appendage using an automatic surgical stapler. *Ann Thorac Surg* 1988;46(6):652-653.

24. Nakai T, Lesh MD, Gerstenfeld EP, et al. Percutaneous left atrial appendage occlusion (PLAATO) for preventing cardioembolism: first experience in canine model. *Circulation* 7 2002;105(18):2217-2222.

25. Ostermayer SH, Reisman M, Kramer PH, et al. Percutaneous left atrial appendage transcatheter occlusion (PLAATO system) to prevent stroke in high-risk patients with non-rheumatic atrial fibrillation: results from the international multi-center feasibility trials. *J Am Coll Cardiol* 5 2005;46(1):9-14.

26. Sick PB, Shuler G, Hauptmann KE, et al. Initial worldwide experience with the WATCHMAN left atrial appendage system for stroke prevention in atrial fibrillation. *J Am Coll Cardiol* 2007;49(13):1490-1495.

27. Möbius-Winkler S, Shuler GC, Sick PB. Interventional treatments for stroke prevention in atrial fibrillation with emphasis on the WATCHMAN device. *Curr Opin Neurol* 2008;21:64-69.

28. Fountain RB, Holmes DR, Chandrasekaran K, et al. The PROTECT AF (WATCHMAN Left Atrial Appendage System for Embolic PROTECTion in Patients with Atrial Fibrillation) trial. *Am Heart J* 2006;151(5):956-961.

29. Holmes DR, Reddy VY, Turi ZG, et al. Percutaneous closure of the left atrial appendage versus warfarin therapy for prevention of stroke in patients with atrial fibrillation: a randomised non-inferiority trial. *Lancet* 2009;374(9689):534-542.

SHELDON M. SINGH, VIVEK Y. REDDY

Transseptal catheterization was first described by Ross in 1959[1] to provide access to the left atrium (LA) during diagnostic left heart catheterization. Although initially popular, the development of pulmonary artery flotation catheters and of the retrograde aortic approach to accessing the left ventricle resulted in a diminished need for transseptal catheterization. However, there is now a resurgence of interest in this procedure due to the increasing numbers of "left-sided" electrophysiological and interventional cardiac procedures, including catheter ablation of cardiac arrhythmias such as atrial fibrillation, implantation of left atrial appendage occlusion devices, percutaneous cardiac valvular procedures, and placement of percutaneous ventricular assist devices. Despite a high success rate (>99%) and a low (0.8%)

complication rate[2] in experienced hands, variations in the position and structure of the interatrial septum may result in challenging punctures and increase the risk of inadvertent perforation of adjacent structures, such as the aortic root, the coronary sinus, and the posterior right atria wall. Although the current technique for transseptal access has changed little since first described, tools are being developed to improve the ease and safety of this procedure. This chapter will review these novel approaches with specific attention to innovative methods of visualizing and perforating the fossa ovalis.

Current Approach to Transseptal Catheterization

Venous access is typically obtained from the right femoral vein, and a long guidewire

Transseptal Catheterization and Interventions.
© 2010 Ranjan Thakur MD and Andrea Natale MD, eds.
Cardiotext Publishing, ISBN 978-0-9790164-1-7.

(generally, 150-180 cm long and 0.032 inch wide, or smaller) is advanced into the region of the superior vena cava (SVC) over which the transseptal sheath-dilator system (generally, 59-63 cm long) is advanced. The guidewire is removed and the sheath-dilator system is flushed to remove any coagulum. A standard 71-cm Brockenbrough transseptal needle is inserted into the dilator and positioned just proximal to its tip. A 10-cc syringe with radiopaque contrast is then attached to the end of the transseptal needle. A three-way stopcock may be connected to the hub of the needle to permit hemodynamic monitoring during the puncture. Once in the SVC, the entire transseptal apparatus (sheath-dilator-needle) is placed in a septal position based upon the fluoroscopic left anterior oblique (LAO) and right anterior oblique (RAO) views. Generally, the needle hub is oriented between 4 o'clock and 6 o'clock.

The transseptal apparatus is withdrawn inferiorly, watching for the first dilator jump, which occurs as the system falls off the torus aorticus, followed by a second jump as the system falls off the limbus of the fossa ovalis. At this point, the transseptal apparatus is then advanced slightly (1-2 mm) to ensure it is in contact with the fossa ovalis. To stain the fossa ovalis and demonstrate tenting, 3 cc to 5 cc of contrast may be injected. Once anticoagulation is administered (150 U/kg heparin bolus), the needle is advanced across the interatrial septum and into the LA. Crossing of the interatrial septum may be confirmed with contrast injection into the LA, analysis of blood oxygen saturation, or with pressure monitoring. A 0.014-inch angioplasty wire may be inserted through the lumen of the Brockenbrough needle into a pulmonary vein; this technique may both confirm the location of the needle in the LA and theoretically minimize inadvertent movement and puncturing of adjacent structures by

the transseptal system. On the other hand, because of the extreme thrombogenicity of metal, it is advisable to minimize the time the wire is in contact with the blood pool.

Once the needle has crossed the interatrial septum, the transseptal system is rotated anteriorly (ie, counterclockwise to approximately 3 o'clock) to avoid puncturing the posterior LA. The dilator is advanced over the needle, followed by the sheath over the dilator; a stained fossa ovalis allows the operator to gauge the depth of the sheath within the LA. The sheath is then stabilized, and the dilator and needle are removed as a unit.

Many electrophysiology laboratories perform transseptal punctures solely with the aid of fluoroscopy. A pigtail is often placed in the aortic root to mark the level of the aortic valve. Alternatively, a catheter may be placed at the level of the His bundle to approximate the inferior aspect of the aortic valve. The posterior and lateral borders of the atria are identified on the RAO and LAO views, respectively. Generally speaking, the fossa ovalis lies approximately 1 cm to 3 cm inferior to the level of the aortic valve. In the RAO view, the fossa ovalis is *en face*. Thus, this view is useful to tailor the anterior-posterior septal location of the puncture according to the clinical need; for example, for catheter ablation of atrial fibrillation, a posterior puncture is preferred, but during left atrial appendage occlusion, a more anterior septal puncture is preferred. Although fluoroscopy provides excellent spatial resolution to allow real-time visualization of the needle and sheath assembly, it is limited in its ability to resolve soft tissue. In addition, traditional fluoroscopic landmarks may not hold for all groups of patients; for example, the successful transseptal puncture position has been shown to be fluoroscopically posterior and higher in older individuals.[3]

Methods to Visualize the Fossa Ovalis During Transseptal Catheterization

The inability to identify the fossa ovalis may be responsible for approximately half of all failures to enter the left atrium during transseptal catheterization.[4] Imaging techniques including the use of echocardiography, magnetic resonance imaging (MRI), computed tomography (CT), electroanatomic mapping and direct endoscopic visualization of the fossa ovalis can complement traditional fluoroscopic approaches to identifying the fossa ovalis.

Echocardiography

The use of echocardiography to guide transseptal catheterization has been extensively studied.[5-8] While transthoracic echocardiography (TTE) may permit visualization of the interatrial septum and adjacent structures, its role in guiding transseptal catheterization is limited due to poor image quality, disruption of the sterile field, and the requirement of a second operator. Concomitant transesophageal echocardiography (TEE) can be performed with the use of fluoroscopy without disruption of the sterile field; however, this technique also requires a separate operator. In many centers, intracardiac echocardiography (ICE) is routinely used, given its ability to delineate the anatomy of the interatrial septum and adjacent structures without the need for a separate operator.

Intracardiac Echocardiography

Currently 2 types of ICE catheters are available for use: (1) 64-element phased array ultrasound systems, which allow imaging of a sector in the plane of the ICE catheter (either ACUSON AcuNav [Siemens Healthcare, Mountain View, CA] or ViewFlex [EP MedSystems, Inc, West Berlin, NJ]), and (2) an ultrasound transducer with a single rotating crystal that provides a circumferential field of view (Ultra ICE [Boston Scientific, Inc, Natick, MA]). Via femoral venous access, the ICE catheter is placed in the mid-right atrium, and the fossa ovalis is identified. The transseptal system may be identified when it is positioned in the area of the fossa ovalis. With gentle advancement of the transseptal system, tenting of the fossa may be demonstrated with ICE (Figure 14.1). Once the interatrial septum is punctured, contrast or saline is injected through the transseptal needle and is visualized in the LA with ICE. For atrial fibrillation ablation procedures the fossa is punctured at a mid-low level with the left pulmonary veins in the ultrasound plane; this seems to provide the ideal access to the LA sites targeted during this ablation procedure.

In addition to identifying normal fossa anatomy, ICE can be quite helpful in iden-

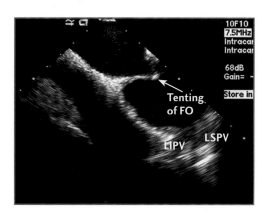

FIGURE 14.1   Intracardiac echocardiography demonstrating tenting of the fossa ovalis. FO = fossa ovalis; LIPV = left inferior pulmonary vein; LSPV = left superior pulmonary vein.

tifying anatomic variants, including septal thickening, septal aneurysms, and congenital anomalies, such as the presence of a double-layered fossa (Figure 14.2). Of note, care must be taken when interpreting the position of the transseptal apparatus with ICE, due to the reverberation artifact from the transseptal needle. Finally, ICE is extremely useful to assess for possible complications related to the transseptal procedure, such as (1) inadvertent posterior puncture resulting in pericardial effusion, (2) inadvertent puncture of the aorta, (3) inadvertent puncture of the posterior LA wall, resulting in an LA wall hematoma, or (4) formation of a thrombus related to transseptal apparatus or septal puncture site.[9,10]

Three-Dimensional Transesophageal Echocardiography

Three-dimensional (3-D) ultrasound is now available with transesophageal imaging probes, allowing for high-resolution, real-time volume imaging of cardiac structures. The greatest potential advantage that 3-D

TEE has over traditional 2-D TEE is its easy-to-understand volumetric image of the fossa ovalis and transseptal apparatus (Figure 14.3).[11,12] One limitation of 3-D TEE is the somewhat increased time required to properly segment and present the image to the operator in a clinically useful and timely manner. However, with increased availability and experience, this imaging modality is likely to have a more widespread role in guiding transseptal catheterization.

Real-time MRI

Echocardiography is frequently limited by acoustic shadowing and the inability to obtain adequate imaging windows. Despite this, the strength of echocardiography lies in its ability to provide real-time visualization of the fossa ovalis and transseptal system during transseptal catheterization. Recently, Raval et al[13] reported their experience with real-time MRI guidance of transseptal punctures in swine. Using custom designed MRI-compatible transseptal needles and sheaths, atrial septal punctures and balloon atrial septotomies were performed in a 1.5-tesla MRI interventional suite. Clear visualization of the fossa ovalis

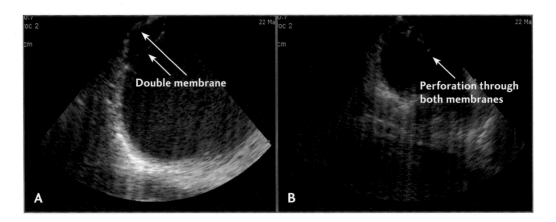

FIGURE 14.2   **A.** A double membrane fossa ovalis. **B.** Perforation of both membranes.

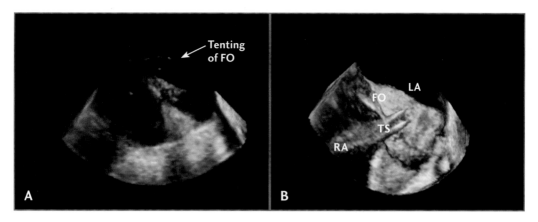

FIGURE 14.3   A 3-D echocardiographic localization of the fossa ovalis (FO). **A.** Demonstration of tenting of the fossa. **B.** Placement of 2 transseptal sheaths across the FO.
LA = left atrium; RA = right atrium; TS = transseptal sheath.

and transseptal apparatus was observed with MRI imaging. Atrial septal puncture was successful in all animals; however, catheter malfunction lead to hemorrhage in one animal. With the development of human-grade MRI compatible catheters, real-time MRI-guided transseptal puncture may be possible in clinical practice.

Image Integration

Image integration techniques may also guide transseptal catheterization.[14,15] Specifically, the fossa ovalis may be identified on pre-procedural volume rendered CT images of the left atrium obtained in patients undergoing complex electrophysiology ablation procedures. Using standard fluoroscopic views and additional landmark points, the pre-acquired CT image may be oriented to, and superimposed upon, the fluoroscopic image, allowing one to approximate the location of the fossa ovalis with fluoroscopy (Figure 14.4). Although the spatial accuracy of this approach has yet to be defined, it seems likely to provide an advantage over transseptal puncture guided solely by fluoroscopic landmarks.

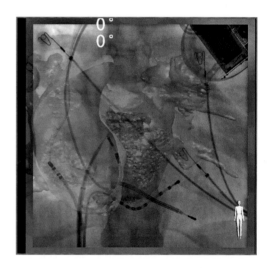

FIGURE 14.4   Use of CT (computed tomography) localization of the fossa ovalis to guide fluoroscopic transseptal puncture. Courtesy of Pierre Jaïs, Bordeaux, France.

Electroanatomical Mapping

The EnSite NavX electroanatomic mapping system (St. Jude Medical, Inc, St. Paul, MN) can provide an additional nonfluoroscopic method of localizing the position of the transseptal needle during transseptal catheterization (Figure 14.5).[16,17] Configuring the transseptal needle as a unipolar electrode allows it to be displayed on the 3-D electro-anatomic reconstruction of the right atrium once the needle is exposed beyond its sheath. In order to avoid inadvertent cardiac perfo-ration with an exposed needle, the superior aspect of the transseptal dilator can be modi-

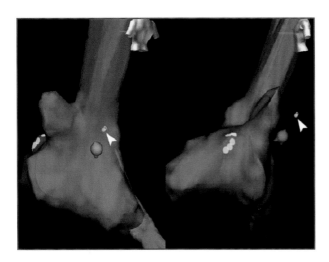

FIGURE 14.5   Identification of the transseptal needle (arrowhead) using the EnSite NavX mapping system (St. Jude Medical, Inc, St. Paul, MN). With kind permission from Springer Science+Business Media: *J Interv Cardiac Electrophysiology* 22(3) Sept 2008, 185, Ewan J Shepherd, Stott A. Gall, Stephen S. Furniss, Figure 4.

fied, allowing the needle to be exposed yet remain within the sheath.[17] There is minimal clinical experience with this approach, but the early experience suggests a good corre-lation with fluoroscopic images. However, it is important to recognize that these elec-troanatomic images are static, and patient respiration and movement can degrade the quality of the spatial resolution. Nevertheless, further refinements with this approach and additional experience may permit nonfluoro-scopic mapping systems to play an important role in guiding transseptal puncture.

Direct Visualization

Direct visualization of the fossa ovalis during transseptal procedures is now possible with a novel fiber-optic catheter (IRIS [Voyage Med-ical, Inc, Campbell, CA]) (Figure 14.6).[18,19] This 70-cm, 12 F catheter with controls for flexion and axial position consists of a 10,000-pixel fiber-optic scope to visualize intracardiac tissues. A collapsible hood located at the distal end of the catheter receives an infu-sion of saline, which effectively excludes blood from the field of view, thereby optimizing visualiza-tion of intracardiac structures. In additional, a 21-gauge transseptal needle may be advanced for trans-septal puncture through a proxi-mal port with a working lumen. Thiagalingam et al[18,19] studied this device in 6 swine. The fossa was identified as a non-contracting region surrounded by fibrous tis-sue (white); in some animals, the thinnest portion of the fossa was red in color because blood from the left atrium was visible through the thin, translucent fossa. In all swine, punc-ture sites were confirmed to be located at the fossa ovalis on pathological specimens. In addition to guiding the initial transsep-tal puncture, direct fossa visualization also permitted operators to cannulate previous puncture sites with an 0.035" guidewire. The initial human experience with this technol-ogy has confirmed the safety and feasibility of this promising technology.[20]

The SiteSeekir fiber-optic catheter (CardioOptics, Inc, Boulder, CO) may also allow direct visualization of the fossa ovalis. By "looking" only in certain infrared frequen-cies of the light spectrum, through-blood endoscopic visualization of the fossa is pos-sible. But to date, this catheter has also only

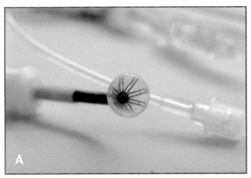

FIGURE 14.6 Direct visualization of the fossa ovalis with the fiber optic IRIS Catheter System (Voyage Medical, Inc, Campbell, CA). **A.** Collapsible hood at distal end of catheter. Courtesy of Voyage Medical, Inc. **B.** Intracardiac echocardiography visualization of the catheter hood at the fossa ovalis. **C.** Endoscopic view of the fossa ovalis.

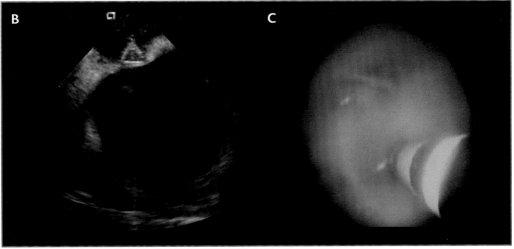

been tested in animals for general visualization, and there is no published feasibility data on transseptal puncture in animals, much less in humans.

Voltage Mapping

In addition to direct visualization, one may indirectly localize the fossa by exploiting its electrophysiological properties. As the fossa ovalis is essentially a fibrotic membrane, its electrophysiological properties are dissimilar to the adjacent atrial myocardium and demonstrate uni- and bipolar voltage reduction, fractionation electrograms with broadened signals and reduced slew rate, and increased pacing threshold. Thus, conventional voltage mapping with commercially available electroanatomical mapping systems may localize

the fossa. In addition, a transseptal system with 2 electrodes on the distal portion of the catheter is under development[21] and may also allow operators to determine the location of the fossa based on its electrophysiological properties.

Puncturing the Fossa Ovalis

On occasion, operators are unable to cross the interatrial septum despite adequate visualization of the fossa. This often arises in the presence of a thickened, heavily fibrotic septum (most commonly seen after repeated transseptal procedures[22]) or conversely, with a thin, aneurysmal, highly mobile septum. In these situations the force applied to cross the septum may lead to sudden uncontrollable motion of the transseptal assembly resulting in inadvertent cardiac perforation. When such conditions exist, the use of either radiofrequency[22-26] or laser[27] energy during transseptal puncture may allow for safe penetration of the septum.

Radiofrequency Energy

Radiofrequency (RF) energy can safely facilitate transseptal puncture. Unlike RF energy applied during the creation of ablation lesions, perforating RF ablation employs higher voltages (150-180 V compared to 30-50 V) with lower power delivered for shorter periods of time. When RF energy is applied to the fossa, a rise in tissue temperature occurs with protein denaturation, intracellular water vaporization, cell membrane rupture, and, ultimately, perforation of the interatrial septum (when tissue temperatures exceed $100°C$).

Commercial RF transseptal puncture systems are now available (Toronto Transseptal Catheter [Baylis Medical Company, Inc, Montreal, Canada]) (Figure 14.7). This system is delivered through an 8 F guiding sheath with a fixed dilator (TorFlex Transseptal Guiding Sheath [Baylis Medical Company, Inc, Montreal, Canada]). The distal aspect of the transseptal perforation catheter is flexible with an atraumatic tip; perforation does not result without the application of RF energy. Compared to a traditional hollow-bore transseptal needle, the atraumatic tip of the perforation catheter prevents boring of the interatrial septum (with possible tissue embolization) during the puncture. Four side holes are located approximately 1 mm to 1.4 mm from the distal aspect of the catheter, and allow for contrast infusion or pressure monitoring. The curved distal end of the RF catheter allows one to safely advance the system into the LA without the need to direct the system anteriorly (to avoid posterior LA trauma) or posteriorly (to avoid LA appendage trauma).

Using ICE or fluoroscopic guidance, the RF transseptal catheter is positioned and RF

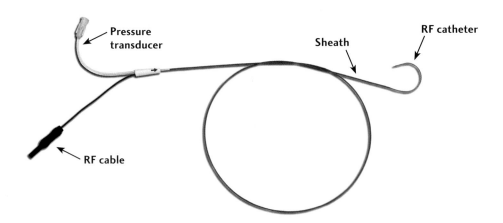

FIGURE 14.7   Components of the Toronto Transseptal Catheter (Baylis Medical Company, Inc, Montreal, Canada). The radiofrequency (RF) catheter passes through the dilator and sheath. An RF cable is connected to the catheter. Pressure monitoring from 4 side holes from the distal portion of the catheter is possible via a pressure transducer. Printed with permission from Baylis Medical Company.

energy delivered once the fossa is engaged. Generally, short 2- to 5-second pulses of 5 W to 10 W may be applied. Once the operator has perforated the septum, RF power application is stopped to avoid perforation of other LA structures. Generally, the septum can be punctured with the application of 1 to 4 pulses of RF.

As an alternative to this commercial system, a number of investigators have reported the use of RF energy transmitted through a conventional Brockenbrough transseptal needle. The energy is applied to the hub at the back end of the needle, using either an ablation catheter or a Bovie surgical electrocautery tip (in "cut" mode). The RF energy required for transseptal puncture is not well defined with this approach. In general, higher RF energy is applied because, unlike commercial RF transseptal catheters, which are insulated to minimize current leakage, conventional transseptal needles are not insulated. In our experience, 20 W to 30 W of unipolar RF energy applied for 1 to 3 seconds is often sufficient to perforate the fossa. In one published experience with 15 patients, Knecht et al reported successful transseptal access using 30 W of unipolar RF energy, applied for a median of 1 second in duration.[22] It is of paramount importance to ensure proper needle positioning prior to the application of RF energy in order to avoid inadvertent puncture of collateral structures. Attention must be paid to ICE, fluoroscopy, and/or hemodynamic waveforms to identify when the perforating catheter has crossed the septum.

There is currently minimal published data on the thrombotic potential of RF transseptal puncture. Histologic studies demonstrate the acute deposition of mural thrombus similar to that with conventional transseptal puncture.[25] In our own clinical experience, thrombus has been noted on the needle during RF transseptal puncture, particularly with prolonged applications of RF energy delivery. One advantage of ICE guidance is the ability to visualize microbubbles during energy delivery. While initially seen in the right atrium only, these microbubbles are then visualized within the LA upon successful transseptal puncture (Figure 14.8). It is imperative to immediately cease RF delivery at this point since thrombus/char formation starts to form almost immediately during RF

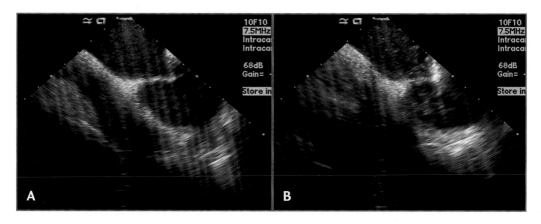

FIGURE 14.8   Microbubble formation during radiofrequency-aided transseptal puncture. **A.** Tenting of the fossa prior to radiofrequency application. **B.** Microbubbles noted in the left atrium with successful radiofrequency-added transseptal puncture.

delivery. Furthermore, we advocate antico-agulation *prior* to any delivery of RF energy. (We also advocate anticoagulation prior to conventional transseptal puncture, but we believe that the import of anticoagulation is even greater in this situation).

Excimer Laser

Excimer laser catheters (0.9 mm CLiRpath X-80 [Spectranetics Corporation, Colorado Springs, CO]) may also be beneficial during difficult transseptal punctures. A laser cath-eter with an inner lumen permitting contrast delivery, pressure transduction, and guidewire insertion can be inserted through a modified Mullins sheath. As the laser catheter has a blunt end, it cannot perforate tissue unless activated. With gentle, continuous pressure, the laser is activated for 2- to 4-second pulses until sep-tal puncture. At this point, laser energy deliv-ery is stopped, and the dilator and sheath are advanced on this "mono-rail" into the LA. As with RF energy, it is important to ensure that the laser catheter engages the fossa appropri-ately, as laser is also capable of perforating col-lateral tissue if incorrectly targeted. In a swine study, an average of 3 seconds of laser time was required for successful transseptal puncture.[27] The force required for laser transseptal punc-ture was 10-fold less than conventional trans-septal puncture, and the punctures sites were 20% to 30% greater in diameter compared to the conventional approach.

mon that electrophysiologists are required to perform transseptal punctures on patients who have undergone device closure of an atrial septal defect (ASD) or patent foramen ovale (PFO). In these patients, fluoroscopic guidance can be employed to guide the trans-septal puncture.[28] However, we prefer to employ ICE to optimize the location of the transseptal puncture site in relation to the LA targets of the ablation procedure. Typi-cally, one targets the thin rim of the septum primum located 2 cm to 4 cm caudal to the inferior margin of the closure device to safely puncture the septum (Figure 14.9).

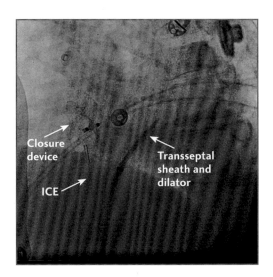

FIGURE 14.9   Safe zone for transseptal puncture inferior to atrial septal defect and patent foramen ovale occlusion devices. ICE = intracardiac echocardiography.

Special Circumstances

Post–Atrial Septal Defect/ Patent Foramen Ovale Device Closure

Given the association between atrial arrhyth-mias and atrial septal defects, it is not uncom-

Superior Approach via the Right Internal Jugular Vein

In certain situations, such as an interrupted inferior vena cava, transseptal access may not be obtained from the femoral veins. In this situation, one may consider access via the right internal jugular vein. The LA-Crosse system (St. Jude Medical, Inc, St. Paul, MN) may aid with the superior approach (Figure 14.10). The system consists of 3 components: a stabilizing sheath with an end hole; a guiding catheter, which is placed though the stabilizing sheath and directed to the fossa ovalis; and an inner catheter with puncture screw. Once the screw has penetrated the LA, a guidewire may be placed in the LA to aid with sheath placement. This sheath system is approved in Europe, but is not yet approved by the Food and Drug Administration for clinical use in the United States; it is currently undergoing clinical investigation as a tool for implantation of LA pressure sensors.

Double Transseptal Access

Double transseptal access is often required for electrophysiology procedures, including atrial fibrillation ablation. Several approaches have been described to avoid performing the second puncture due to its attendant risks.[29] In the first approach, after the first transseptal puncture, (1) the sheath is first withdrawn into the RA over the long guidewire still in the LA, (2) a mapping catheter is advanced through a second transseptal sheath and manipulated into the LA through the original transseptal puncture site, and (3) with the mapping catheter in place, the initial sheath is then readvanced into the LA over the retained guidewire. One disadvantage of this approach is the inevitable physical interaction between both sheaths during LA catheter manipulation. A second approach involves placing 2 guidewires into the LA through the first transseptal sheath. The initial sheath is withdrawn from the body, and 2 transseptal sheaths are reinserted over their respective retained guidewires. In addition to sheath interaction, this latter approach is also limited by the increased bleeding from the single femoral venous puncture site. Because of these limitations, our preference is to perform 2 separate transseptal punctures via sheaths from 2 separate femoral venous puncture sites.

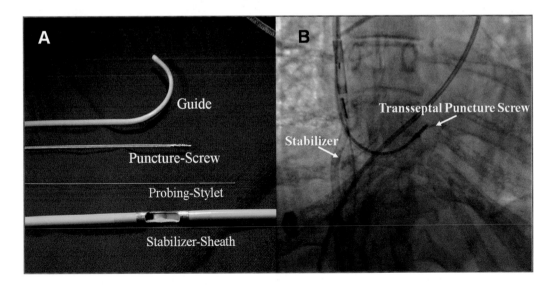

FIGURE 14.10   LA-Crosse system (St. Jude Medical, Inc, St. Paul, MN), allowing for a superior approach to transseptal puncture.

Conclusion

With the increasing frequency of left-sided cardiac procedures, transseptal access will continue to be an indispensable skill for invasive cardiologists. Awareness and familiarity with the various approaches and tools being developed to facilitate this procedure should improve its feasibility. Furthermore, because complications associated with transseptal puncture are potentially life-threatening, we advocate that one should accept nothing short of a zero-complication rate. With proper experience and judicious use of novel approaches and tools, we firmly believe that this is an achievable goal.

References

1. Ross J. Transseptal heart catheterization: a new method of left atrial puncture. *Ann Surg* 1959;140:395-401.

2. De Ponti R, Cappato R, Curnis A, Della Bella P, Padeletti L, Raviele A, Santini M, Salerno-Uriarte JA. Trans-septal catheterization in the electrophysiology laboratory: data from a multicenter survey spanning 12 years. *J Am Coll Cardiol* 2006;47:1037-1042.

3. Hu YF, Tai CT, Lin YJ, Chang SL, Lo LW, Wongcharoen W, Udyavar AR, Tuan TA, Chen SA. Does the age affect the fluoroscopy guided trans-septal puncture in catheter ablation of atrial fibrillation? *Pac Clin Electrophysiol* 2007;30:1506-1510.

4. Lew AS, Harper RW, Federman J, Anderson ST, Pitt A. Recent experience with transseptal catheterization. *Cathet Cardiovasc Diagn* 1983;9:601-609.

5. Daoud EG, Kalbfleisch SJ, Hummel JD. Intracardiac echocardiography to guide transseptal left heart catheterization for radiofrequency catheter ablation. *J Cardiovasc Electrophysiol* 1999;10:358-363.

6. Hurrell DG, Nishimura RA, Symanski JD, Holmes DR Jr. Echocardiography in the invasive laboratory: utility of two-dimensional echocardiography in performing transseptal catheterization. *Mayo Clin Proc* 1998;73:126-131.

7. Ren JF, Marchlinski FE, Callans DJ, Herrmann HC. Clinical use of AcuNav diagnostic ultrasound catheter imaging during left heart radiofrequency ablation and transcatheter closure procedures. *J Am Soc Echocardiogr* 2002;15:1301-1308.

8. Epstein LM, Smith T, TenHoff H. Nonfluoroscopic transseptal catheterization: safety and efficacy of intracardiac echocardiographic guidance. *J Cardiovasc Electrophysiol* 1998; 9:625-630.

9. Maleki K, Mohammadi R, Hart D, Cotiga D, Farhat N, Steinberg JS. Intracardiac ultrasound detection of thrombus on transseptal sheath: incidence, treatment, and prevention. *J Cardiovasc Electrophysiol* 2005;16:561-565.

10. Martelo S, d'Avila A, Ferreira F, Saad EB. Implantation of bilateral carotid artery filters to allow safe removal of left atrial thrombus during ablation of atrial fibrillation. *J Cardiovasc Electrophysiol* 2006;17:1140-1141.

11. Suk Yang H, Srivathsan K, Wissner E, Chandrasekar K. Real-time 3-dimensional transesophageal echocardiography: novel utility in atrial fibrillation ablation with a prosthetic mitral valve. *Circulation* 2008;117:e304-305.

12. Lim KK, Sugeng L, Lang R, Knight BP. Double transseptal catheterization guided by real time 3-dimensional transesophageal echocardiography. *Heart Rhythm* 2008;5:324-325.

13. Raval AN, Karmarkar PV, Guttman MA, Ozturk C, Desilva R, Aviles RJ, Wright VJ, Schenke WH, Atalar E, McVeigh ER, Lederman RJ. Real-time MRI guided atrial septal puncture and balloon septostomy in swine. *Catheter Cardiovasc Interv* 2006;67:637-643.

14. Graham LN, Melton IC, MacDonald S, Crozier IG. Value of CT localization of the fossa ovalis prior to transeptal left heart cath-

eterization for left atrial ablation. *Europace* 2007;9:417-423.

15. Knecht S, Skali H, O'Neill MD, Wright M, Matuso S, Nault I, Lim K-T, Sacher F, Derval N, Deplange A, Montaudon M, Corneloup O, Bordachar P, Hocini M, Clementy J, Haïssaguerre M, Orlov MV, Jaïs P. Real-time high resolution imaging of the left atrium using CT-fluoroscopy overlay to assist AF ablation [Abstract]. *Heart Rhythm* 2008;5(5) (suppl):S225.

16. Verma S, Borganelli M. Real-time, three-dimensional localization of a Brockenbrough needle during transseptal catheterization using a nonfluoroscopic mapping system. *J Invasive Cardiol* 2006;18:324-327.

17. Shepherd EJ, Gall SA, Furniss SS. Interatrial septal puncture without the use of fluoroscopy-reducing ionizing radiation in left atrial ablation procedures. *J Inter Card Electrophysiol* 2008;22:183-187.

18. Thiagalingam A, d'Avila A, Foley L, Miller D, Rothe C, Saadat V, Ruskin JN, Reddy VY. Direct visualization of the fossa ovalis for transeptal puncture: *in vivo* evaluation of the IRIS catheter in a porcine model [Abstract 2241]. *Circulation* 2007;116:II_448.

19. Thiagalingam A, d'Avila A, Foley L, Miller D, Rothe C, Saadat V, Ruskin JN, Reddy VY. Full-color direct visualization of the atrial septum to guide transseptal puncture. *J Cardiovasc Electrophysiol* 2008;19:1301-1305.

20. Reddy VY, Neuzil P, Miller D, Rothe C, Malchano ZJ, Robinson R, Sadaat V, d'Avila A. *In vivo* direct visualization of the atrial septum to guide transseptal puncture: results from the first-in-man clinical experience [Abstract] (Submitted for publication).

21. Krishnan, SC, inventor; Dinsmore & Shohl LLP, assignee. Method and apparatus for localizing the fossa ovalis and performing transseptal puncture. http://www.wipo.int/pctdb/en/wo.jsp?wo=2004026134&IA=US2003026776&DISPLAY=STATUS.

22. Knecht S, Jaïs P, Nault I, Wright M, Matsuo S, Madaffari A, Lellouche N, Derval N, O'Neill MD, Deplagne A, Bordachar P, Sacher F, Hocini M, Clementy J, Haïssaguerre M. Radiofrequency puncture of the fossa ovalis for resistant transseptal access. *Cir Arrhythm Electrophysiol* 2008;1:169-174.

23. Casella M, Dello Russo A, Pelargonio G, Martino A, De Paulis S, Zecchi P, Bellocci F, Tondo C. Fossa ovalis radiofrequency perforation in a difficult case of conventional transseptal puncture for atrial fibrillation ablation. *J Interv Card Electrophysiol* 2008;21:249-253.

24. Sherman W, Lee P, Hartley A, Love B. Transatrial septal catheterization using a new radiofrequency probe. *Catheter Cardiovasc Interv* 2005;66:14-17.

25. Veltdman GR, Wilson GJ, Peirone A, Hartley A, Estrada M, Norgard G, Leung RK, Visram N, Benson LN. Radiofrequency perforation and conventional needle percutaneous transseptal left heart access: pathologic features. *Catheter Cardiovasc Interv* 2005;65:556-563.

26. Veltdman GR, Hartley A, Visram N, Benson LN. Radiofrequency applications in congenital heart disease. *Expert Rev Cardiovasc Ther* 2004;2:117-126.

27. Elagha AA, Kim AH, Kocaturk O, Lederman LJ. Blunt atrial transseptal puncture using excimer laser in swine. *Catheter Cardiovasc Interv* 2007;70:585-590.

28. Zakar-Sharak R, Fuhrer J, Meier B. Transseptal puncture for catheter ablation of atrial fibrillation after device closure of a patent foramen ovale. *Catheter Cardiovasc Interv* 2008;71:551-552.

29. Yamanda T, McElderry HT, Epstein AE, Plumb VJ, Kay GN. One-puncture, double transseptal catheterization manoeuvre in the catheter ablation of atrial fibrillation. *Europace* 2007;9:487-489.

Complications of
Transseptal Catheterization

Mehul B. Patel, Khyati Pandya,
Atul Khasnis, Ranjan Thakur

*If you don't know where you are going,
you will wind up somewhere else.*

—Yogi Berra

In the early days of cardiac catheterization, the diagnosis of valvular and congenital heart disease required measurement of pressures in the left heart chambers. The initial approaches to obtaining left heart pressure measurement included the right paravertebral technique described by Bjork[1] and the left bronchial puncture technique by Allison in 1953,[2] followed by the direct left ventricular puncture procedure by Ponsdomenech and Brock in 1956.[3,4] Transseptal puncture (TSP) for left heart catheterization (LHC) was first introduced by Cope and Ross in 1959[5,6] and later modified by Brockenbrough and Braunwald in 1960.[7] Mullins further modified this

Transseptal Catheterization and Interventions.
© 2010 Ranjan Thakur MD and Andrea Natale MD, eds.
Cardiotext Publishing, ISBN 978-0-9790164-1-7.

technique using a long sheath and dilator in 1983, and since then there has been very little change.[8]

Amongst transbronchial, transthoracic, and transventricular techniques for the assessment of left heart pressures, TSP has emerged as the most practical method.[9] TSP also allows therapeutic intervention, which is not possible using the other methods. As the decades have elapsed, TSP has emerged as one of the most significant procedural developments in the field of interventional cardiology. In the late 1960s, however, this technique was associated with an aura of "danger and intrigue," leading to a worldwide decline in the number of procedures. The advent of percutaneous transvenous mitral commissurotomy (PTMC) by Kanji Inoue, MD, in 1984 required transseptal catheterization (TSC) to reach the left atrium via TSP.[10] With this development, TSP reclaimed its importance and became the pivotal component of access to the left side of the heart for complex structural interventions.[11] TSP became important to the electrophysiologist for ablation of left-sided accessory pathways and left atrial tachycardias starting in the early 1990s. However, it wasn't until Haïssaguerre showed that atrial fibrillation (AF) is often caused by a rapidly firing focus in one of the pulmonary veins, thus ushering in the present era of AF ablation, that the TSP technique saw a worldwide resurgence.[12] Commonly used indications for transseptal catheterization are listed in Table 15.1. Although safe in experienced hands, TSP can be a challenging and an unforgiving procedure. As there are very few large studies on TSP,[13] most of the reported complications are from anecdotal case reports. In one series, the reported complication rate from TSC was 0.74% to 0.79%.[14] This chapter describes many of the potential complications associated with TSP and offers important tips for anticipating, preventing, assessing, and managing those complications.

Anatomy: The Roadmap

Fossa Ovalis

The right and left atria are not lateral to each other; the right atrium (RA) is located antero-lateral to the left atrium (LA). The LA is the most posterior cardiac chamber and forms two-thirds of the base of the heart. The inter-atrial septum (IAS) is therefore not a vertical midline structure, but rather slanted in the posterior-anterior plane from the right to the left, at a 65° angle (Figure 15.1). Embryologically, the IAS is formed by overlap of the septum primum and secundum; the gap in between, called the foramen ovale, is represented by the fossa ovalis component of the IAS in adulthood.

The fossa ovalis comprises about 28% of the total interatrial septal area, which measures about 240 mm² in adults.[15] Though usu-

ally located posteriorly at the junction of the mid and lower third of the RA, its position can vary in hearts where the anatomy has been distorted by concomitant valvular or congeni-

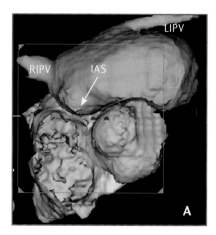

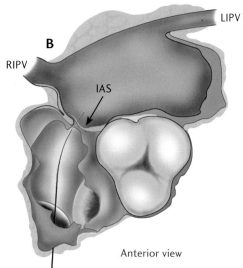

FIGURE 15.1   *Schematic Representation of the Ideal Transseptal Puncture Site*

A. A computed tomography image of the heart is shown in the transverse plane at the level of the fossa ovalis and the inferior pulmonary veins. LIPV = left inferior pulmonary vein; RIPV = right inferior pulmonary vein. **B.** A schematic of the same image is shown. Note that the interatrial septum (IAS) (arrow) runs at an angle from right to left. Courtesy of Mehul B. Patel, MD, and Delilah Cohn, MFA, CMI.

tal heart disease. The muscular border of the fossa ovalis is 2-layered and formed by the folding of both the atrial walls. The anatomy of the inferior rim of the fossa ovalis also deserves attention. Anteroinferior to the fossa ovalis is the opening of the coronary sinus into the right atrium. The posterior aspect of the atrioventricular (AV) groove separating the LA from the left ventricle contains fibro-adipose tissue, and the AV nodal artery supplying the AV node (which lies in the triangle of Koch) runs through this section of the posteroinferior IAS.[16] Excessive manipulation of the transseptal needle in this anatomical region can result in compromised AV nodal circulation. The artery to the sinus node (SN) originates from the right coronary artery in 55% cases and runs in the area around the superior vena cava (SVC)-RA junction.[17] Though the RA is usually accessed through the inferior vena cava (IVC), in cases where the SVC is the route of entry, the anatomical location of the artery to the SN has important implications

The LA has 3 components: a smooth-walled venous chamber, an atrial appendage lined by pectinate muscles, and a vestibule supporting the attachments of the leaflets of the mitral valve. The pulmonary veins (PVs) enter the LA at the 4 "corners" of the venous chamber, enclosing a prominent atrial dome. The anterosuperior aspect of the fossa ovalis is related to the aortic root, and inadvertent puncture of this part of the IAS can result in a catastrophic aortic entry.

Atrial Septal Neighborhood

The IAS is a blade-like structure with a concave anterior curve formed by the ascending aorta and a convex posterior border. The posterior border is formed by the narrow expanse of the right atrial wall on the right and by the right pulmonary veins on the left. The tip of

the blade is formed by the SVC on the right and by the right superior pulmonary vein on the left. The inferior margin is formed by the right atrial endocardium overlying the membranous interventricular septum (IVS) on the right and the mitral annulus on the left[18-20] (Figure 15.2).

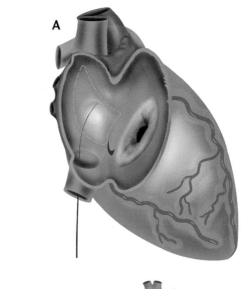

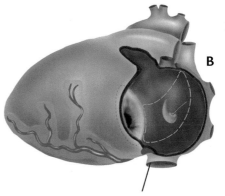

FIGURE 15.2 *The Interatrial Septum Neighborhood Viewed from the Right Atrium and Left Atrium*
A: RA.The blade-like IAS and the fossa ovalis are outlined in yellow. The needle tip is seen resting against the limbus in the fossa ovalis. **B:** LA.This view of the IAS neighborhood shows the ideal site of puncture, with the needle penetrating through the fossa into the LA. Courtesy of Mehul B. Patel, MD, and Delilah Cohn, MFA, CMI.

TSP Procedure

Originally, TSC was performed with only fluoroscopic guidance. As echocardiography came into use, transesophageal echocardiography (TEE) and intracardiac echocardiography (ICE) were integrated to improve safety and success rate. We describe some landmarks that can be useful for the fluoroscopy-guided procedure.

Though biplane fluoroscopy is preferable for TSP, single-plane fluoroscopy is usually sufficient. The instruments used for the procedure include a Brockenbrough needle, a 70-cm 14 F tapered tip polyethylene dilator, and a 7 F or 8 F transseptal sheath. A 5-mL or 10-mL syringe containing pure contrast medium is connected to the manifold, which is attached to the hub of the transseptal needle for constant pressure monitoring and also for contrast injection when needed. The anatomic and fluoroscopic landmarks, along with the "septal flush" or the "septal stain" method, can identify the IAS and fossa ovalis.

To identify the ideal site for TSP, the following steps can be helpful.

Steps and Landmarks for Optimal TSP

1. After obtaining a diastolic still frame of the left ventriculogram in the 30° right anterior oblique (RAO) view, draw a horizontal line from the center of the mitral valve (M line). (Figure 15.3a)

2. Take a cineangiogram with the pigtail sitting on the aortic valve in the frontal view. Draw a horizontal line from the lowest point of the pigtail horizontally to the right outmost border of the LA. Draw a perpendicular line from the midpoint of this line. (A horizontal line drawn from the summit of the His-bundle catheter recording a His-bundle electrocardiogram would also serve as a similar reference for the M line.) (Figure 15.3b)

3. The point of intersection of this perpendicular midline to the horizontal M line is the ideal site of puncture (P). It is assumed that the vertical midline divides the IAS into anterior and posterior halves ("midline") (Figure 15.3c).

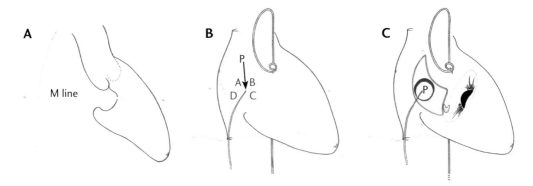

FIGURE 15.3   *Understanding the Steps of Transseptal Puncture*
A. Diastolic still frame of left ventriculogram in the right anterior oblique (RAO) view with the M line. The M line is a horizontal line drawn at the center of the mitral annulus. **B.** The midline with the ideal site of puncture (P). **C.** Superimposition of the atrial neighborhood on the fluoroscopic anatomy for transseptal puncture. Courtesy of Mehul B. Patel, MD.

Contraindications to TSP

Few conditions constitute absolute contraindications for TSC.

LA Thrombus or Mass

Patients with mobile thrombi in the LA are at a high risk of systemic embolism, and TSP should be deferred in such patients. Patients with non-mobile thrombi in the LA cavity should be treated with long-term anticoagulation therapy to maintain an international normalized ratio (INR) between 2 to 3, and resolution of the thrombus should be ascertained before proceeding with LA cannulation and catheter manipulation. Presence of thrombi confined to the LA appendage (without protrusion into the LA cavity) is not a contraindication for PTMC.[21-24] However, catheter ablation for AF should be deferred until patient has been anticoagulated for an adequate length of time and resolution of thrombus is documented.

Bleeding Diathesis or Conditions Necessitating Anticoagulation

Patients undergoing TSC should be anticoagulated before TSP is done or immediately after the LA is entered. Within minutes of entering the LA, a thrombus may form in and around the sheath and lead to an embolic event, as shown in Figure 15.4. Thus, inability to anticoagulate a patient because of a bleeding diathesis or another contraindication, such as intracranial bleeding or gastrointestinal bleeding, constitutes an absolute contraindication for TSC.

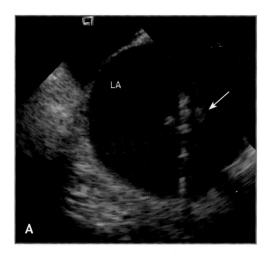

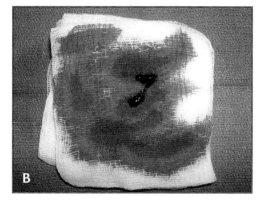

FIGURE 15.4   *Thrombus Formation on a Transseptal Sheath*

A. An intracardiac echocardiography (ICE) image is shown of a 72-year-old man who underwent transseptal catheterization (TSC) for ablation of atrial fibrillation (AF). After the first transseptal sheath was placed, the patient was not heparinized while attempting the second transseptal puncture (TSP). A mobile density (arrow) was noted at the tip of the first sheath before the second TSP could be completed. **B.** Blood was aspirated from the sheath, and the thrombus was aspirated. The patient was heparinized to achieve an activated clotting time (ACT) >300 seconds, and the procedure was completed uneventfully.

Complications of TSC: What the Mind Does Not Know the Eye Does Not See

TSC is generally a safe procedure in experienced hands. Most complications have been reported from the days of fluoroscopy-guided procedures. It may be reasonable to conclude that availability of ICE and TEE will reduce the risk of complications, as evidenced by the example illustrated in Figure 15.4.

An arbitrary classification of potential complications is provided in Table 15.2.

I. Related to TSP

A. Puncture-Related

1. Puncture of Sites Other Than IAS

This is a major complication of TSP, if not recognized early. Having a high index of suspicion for cardiac perforation is crucial for preventing catastrophic outcomes. Cardiac perforation may result in chest pain and may be accompanied by a decline in the arterial pressure, an increase in cardiac size on fluoroscopy, and loss of cardiac motion on fluoroscopy. Uncomplicated needle or catheter perforation is usually due to RA puncture. Such punctures cause chest pain, generally without any major sequelae.

a. Perforation of Aorta

Diagnosis Needle puncture of the aortic wall may lead to pericardial effusion. Low magnification fluoroscopy in left anterior oblique (LAO) view may show loss of cardiac pulsations at the costophrenic angle with or without an appreciable increase in the cardiac size.

Management Inform the surgical team and withdraw the needle. Watch for changes in heart rate and blood pressure for a substantial period of time on the catheterization table. Needle-only perforations usually seal off without need for surgery. In the absence of hemodynamic changes, a decision should be made whether the procedure should be continued or abandoned because the patient will require full intraprocedural anticoagulation. If the risk is unknown or deemed high, it may be best to abort the procedure. All such patients should be watched and monitored carefully for several hours in the intensive care unit. In case of hemodynamic compromise with effusion on echocardiography, the patient should be emergently wheeled to the operating room. If it is determined that the aorta is definitely punctured with the dilator and/or the transseptal sheath, it is best to leave the instrument in place to seal the entry site rather than withdrawing it and risking hemodynamic collapse.

Prevention It is a good practice to check the aortic root size before TSP. Have a high index of suspicion if the aortic root is dilated. Avoiding punctures medial to the midline (zones B and C of Figure 15.3b) could potentially prevent most inadvertent aortic punctures. Also, it is vital to feel the transmitted pulsations with the right-hand fingertips holding the needle hub. Importantly, it should be remembered that the aorta can be punctured even after successful entry into the LA if the needle is pointed anteriorly. Hence, continuous needle pressure monitoring is crucial. Recording a left ventricular (LV) pressure waveform could mean that the needle has punctured the aorta and entered the left ventricle retrogradely. (See Figures 15.5 and 15.6.)

b. Perforation of RA, LA, or LV

Diagnosis of Tamponade Asymptomatic pericardial effusion not requiring intervention is reported in 2.5% of cases.[25] Pericardial tamponade requiring intervention is reported

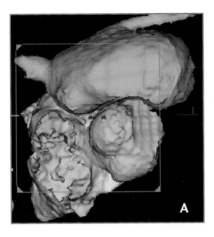

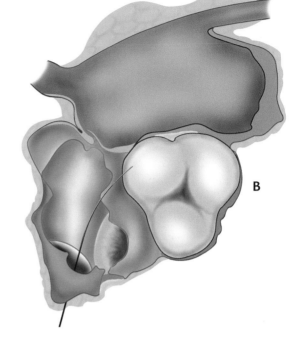

FIGURE 15.5   *Accidental Aortic Puncture*

A. Computed tomography (CT) reconstruction image of the heart with a transverse cut made at the level of the fossa ovalis showing the inferior pulmonary veins. **B.** A schematic of the same figure. Aortic puncture secondary to uncontrolled counterclockwise or anterior movement of the needle tip is illustrated. Courtesy of Mehul B. Patel, MD, and Delilah Cohn, MFA, CMI.

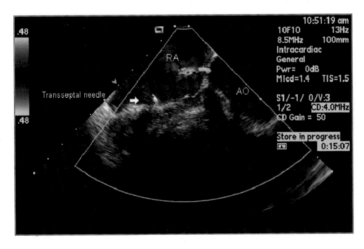

FIGURE 15.6   *A Doppler Image after Aortic Puncture*

A small jet is shown at the base of the aorta, from the aorta (AO) to the right atrium (RA). Reprinted with permission from Deborah Creighton, Biosense Webster.

in 1% of all cases undergoing TSP.[25] Loss of cardiac borders on fluoroscopy with loss of cardiac pulsations generally precedes the hemodynamic signs; one should *never* wait for the classical Beck's triad of hemodynamic collapse.[26] Acute cardiac tamponade due to perforation during cardiac intervention is a potentially lethal complication with a mortality rate as high as 42%.[27] Hypotension is usually the first hemodynamic sign. Bradycardia is another important early sign of perforation. These hemodynamic clues should alert the operator to the possibility of tamponade, but these changes are not very specific and may be related to a variety of other causes, such as sedation and alteration of autonomic tone. Furthermore, it is extremely crucial to realize that tamponade can occur even in the absence of elevated venous pressures. Blood accumulates first in the posterolateral pericardial sac as the pericardium is attached anteriorly to the sternum and posteriorly to the spine. This region is best visualized as the lateral heart border in the LAO view. An emergency transthoracic echocardiogram (TTE) is also crucial to diagnose a global or a localized effusion. In rare cases, there may be serious significant bleeding into the posterior pericardial space, leading to the missed diagnosis of tamponade with a "dry" tap on pericardiocentesis.

Uncontrolled posterosuperior movement of the needle can cause puncture of the right atrial and left atrial walls in the transverse sinus, permitting needle entry from the RA into the LA cavity. This "phenomenon of stitching" can be catastrophic if the passage is subsequently dilated with the dilator and the sheath. As long as the sheath is in place, the patient may remain asymptomatic. However, once the sheath is removed, rapid hemodynamic collapse may ensue because large rents are created in both the RA and LA (Figure 15.7; see also Figure 15.8).

Further posterosuperior movement of the needle can cause puncture of the RA in the transverse sinus (Figure 15.9).

Steady advancement of the needle after transseptal puncture can cause puncture of the LA roof or the left superior pulmonary vein (Figure 15.10).

For procedures such as PTMC, LV perforation is a potential complication. Left ventricular hypertrophy does not attenuate the risk of LV perforation. In fact, perforation of a hypertrophied ventricle appears to occur just as readily as a normal ventricle.

Joseph et al investigated mechanisms underlying 10 cases of cardiac perforation with tamponade among 903 balloon mitral valvuloplasty procedures. Two mechanisms of hemopericardium related to TSC were proposed: (1) perforation of the aortic root and adjacent RA by upward displacement of the transseptal apparatus, (2) tear of the posterior RA wall by dilatation of the track produced by very low IAS punctures. Operator experience (inversely related) and patient age (directly related) were predictors of cardiac perforation in this study.[28]

Management of Tamponade There is no compelling evidence based on interventional cardiology procedures that an uncomplicated atrial perforation contraindicates continuation of the procedure. In the absence of effusion and hemodynamic changes, the procedure may be completed using an alternate TSP site. However, interventional electrophysiology procedures, such as mapping and ablation of left atrial tachycardias or atrial fibrillation, may be lengthy procedures, and full anticoagulation may be associated with increased risk of pericardial effusion. Pericardiocentesis may be required to decompress the pericardial sac in the setting of hypotension and/or moderate effusion by echocardiogram. Vasopressor agents to elevate the systemic blood pressure and fluid infusion to increase preload to prevent ventricular collapse should be started immediately. Blood transfusion or auto transfusion may be needed to maintain the oxygen-carrying capacity. The rent thus created in the atrium has to be sealed by either a percutaneous intervention or an open thoracotomy procedure. Interventional techniques to seal the rent by using the fast-acting sterile cyanoacrylate glue applied close to the rent from the pericardial surface has been described.[29] Patients undergoing open pericardiotomy should also undergo definitive surgery if indicated.

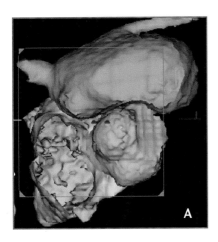

FIGURE 15.7 *Posterior Transseptal Catheterization Resulting in the "Stitching" Phenomenon*

A. Computed tomography (CT) reconstruction image of the heart with transverse cut made at the level of the fossa ovalis showing the inferior pulmonary.
B. A schematic of the CT image illustrating postero-superior movement of the needle causing the "stitching" phenomenon. Courtesy of Mehul B. Patel, MD, and Delilah Cohn, MFA, CMI.

FIGURE 15.8 *Transseptal Puncture of the Posterior Right Atrium*

A. Computed tomography (CT) reconstruction image of the heart with transverse cut at the level of the fossa ovalis showing the inferior pulmonary veins.
B. A schematic of the same image demonstrating how extreme posterosuperior movement of the needle causes puncture of the right atrium (RA) into the transverse sinus. Courtesy of Mehul B. Patel, MD, and Delilah Cohn, MFA, CMI.

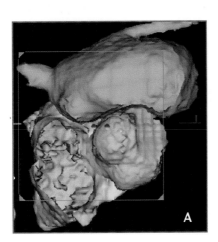

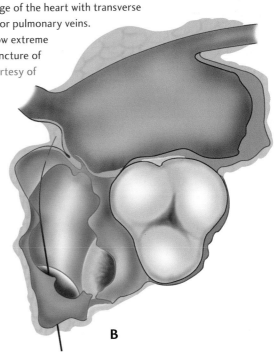

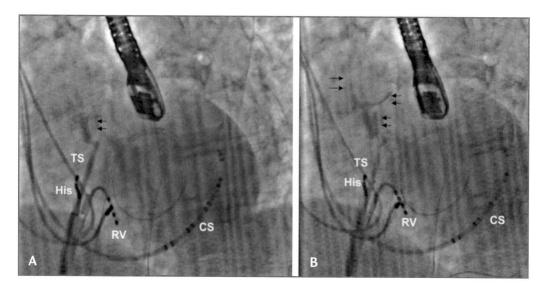

FIGURE 15.9   *Fluoroscopic Images*
from a Transseptal Catheterization Procedure

A. The first transseptal puncture (TSP) was followed by introduction of a guidewire into the left atrium (LA).
B. This was followed by a second TSP, which perforated the right atrium (RA) posteriorly. CS = coronary sinus catheter; His = His-bundle catheter; RV = right ventricular catheter; TS = transseptal dilator. Courtesy of Dr. Kalyanam Shivkumar.

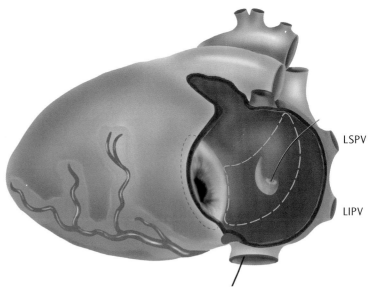

FIGURE 15.10   *The Interatrial Septum from the Left Atrium*

The transseptal needle is seen coming through the fossa and being advanced through the roof of the LA. If the LA is small, the needle may reach all the way to the left superior pulmonary vein. LIPV = left inferior pulmonary vein; LSPV = left superior pulmonary vein Courtesy of Mehul B. Patel, MD, and Delilah Cohn, MFA, CMI.

Prevention of Tamponade Continuous pressure monitoring is of utmost importance to prevent this potentially fatal complication. Recording of unusually low-pressure pulse with dips below 0 mm or aspiration of yellow or blood-tinged fluid through the transseptal needle or sheath clearly identifies the needle tip in the pericardial cavity.

Avoiding a puncture medial to midline (zones B and C of Figure 15.3b) prevents inadvertent puncture of the adjacent structures, such as the tricuspid valve and coronary sinus. Use of ICE or TEE may reduce, but does not necessarily eliminate, the risk of cardiac perforation.[30]

c. Atrial Tear

This is a rare complication of TSP seen during high pressure IAS balloon dilation after septal puncture. The tear extends from the IAS to the atrial free wall to cause tamponade. This complication was reported after an internal jugular vein approach for TSP due to an unusual angle in the dilated atrium.[31]

Prevention Atrial tear can be prevented easily by avoiding balloon dilation of the IAS. It is unclear whether controlled cuts using blade balloon dilation can reduce the incidence of this complication.

d. Coronary Sinus

Diagnosis During fluoroscopy-guided TSP, it may be possible to enter the LA via a dilated coronary sinus (CS). Puncture of the roof of a dilated CS can lead to uneventful entry of the needle into the LA. Subsequent dilation caused by the dilator-sheath assembly may create a permanent passage of deoxygenated blood into the LA, causing systemic desaturation. Puncture of the posterior wall of the CS can cause pericardial effusion with or without tamponade.

Prevention (1) Avoid medial to midline punctures (zones B and C of Figure 15.3b).

(2) A detailed echocardiogram before the TSP procedure may define a persistent left superior vena cava (LSVC) and a dilated CS. Presence of LSVC on the echocardiogram, should prompt the interventionalist to do a left-arm venous angiogram to fluoroscopically define the borders of the dilated CS. Alternatively, the TSP procedure can be done with ICE or TEE guidance.

e. Coronary Artery Atrial Fistula

This complication has been reported in a 46-year-old woman with mitral stenosis undergoing a diagnostic cardiac catheterization. TSC led to a fistula formation between the left circumflex coronary artery and right atrium. Fortunately, the patient did not experience any clinical or hemodynamic consequences of this complication.[32]

2. Puncture of IAS

a. Limbus

Diagnosis This is characterized by a difficult puncture requiring considerable force with damped needle pressure. One can use the septal flush method to characterize the septal stain. An oblique stain would mean septal stain due to needle entrapment in a thick septum or the limbus, and a prolonged vertical stain would suggest septal dissection. Excessive manipulation of the transseptal needle in this region may cause a hematoma or edema in the IAS (Figure 15.11).

Management Use the septal flush method to define the septum and proceed with puncture.

Prevention Continuous needle pressure monitoring fails to differentiate septal entrapment versus septal dissection.

b. IAS Dissection

This can be seen with forceful contrast injection in the IAS to stain the septum. It is usually benign, and one can proceed with

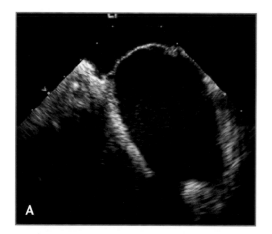

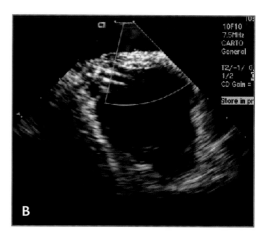

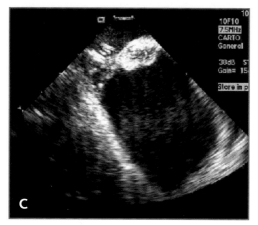

FIGURE 15.11   *Intracardiac Echocardiographic Images from a Transseptal Catheterization Procedure* **A.** View of the fossa before transseptal puncture is attempted. **B.** View after the first transseptal puncture. The interatrial septum (IAS) above the limbus appears thickened, probably due to trauma. **C.** This image was obtained a few minutes later, showing even more swelling. Reprinted with permission of Kathleen Dutton, Biosense Webster.

TSP in the absence of hemodynamic compromise.

c. Pulmonary Vein Puncture

In patients with a floppy or aneurysmal IAS (Figures 15.12 and 15.13), it may be difficult to engage the fossa. Furthermore, once the fossa is engaged, the needle may drag the floppy IAS along with it to the roof or to the lateral wall of the LA and can cause puncture of the LA or of the left superior pulmonary vein.

d. Avulsion of IAS

In patients with a resilient IAS, avulsion of the IAS can occur during septal puncture. The septal-stain method or ICE can identify the cause of resistance. The absence of IAS

tenting with needle advancement and the en bloc movement of the septum is a harbinger of IAS avulsion. This is usually painful. Any pain during any step of the procedure should be respected and diligent care taken to evaluate the cause of pain before proceeding.

The IAS may be very difficult to cross using the Brockenbrough needle. The radiofrequency ablation (RFA) needle (Baylis Medical Company, Inc, Montreal, Canada) avoids the use of mechanical force on the IAS during puncture and thus reduces the likelihood of complications. However, while the RF needle can penetrate the IAS, it may still be difficult to advance the dilator and the sheath. The phenomenon of mechanical needle skiving and plastic material embolization, which may both happen with the Brockenbrough needle, is unlikely with the RFA needle (Figure 15.14).

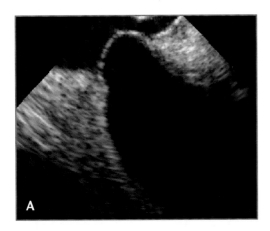

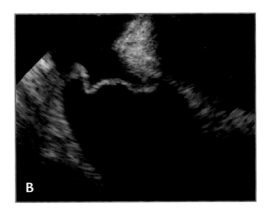

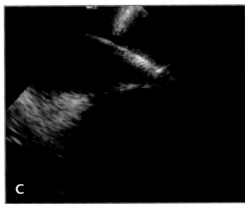

FIGURE 15.12   *Intracardiac Echocardiography of a Floppy Fossa Ovalis*

A, B. The fossa ovalis. **C.** The fossa ovalis being stretched deep into the left atrium (LA) during transseptal puncture.

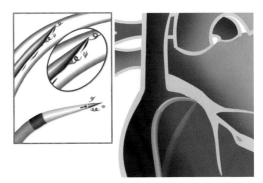

FIGURE 15.14   *Mechanical Needle Skiving with Regular Brockenbrough Needle*

As the needle is advanced through the dilator, it may shave off small fragments, which may embolize. To prevent this, it is recommended that the fine-wire stylet that comes with the transseptal needle be kept in place while the needle is advanced through the dilator and removed once the needle has reached within a few centimeters of the dilator tip. The figure shows bowing of the transseptal assembly because the interatrial septum (IAS) is too thick to puncture. A radiofrequency (RF) needle can be used to puncture the resilient IAS and cross it. Reprinted with permission from Baylis Medical Company, Inc, Montreal, Canada.

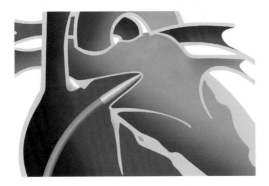

FIGURE 15.13   *Using Radiofrequency Needle to Prevent Problem of Stretching the Floppy Fossa Ovalis Deep into the Left Atrium*

The problem of stretching the floppy fossa deep into the LA can be prevented by using the radiofrequency (RF) needle. Reprinted with permission from Baylis Medical Company, Inc, Montreal, Canada.

B. Inherent to the Procedure

1. Systemic Embolism

The most common sites for embolization include coronary and cerebral circulation. The reported incidence of transient ischemic attack during or after TSP is about 0.4%.[33]

a. Air Embolism

Air embolism may be silent, or symptoms may be attributable to the vascular bed that receives the embolus. Embolism to high-demand vascular beds, such as the coronary and cerebral circulations, are the most readily recognized and reported (Figures 15.15 and 15.16).

Prevention (1) Always keep the assembly airtight and the inflation pressure as low as

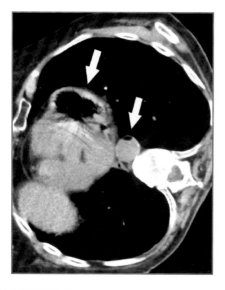

FIGURE 15.15   *Massive Air Embolism Filling the Left Ventricle and the Descending Thoracic Aorta*
Arrows point to air (black) within the left ventricle and the descending aorta. Ghaye, B., Bruyère PJ, Dondelinger RF. Nonfatal systemic air embolism during percutaneous radiofrequency ablation of pulmonary metastasis. *Am J Roentgenol* 2006;187: W327-W328. Reprinted with permission from the *American Journal of Roentgenology.*

possible in order to visualize the "back bleed." (2) Withdraw the needle and dilator from the sheath slowly to prevent any air in the sheath getting sucked into the LA. (3) Always check the hemostatic valve on the sheath. A leaky valve may cause inadvertent air embolism during heavy respiration, coughing, or sneezing. (4) Ensure adequate hydration prior to the procedure to prevent a low or subzero central venous pressure to prevent negative pressure in the system.

b. Thromboembolism

Thrombus may either be preexisting or can form de novo during the procedure. It may manifest either immediately during the procedure or may be delayed for hours to days after the procedure.

Prevention (1) TEE before the procedure or ICE-guided TSP is extremely useful. (2) Withdraw, aspirate, and flush the system after each step. (3) Reduce procedure time by adequate preplanning.

c. Thrombus on the Sheath or Guidewire

Guidewires should be kept in the endovascular system for as short a duration as possible to prevent thrombus formation on the wire.

2. Pulmonary Embolism

This, too, may be due to air or thrombus. Late pulmonary embolism (PE) is directly related to the trauma inflicted on the femoral vein due to instrumentation. The resultant thrombophlebitis of the femoral vein may cause deep venous thrombosis (DVT) and thrombus propagation; the thrombus may fragment and embolize to the pulmonary arteries. This may occur acutely or may be delayed. Braunwald et al reported a high incidence of PE in patients who developed thrombophlebitis due to difficult femoral vein entry requiring mul-

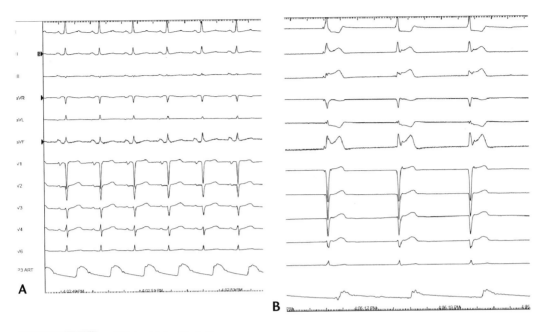

FIGURE 15.16   *Clinical Manifestations of Air Embolism*

A 61-year-old man was referred for atrial fibrillation (AF) ablation (no coronary artery disease on cardiac catheterization). He underwent an uneventful double transseptal puncture (TSP). An ablation catheter and a circular mapping catheter were placed in the left atrium (LA). The left panel shows the baseline 12-lead ECG and the arterial pressure tracing (bottom). He developed sudden, hyperacute ST-segment elevation, hypotension, and junctional rhythm (right panel); note ST segment elevation in leads II, III, and aVF as well as junctional rhythm and hypotension evident on the arterial pressure tracing. This finding was seen just prior to ablation at the left superior pulmonary vein (LSPV). Immediate right coronary artery (RCA) angiogram showed air embolus in the right coronary artery; this resolved spontaneously without myocardial infarction. Courtesy of Dr. Kalyanam Shivkumar.

tiple punctures.[13] Usually, small pulmonary emboli are uneventful.

3. Residual Shunt

Residual shunting produced by transseptal catheterization for valvular disease has been described[34,35] even with cases of documented persistence.[36] In a study of 27 patients who underwent TSC and RF ablation for AF, 8 patients had an atrial septal defect (ASD), and 6 of those demonstrated residual shunting (right to left) at 9 months follow-up. The development of a persistent residual shunt was more common in patients with elevated pre-procedural pulmonary artery pressures.[37]

C. Other Rare But Serious Complications

Infective endocarditis from *Streptococcus viridans* in a patient with pre-existing mitral regurgitation, bacterial pneumonia, pneumothorax, hemothorax, pleural effusion, serious cardiac arrhythmias (ventricular fibrillation, ectopic atrial beats), and acute pulmonary edema have all been reported as complications of left heart catheterization using TSC.[38]

II. Possibly, But Not Definitely, Related to TSP

A. Pulmonary Edema

Possibly neurogenic, this complication may be due to stimulation of nerve fibers in the IAS. The exact mechanism, however, is unclear.

B. Hypotension Unrelated to Perforation

This complication may be due to excess autonomic stimulation of IAS nerve fibers, causing vagal discharge.

C. Arrhythmia

This is a rare complication. Two dreaded arrhythmias noted during TSP include:

1. Complete Heart Block

Traction on the IAS can cause traction on the conduction system, and complete heart block (CHB) may result. This development is usually transient and self-recovering. CHB may also occur when the TSP assembly inadvertently enters the RV or hits the membranous interventricular septum. As noted above, the blood supply to the structures of the key conduction system lie in the region of access to the RA (especially with entry through the SVC) and in the posterior region of the IAS during routine TSC, and these structures can be damaged. The superior transseptal approach to mitral valve disease has been associated with a higher likelihood (hazard ratio 2.2) of need for pacemaker implantation compared to the LA approach

in surgical literature.[39] A similar study is not available from the catheter-based RF ablation literature.

2. Ventricular Tachycardia or Fibrillation

This can be caused by mechanical stimulation from the needle or transseptal sheath in the ventricle.

D. Fever

This complication likely results from the accumulation of asymptomatic fluid or blood in the pericardial sac, causing inflammation and pyrogenesis. Fever may be seen the day after the procedure.

E. Transient ST-segment Elevation

Transient ST-segment elevation mimicking ST-elevation myocardial infarction has been reported during transseptal puncture for radiofrequency catheter ablation of atrial fibrillation. Symptoms and electrocardiographic findings usually resolve spontaneously. The possible hypothesis for this phenomenon include a neurally mediated mechanism, activated by the mechanical effects of the transseptal puncture on the interatrial septum or coronary artery spasm or coronary air embolism. The occurrence of ST elevation in anesthetized patients, however, refutes the neural theory. Some believe that ST elevation during TSP is predominantly due to air embolism occurring preferentially in the right coronary artery due to its superior location in the recumbent position[40,41] (Figure 15.15).

Fagundes et al reported transient ST elevation in 8 of 1150 patients undergoing atrial fibrillation ablation (0.6%) right after puncturing the interatrial septum.[42] A sudden ST-segment elevation in the inferior leads was documented, accompanied by diaphoresis, hypotension, and chest discomfort. Coronary angiogram failed to show obstruction in the epicardial coronary circulation. The phenomenon spontaneously receded in 5 minutes to 10 minutes without any sequelae. Although typical Bezold-Jarisch-like reflex secondary to stimulation of autonomic nerve fibers of the IAS has been suggested, air embolism cannot be excluded.[43]

III. Unrelated to TSP

A. Concomitant Procedures

1. Vascular
  a. Arterial
  i.   Hematoma
  ii. Arteriovenous Fistula
  iii. Pseudoaneurysm
  iv. Thrombosis
  v.   Vascular Closure Device–related Complications

Prevention A single anterior wall puncture in the common femoral artery can eliminate most arterial complications.

  b. Venous
  i.   Hematoma
  ii. Thrombosis
  iii. Tear

Prevention The Braunwald series[13] clearly depicted a low complication rate with fewer venous punctures. Also, while dilating the vein, it is important to keep in mind that the tract should snuggly accept the TSP assembly.

IV. Special Circumstances

Certain anatomic variations require stringent precautions, which deserve special attention.

A. Scoliosis with Rotated Heart
Cardiac anatomy can be quite distorted. Ideally, TSP should be performed using ancillary imaging techniques, such as ICE or TEE.

B. Large LA
This greatly distorts the atrial septal geometry, leading to a more horizontal septum; in such a case, the puncture should be more posterior and inferior, at about a 5 o'clock or 6 o'clock position (zone D of Figure 15.3). A slight counterclockwise twist of the needle and firm pressure on the IAS before puncture helps. A few operators like to reshape the needle tip angle to prevent dissection/abrasion of the IAS. An oral contrast esophagogram may show the left atrial impression on the esophagus and significantly improve the success rate of TSP. This is especially helpful in cases where the left atrial silhouette is not clearly seen by fluoroscopy.[44]

C. Small LA
In cases with a very small pulmonary venous atrium, the target for the transseptal puncture is both small and shallow, permitting less room for error. This usually leads to a vertical septum, and thereby warrants a more anterior and superior puncture at 3 o'clock (zone B of Figure 15.3b).

D. Low BMI
The area of the fossa ovalis is directly related to body weight.[19] Thus a thin patient is likely to have a small area of fossa ovalis, an inconspicuous limbus, and a small LA. Slight lateral puncture is permissible to avoid puncture close to the mitral valve (zone A of Figure 15.3b).

E. Tall Patient with Vertical Heart
This would warrant a higher puncture site at the 3 o'clock position (zone B of Figure 15.3).

F. Left Persistent Superior Vena Cava

Contrast injection in the left upper limb vein to define the LSVC and the CS anatomy before puncture helps prevent inadvertent CS punctures.

G. CS Aneurysm

Left coronary injection with a prolonged cineangiogram for the venous phase to define the CS helps in this situation.

H. Absent IVC

An internal jugular vein (IJV) approach can be used. For the IJV approach, the curve of the transseptal needle has to be increased to avoid oblique passage of the needle through the IAS. This is an excellent approach for difficult access from the lower limbs in situations such as thrombosed femoral veins, azygos continuation of the IVC, IVC webs, or thrombosed IVC filters. This technique is rarely required; so, even operators who are very adept at trans-femoral TSC are relatively inexperienced in this technique. Complications of this technique include injury to the SVC and the carotid artery.

I. Dilated Aortic Root

A dilated aortic root is likely to exaggerate the aorto-septal groove and distort landmarks posteriorly, thereby distorting the stepladder feel during positioning of the needle. Avoid medial to midline punctures. Adjunctive echocardiography (ICE or TEE) should definitely be used.

J. Interatrial Baffles/Conduit and Patches

El-Said et al reported a study of TSP in 39 patients with an intraatrial patch and concluded that TSP through patches are safe and effective for accessing the pulmonary venous atrium and avoiding femoral artery trauma associated with retrograde catheterization.[45] The material used to create the intraatrial patch does not affect the success of the transseptal procedure. The transseptal puncture can be performed both in the early and late postoperative period and does not create residual atrial level shunts as assessed by echocardiography.[45,46]

K. Breathless Patient in a Propped-up Position

A patient who has difficulty lying flat because of shortness of breath or severe kyphosis may require TSC while he/she is propped up at an angle. In such a situation, the image intensifier can be tilted caudally, so that it is perpendicular to the patient's chest. In this situation, ICE should be used to guide TSC in order to prevent a complication.

L. IVC Filter

The presence of an IVC filter is not a contraindication for transseptal catheterization. In fact, sheaths as large as 21 F can be inserted through the IVC filter.

M. ASD or Patent Foramen Ovale (PFO) Closure Device

Contrary to popular belief that device closure for IAS septal defects constitutes a contraindication for TSP, the ASD/PFO occluder provides a handy landmark (Figure 15.17). There is usually a safe area for puncture of 2 cm to 4 cm of thin septum primum below the caudal rim of the device. This corresponds to the zone C of the IAS neighborhood (Figure 15.3). There is no reason to avoid a TSP in such patients. Moreover, in patients with a valid indication for PFO closure, it may be prudent to close it after the necessary intervention in the left atrium; this can be done

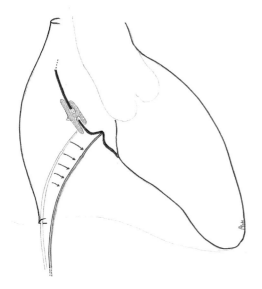

FIGURE 15.17   *Puncture Site in Patient with Atrial Septal Defect (ASD) Device Closure* Courtesy of Mehul B. Patel, MD.

without any fear of complication from the subsequent TSP, if required.[47,48]

N. Pregnant Patient

Intervention requiring radiation should be avoided in pregnant patients. In patients with life-threatening mitral stenosis, balloon mitral valvuloplasty has been reported without the use of X-ray, entirely under echocardiographic guidance. While this is technically feasible, it will not be the clinical practice in most laboratories. Internal jugular vein (IJV) technique may be the best fluoroscopic approach to reduce radiation for pregnant women. Fetal radiation can be prevented by using lead aprons wrapped over the abdomen, pelvis, and groin to prevent scatter effects. The patient can flex the hips and knees during the procedure to avoid the discomforts of prolonged immobility.

V. Miscellaneous
A. Instrument Breakage
1. Brockenbrough Needle Fracture in the Iliac Vein

2. Fracture of the Seldinger Guidewire Tip
Snaring and retrieving the broken fragment is the first option, if the remains are not sharp. Should this fail, an open surgical procedure may be required.

Long-Term Outcomes of Complications: Looking Ahead

The most common long-term outcome of TSC is the presence of a residual shunt. In a study of 184 TSC procedures performed in 176 patients, the group of patients undergoing valvuloplasty had a significantly higher prevalence of residual ASD after TSC, especially in those with more severe mitral stenosis and less valvuloplasty success; however, the presence of an ASD did not affect the 1.5-year prognosis.[49] TSC has stood the test of time as a practical and useful means of access to the left side of the heart. Complications and adverse outcome related to TSC can be best prevented when the procedure is performed by an experienced operator with a sound knowledge of cardiac anatomy, when imaging is used to guide the operator, and when a low threshold is maintained for detecting complications with timely management, if they do occur. As noted above, although TSC is a relatively safe procedure, complications ranging from benign to fatal can happen. Now that we know the road we have to travel, using available means to make the journey safer will only lead to more trips and better outcomes.

Summary

While transseptal catheterization remains "cloaked in intrigue" because of its potentially life-threatening complications, this technique has become essential for interventional cardiologists and electrophysiologists. Our understanding of the potential complications comes from the days of fluoroscopic-guided procedures. While the technique has essentially remained unchanged from the pioneering descriptions contributed by Ross, Braunwald, Brockenbrough, and Mullins, technologic innovations have made this a safe and widely used procedure.[50] Advances in needle and sheath design and in the manufacturing and use of echocardiographic imaging have increased the safety of this procedure, and it has entered the domain of routine electrophysiology fellowship training. It is essential that operators know the potential complications of this procedure and the expeditious measures to deal with them.

Acknowledgments

We wish to thank many colleagues who contributed figures for this chapter, but especially Dr. Kalyanam Shivkumar and Dr. Rahul Sakhuja.

TABLE 15.1

Current Uses of Transseptal Puncture

I. **Interventional cardiology**
   A. Diagnostic
      1. For accurate assessment of left heart pressures
   B. Interventional
      1. Percutaneous transvenous mitral commissurotomy (PTMC)
      2. Antegrade balloon aortic valvuloplasty
      3. Antegrade percutaneous aortic valve replacement
      4. Temporary percutaneous left ventricle assist devices (eg, TandemHeart, Cardiac Assist, Inc, Pittsburgh, PA)
      5. Extensive 4-limb peripheral arterial disease with no arterial access for intervention

II. **Invasive electrophysiology**
   A. Ablation of left-sided accessory pathways
   B. Ablation of left atrial flutter
   C. Ablation of left atrial tachycardia
   D. Pulmonary vein isolation for atrial fibrillation
   E. Percutaneous insertion of left atrial appendage occluder

TABLE 15.2

Transseptal Puncture Complications

I. Related to TSP
  A. Puncture
    1. Puncture other than interatrial septum (IAS)
      a. Perforation of aorta
      b. Perforation of right atrium (RA), left atrium (LA), or left ventricle (LV)
      c. Atrial tear
      d. Coronary sinus (CS) perforation
    2. Puncture of IAS
      a. Limbus
      b. IAS dissection
      c. Pulmonary vein (PV) puncture
      d. Avulsion of IAS
  B. Inherent to the procedure
    1. Systemic embolism
      a. Air embolism
      b. Thromboembolism
      c. Thrombus on sheath or guidewire
    2. Pulmonary embolism
    3. Residual shunt
  C. Other rare but serious side effects
    1. Infective endocarditis
    2. Pneumothorax

II. Possibly, but not definitely, related to TSP
  A. Pulmonary edema
  B. Hypotension unrelated to perforation
  C. Arrhythmia
    1. Complete heart block (CHB)
    2. Ventricular tachycardia or fibrillation
  D. Fever
  E. Transient ST-elevation

III. Unrelated to TSP
  A. Concomitant procedures
    1. Vascular
      a. Arterial
        i. Hematoma
        ii. Arteriovenous fistula
        iii. Pseudoaneurysm
        iv. Thrombosis
        v. Vascular closure device–related complications
      b. Venous
        i. Hematoma
        ii. Thrombosis
        iii. Tear
        iv. Deep-venous thrombosis and delayed pulmonary embolism

IV. Special Circumstances
  A. Scoliosis with rotated heart
  B. Large LA
  C. Small LA
  D. Low body mass index (BMI)
  E. Tall patient with vertical heart
  F. Left persistent superior vena cava (SVC)
  G. CS aneurysm
  H. Absent inferior vena cava (IVC)
  I. Dilated aortic root
  J. Interatrial baffles/conduit and patches
  K. Breathless patient in a propped-up position
  L. IVC filter
  M. ASD or patent foramen ovale (PFO) closure device
  N. Pregnant patient

V. Miscellaneous
  A. Instrument breakage
    1. Brockenbrough needle fracture in the iliac vein
    2. Fracture of the Seldinger guidewire tip

References

1. Bjork VO, Malmstrom G, Uggla LG. Left auricular pressure measurements in man. *Ann Surg* 1953;138:718-725.

2. Allison PR, Linden RJ. The bronchoscopic measurement of left auricular pressure. *Circulation* 1953;7:669.

3. Ponsdomenech ER, Nunez VB. Heart puncture in man for Diodrast visualization of ventricular chambers and great arteries. *Am Heart J* 1951;41:643.

4. Brock R, Milstein BB, Ross DN. Percutaneous left ventricle puncture in the assessment of aortic stenosis. *Thorax* 1956;11:163.

5. Cope C. Technique for TSP of the left atrium: preliminary report. *J Thorac Surg* 1959;37:482-486.

6. Ross JJ, Braunwald E, Morrow AG. Transseptal left atrial puncture; new technique for the measurement of left atrial pressure in man. *Am J Cardiol* 1959;3:353-355.

7. Brockenbrough EC, Braunwald E. A new technique for left ventricular angiocardiography and transseptal left heart catheterization. *Am J Cardiol* 1960;6:1062.

8. Mullins CE. Transseptal left heart catheterization: experience with a new technique in 520 pediatric and adult patients. *Pediatr Cardiol* 1983;4:239-246.

9. Brock R, Milstein BB, Ross DH. Percutaneous left ventricular puncture in the assessment of aortic stenosis. *Thorax* 1956;11:163-171.

10. Inoue K, Owaki T, Nakamura T, et al. Clinical application of transvenous mitral commissurotomy by a new balloon catheter. *J Thorac Cardiovasc Surg* 1984;87:394-402.

11. Clugston R, Lau FY, Ruiz C. Transseptal catheterization update 1992. *Cathet Cardiovasc Diagn* 1992;26:266-674.

12. Haïssaguerre M, Jaïs P, Shah D, et al. Spontaneous initiation of atrial fibrillation by ectopic beats originating in the pulmonary veins. *N Engl J Med* 1998;339:659-666.

13. Braunwald E. Cooperative study on cardiac catheterization. Transseptal left heart catheterization. *Circulation* 1968;37:(5 suppl):III74-79.

14. De Ponti R, Cappato R, Curnis A, et al. Trans-septal catheterization in the electrophysiology laboratory: data from a multicenter survey spanning 12 years. *J Am Coll Cardiol* 2006;47:1037-1042.

15. Sweeney LJ, Rosenquist GC. The normal anatomy of the atrial septum in the human heart. *Am Heart J* 1979;98:194-199.

16. Anderson RH, Webb S, Brown NA. Clinical anatomy of the atrial septum with reference to its developmental components. *Clin Anat* 1999;12:362-374.

17. Anderson RH, Ho SY, Becker AE. The surgical anatomy of the conduction tissues. *Thorax* 1983;38:408-420.

18. Bloomfield DK, Sinclair-Smiths BC. The limbic ledge. *Circulation* 1965;31:103.

19. Sweeney LJ, Rosenquist GC. The normal anatomy of the atrial septum in the human heart. *Am Heart J* 1979;98:194-199.

20. Reig J, Mirapeix R, Jornet A, et al. Morphologic characteristics of the fossa ovalis as an anatomic basis for TSP. *Surg Radiol Anat* 1997;19:279-282.

21. Hung JS. Mitral stenosis with left atrial thrombi: Inoue balloon catheter technique. In: Cheng TO, ed. *Percutaneous Balloon Valvuloplasty.* New York: Igaku-Shoin; 1992:280-293.

22. Hung JS, Lau KW. Pitfalls and tips in Inoue balloon mitral commissurotomy. *Cathet Cardiovasc Diagn* 1996;37:188-199.

23. Yeh KH, Hung JS, Wu CJ, et al. Safety of Inoue balloon mitral commissurotomy in patients with left atrial appendage thrombi. *Am J Cardiol* 1995;75:302-304.

24. Hung JS, Lau KW, Lo PH, et al. Complications of Inoue balloon mitral commissurotomy: impact of operator experience and evolving technique. *Am Heart J* 1999;138:114-121.

25. Hammersting C, Lickfett L. Safety of single transseptal puncture for ablation of atrial fibrillation: retrospective study from a large cohort of patients. *J Cardiovasc Electrophysiol* 2007;18:1277-1281.

26. Fejka M, Dixon SR, Safian RD, et al. Diagnosis, management, and clinical outcome of cardiac tamponade complicating percutaneous coronary intervention. *Am J Cardiol* 2002;90:1183-1186.

27. Gorlin R. Perforation and other cardiac complications. *Circulation* 1968;37(suppl III):36-38.

28. Joseph G, Chandy ST, Krishnaswami S, et al. Mechanisms of cardiac perforation leading to tamponade in balloon mitral valvuloplasty. *Cathet Cardiovasc Diagn* 1997;42:138-146.

29. Trehan V, Mukhopadhyay S, Yaduvanshi A, et al. Novel non-surgical method of managing cardiac perforation during percutaneous transvenous mitral commissurotomy. *Indian Heart J* 2004;56:328-332.

30. Goldstein SA, Campbell A, Mintz GS, et al. Feasibility of on-line transesophageal echocardiography during balloon mitral valvulotomy: experience with 93 patients. *J Heart Valve Dis* 1994;3:136.

31. Joseph G, Baruah DK, Kuruttukulam SV, et al. Transjugular approach to transseptal balloon mitral valvuloplasty. *Cathet Cardiovasc Diagn* 1997;42:219-226.

32. Samet P, Bernstein WH, Levine S. Transseptal left heart catheterization. An analysis of 390 studies. *Dis Chest* 1965;48:160-166.

33. Kumaraswamy N, Kay N, Plumb VJ, et al. Decrease in fluoroscopic cardiac silhouette excursion precedes hemodynamic compromise in intraprocedural tamponade. *Heart Rhythm* 2005;2:1224-1230.

34. McCay RG, Lock JE, Safian RD, et al. Balloon dilation of mitral stenosis in adult patients: postmortem and percutaneous mitral valvuloplasty studies. *J Am Coll Cardiol* 1987;9:723-731.

35. Kronzon I, Turick PA, Goldfarb A, et al. Echocardiographic and hemodynamic characteristics of atrial septal defects created by percutaneous valvuloplasty. *J Am Soc Echocardiogr* 1990;3:64-71.

36. Lemmer JH, Winniford MD, Ferguson DW. Surgical implication of atrial septal defect complicating aortic balloon valvuloplasty. *Ann Thorac Surg* 1989;48:295-297.

37. Hammerstingl C, Lickfett L, Jeong KM, et al. Persistence of iatrogenic atrial septal defect after pulmonary vein isolation—an underestimated risk? *Am Heart J* 2006;152:362.e1-5.

38. Pietras RJ, May PC, Gunnar RM, et al. Reappraisal of the posterior percutaneous technique of left heart catheterization. *Dis Chest* 1969;55:471-478.

39. Lukac P, Hjortdal VE, Pedersen AK, et al. Superior transseptal approach to mitral valve is associated with a higher need for pacemaker implantation than the left atrial approach. *Ann Thorac Surg* 2007;83:77-82.

40. Efremidis M, Letsas KP, Xydonas S, et al. ECG findings of acute myocardial infarction and atrioventricular block during a transseptal procedure for left atrial ablation. *Hellenic J Cardiol* 2008;49:284-287.

41. Turi ZG. Puncturing the septum: resurgent technique with inherent risk. *J Invasive Cardiol* 2004;16:3-4.

42. Fagundes RL, Mantica M, De Luca L, et al. Safety of single transseptal puncture for ablation of atrial fibrillation: retrospective study from a large cohort of patients. *J Cardiovasc Electrophysiol* 2007;18:1277-1281.

43. Arita T, Kubota S, Okamoto K, et al. Bezold-Jarish-like reflex during Brockenbrough's procedure for radiofrequency catheter ablation of focal left atrial fibrillation: report of two cases. *J Interv Card Electrophysiol* 2003;8:195-202.

44. Wu TG, Wang LX, Chen SW, et al. Value of radiographic esophageal imaging in deter-

mining an optimal atrial septal puncture site for percutaneous balloon mitral valvuloplasty. *Med Princ Pract* 2008;17:280-283.

45. El-Said HG, Ing FF, Grifka RG, et al. 18-year experience with transseptal procedures through baffles, conduits, and other intra-atrial patches. *Catheter Cardiovasc Interv* 2000;50:434-439.

46. Schneider MB, Zartner PA, Magee AG. Transseptal approach in children after patch occlusion of atrial septal defect: first experience with the cutting balloon. *Catheter Cardiovasc Interv* 1999;48:378-381.

47. Zaker-Shahrak R, Fuhrer J, Meier B. Transseptal puncture for catheter ablation of atrial fibrillation after device closure of patent foramen ovale. *Catheter Cardiovasc Interv* 2008;71:551-552.

48. Lakkireddy D, Rangisetty U, Prasad S, et al. Intracardiac echo-guided radiofrequency catheter ablation of atrial fibrillation in patients with atrial septal defect or patent foramen ovale repair: a feasibility, safety, and efficacy study. *J Cardiovasc Electrophysiol* 2008;19:1137-1142.

49. Liu TJ, Lai HC, Lee WL, et al. Immediate and late outcomes of patients undergoing transseptal left-sided heart catheterization for symptomatic valvular and arrhythmic diseases. *Am Heart J* 2006;151:235-241.

50. Ross J Jr. Transseptal left heart catheterization: a 50-year odyssey. *J Am Coll Cardiol* 2008;51:2107-2115.

INDEX

Figures are indicated by f, *tables by* t,
and charts by c *following the page number.*